Methods in Molecular Biology

Series Editor
John M. Walker
School of Life and Medical Sciences
University of Hertfordshire
Hatfield, Hertfordshire, AL10 9AB, UK

For further volumes:
http://www.springer.com/series/7651

Nanotoxicity

Methods and Protocols

Edited by

Qunwei Zhang

Department of Environmental and Occupational Health Sciences, School of Public Health and Information Sciences, University of Louisville, Louisville, KY, USA

Humana Press

Editor
Qunwei Zhang
Department of Environmental and Occupational Health Sciences
School of Public Health and Information Sciences
University of Louisville
Louisville, KY, USA

ISSN 1064-3745 ISSN 1940-6029 (electronic)
Methods in Molecular Biology
ISBN 978-1-4939-8915-7 ISBN 978-1-4939-8916-4 (eBook)
https://doi.org/10.1007/978-1-4939-8916-4

Library of Congress Control Number: 2018960874

This Humana Press imprint is published by the registered company Springer Science+Business Media, LLC, part of Springer Nature.
The registered company address is: 233 Spring Street, New York, NY 10013, U.S.A.

Preface

Nanotechnology is among the world's most promising new technologies, and it is projected to hold significant importance in the twenty-first century. Nanotechnology has revolutionized areas as diverse as engineering, information technology, and diagnostics. As the prevalence of nanomaterials continues to increase, the risk of environmental contamination by nanoparticles is rising. Consequently, occupational and nonoccupational exposure to nanoparticles is growing, and their health effects cannot be ignored.

The unique physical and chemical properties of solid materials at the nanoscale contribute to serious technical limitations and potentially misleading results using conventional toxicology assays. Due to their high surface area and hydrophobicity, nanoparticles can adsorb vital dyes, cell culture micronutrients, or related cytokines; therefore, the routine methods and protocols for larger-sized particles are unsuitable for nanotoxicology studies. The methods and protocols in *Nanotoxicity: Methods and Protocols* of the successful *Methods in Molecular Biology* series address the recently developed methods for investigating nanotoxicity. These methods and protocols range from routine nanotoxicology assays to genomics and proteomics techniques and include both in vitro and in vivo approaches. We believe this book can serve as a starting point to introduce researchers to the methods and protocols of nanotoxicity, which will expand the work being done in this area.

The target audience for this book comprises researchers and postgraduate students in the fields of toxicology, environmental science, pharmacological science, and clinical medicine.

I am deeply grateful to all contributing authors who devoted their valuable time and effort in writing outstanding state-of-the-art methods and protocols for this book. I also would like to thank the series editor, John Walker, for his valuable suggestions.

Louisville, KY, USA *Qunwei Zhang*

Contents

Contributors

NASSER B. ALSALEH • *Department of Pharmaceutical Sciences, Colorado Center for Nanomedicine and Nanosafety, Skaggs School of Pharmacy and Pharmaceutical Sciences, University of Colorado, Aurora, CO, USA*

SILVANA ANDREESCU • *Department of Chemistry and Biomolecular Science, Clarkson University, Potsdam, NY, USA*

AYNUN N. BEGUM • *College of Veterinary Medicine, Western University of Health Sciences, Pomona, CA, USA*

JARED M. BROWN • *Department of Pharmaceutical Sciences, Colorado Center for Nanomedicine and Nanosafety, Skaggs School of Pharmacy and Pharmaceutical Sciences, University of Colorado, Aurora, CO, USA*

NYMPH CHAN • *College of Veterinary Medicine, Western University of Health Sciences, Pomona, CA, USA*

THEODOROS G. CHATZIMITAKOS • *Department of Chemistry, University of Ioannina, Ioannina, Greece*

NILS DOMMERSHAUSEN • *Department of Chemical and Product Safety, German Federal Institute for Risk Assessment (BfR), Berlin, Germany*

EDUARD DUMITRESCU • *Department of Chemistry and Biomolecular Science, Clarkson University, Potsdam, NY, USA*

MARIA DUSINSKA • *Health Effects Laboratory, Department of Environmental Chemistry, Norwegian Institute for Air Research (NILU), Kjeller, Norway*

THOMAS D. DZIUBLA • *Department of Chemical and Materials Engineering, University of Kentucky, Lexington, KY, USA*

NAOUALE EL YAMANI • *Health Effects Laboratory, Department of Environmental Chemistry, Norwegian Institute for Air Research (NILU), Kjeller, Norway*

ELISABETH ELJE • *Health Effects Laboratory, Department of Environmental Chemistry, Norwegian Institute for Air Research (NILU), Kjeller, Norway*

LINGFANG FENG • *Institute of Occupational Diseases, Zhejiang Academy of Medical Sciences, Hangzhou, P. R. China*

DAGMAR FIEBLINGER • *Department of Chemical and Product Safety, German Federal Institute for Risk Assessment (BfR), Berlin, Germany*

MEIQIN GAO • *Department of Pathology, School of Basic Medical Sciences, Fujian Medical University, Fuzhou, People's Republic of China*

AIHUA GU • *State Key Laboratory of Reproductive Medicine, Institute of Toxicology, Nanjing Medical University, Nanjing, China; Key Laboratory of Modern Toxicology of Ministry of Education, School of Public Health, Nanjing Medical University, Nanjing, China*

ANDREA HAASE • *Department of Chemical and Product Safety, German Federal Institute for Risk Assessment (BfR), Berlin, Germany*

XIAO HE • *CAS Key Lab for Biomedical Effects of Nanomaterials and Nanosafety, Institute of High Energy Physics, Chinese Academy of Sciences, Beijing, P. R. China*

FRANK HERZBERG • *Department of Chemical and Product Safety, German Federal Institute for Risk Assessment (BfR), Berlin, Germany*

J. ZACH HILT • *Department of Chemical and Materials Engineering, University of Kentucky, Lexington, KY, USA*

Yiling Hong • *College of Veterinary Medicine, Western University of Health Sciences, Pomona, CA, USA*
Gary W. Hoyle • *Department of Environmental and Occupational Health Sciences, School of Public Health and Information Sciences, University of Louisville, Louisville, KY, USA*
Alexandra Misci Hudecova • *Health Effects Laboratory, Department of Environmental Chemistry, Norwegian Institute for Air Research (NILU), Kjeller, Norway*
Salik Hussain • *Department of Physiology and Pharmacology, Robert C. Byrd Health Science Center, School of Medicine, West Virginia University, Morgantown, WV, USA*
Mizu Jiang • *Department of Gastroenterology, Affiliated Children's Hospital, Zhejiang University School of Medicine, Hangzhou, Zhejiang Province, China*
Alena Kazimirova • *Health Effects Laboratory, Department of Environmental Chemistry, Norwegian Institute for Air Research (NILU), Kjeller, Norway*
Ali Kermanizadeh • *Nano Safety Research Group, School of Engineering and Physical Science, Institute of Biological Chemistry, Biophysics and Bioengineering, Heriot-Watt University, Edinburgh, UK*
Huangyuan Li • *Fujian Provincial Key Laboratory of Environmental Factors and Cancer, School of Public Health, Fujian Medical University, Fuzhou, P. R. China; Department of Preventive Medicine, School of Public Health, Fujian Medical University, Fuzhou, P. R. China*
Jin Liu • *Fujian Provincial Key Laboratory of Environmental Factors and Cancer, School of Public Health, Fujian Medical University, Fuzhou, People's Republic of China; Department of Preventive Medicine, School of Public Health, Fujian Medical University, Fuzhou, People's Republic of China*
Qian Liu • *State Key Laboratory of Reproductive Medicine, Institute of Toxicology, Nanjing Medical University, Nanjing, China; Key Laboratory of Modern Toxicology of Ministry of Education, School of Public Health, Nanjing Medical University, Nanjing, China*
Yingying Liu • *Department of Raw Material Industry Research, China Center for Information Industry Development, Beijing, People's Republic of China*
Gao Long • *Department of Gastroenterology, Affiliated Children's Hospital, Zhejiang University School of Medicine, Hangzhou, Zhejiang Province, China*
Jianlin Lou • *Institute of Occupational Diseases, Zhejiang Academy of Medical Sciences, Hangzhou, P. R. China*
Andreas Luch • *Department of Chemical and Product Safety, German Federal Institute for Risk Assessment (BfR), Berlin, Germany*
Espen Mariussen • *Health Effects Laboratory, Department of Environmental Chemistry, Norwegian Institute for Air Research (NILU), Kjeller, Norway*
Yiqun Mo • *Department of Environmental and Occupational Health Sciences, School of Public Health and Information Sciences, University of Louisville, Louisville, KY, USA*
Sadiatu Musah • *Department of Environmental and Occupational Health Sciences, School of Public Health and Information Sciences, University of Louisville, Louisville, KY, USA*
Sameera Nallanthighal • *Cancer Research Center, University at Albany, State University of New York, Rensselaer, NY, USA; Department of Biomedical Sciences, University at Albany, State University of New York, Albany, NY, USA*
Ramune Reliene • *Cancer Research Center, University at Albany, State University of New York, Rensselaer, NY, USA; Department of Environmental Health Sciences, University at Albany, State University of New York, Albany, NY, USA*

ELISE RUNDÉN-PRAN • *Health Effects Laboratory, Department of Environmental Chemistry, Norwegian Institute for Air Research (NILU), Kjeller, Norway*
DUSTIN T. SAVAGE • *Department of Chemical and Materials Engineering, University of Kentucky, Lexington, KY, USA*
CONNIE F. SCHLUETER • *Department of Environmental and Occupational Health Sciences, School of Public Health and Information Sciences, University of Louisville, Louisville, KY, USA*
CONSTANTINE D. STALIKAS • *Department of Chemistry, University of Ioannina, Ioannina, Greece*
JULIAN THARMANN • *Department of Chemical and Product Safety, German Federal Institute for Risk Assessment (BfR), Berlin, Germany*
RUIRUI TONG • *Department of Pathology, School of Basic Medical Sciences, Fujian Medical University, Fuzhou, People's Republic of China*
MICHAEL T. TSENG • *Department of Anatomical Sciences and Neurobiology, University of Louisville, Louisville, KY, USA*
KENNETH WALLACE • *Department of Biology, Clarkson University, Potsdam, NY, USA*
RONG WAN • *Department of Pathology, School of Basic Medical Sciences, Fujian Medical University, Fuzhou, People's Republic of China; Department of Environmental and Occupational Health Sciences, School of Public Health and Information Sciences, University of Louisville, Louisville, KY, USA*
YUQIAN WANG • *Key Laboratory of Occupational Safety and Health, Beijing Municipal Institute of Labour Protection, Beijing, People's Republic of China*
CHENG XU • *State Key Laboratory of Reproductive Medicine, Institute of Toxicology, Nanjing Medical University, Nanjing, China; Key Laboratory of Modern Toxicology of Ministry of Education, School of Public Health, Nanjing Medical University, Nanjing, China; Department of Cardiothoracic Surgery, Children's Hospital of Nanjing Medical University, Nanjing, China*
JIN XU • *State Key Laboratory of Reproductive Medicine, Institute of Toxicology, Nanjing Medical University, Nanjing, China; Key Laboratory of Modern Toxicology of Ministry of Education, School of Public Health, Nanjing Medical University, Nanjing, China*
ZHIZHEN XU • *Key Laboratory of Occupational Safety and Health, Beijing Municipal Institute of Labour Protection, Beijing, People's Republic of China*
ROBERT A. YOKEL • *Pharmaceutical Sciences Department, University of Kentucky Academic Medical Center, Lexington, KY, USA*
JUNZHE ZHANG • *CAS Key Lab for Biomedical Effects of Nanomaterials and Nanosafety, Institute of High Energy Physics, Chinese Academy of Sciences, Beijing, P. R. China*
QUNWEI ZHANG • *Department of Environmental and Occupational Health Sciences, School of Public Health and Information Sciences, University of Louisville, Louisville, KY, USA*
WENCHANG ZHANG • *Fujian Provincial Key Laboratory of Environmental Factors and Cancer, School of Public Health, Fujian Medical University, Fuzhou, People's Republic of China; Department of Preventive Medicine, School of Public Health, Fujian Medical University, Fuzhou, People's Republic of China*
YUANBAO ZHANG • *Key Laboratory of Occupational Safety and Health, Beijing Municipal Institute of Labour Protection, Beijing, People's Republic of China*
YUE ZHANG • *Department of Environmental and Occupational Health Sciences, School of Public Health and Information Sciences, University of Louisville, Louisville, KY, USA*

PENG ZHAO • *Key Laboratory of Occupational Safety and Health, Beijing Municipal Institute of Labour Protection, Beijing, People's Republic of China*
FULI ZHENG • *Fujian Provincial Key Laboratory of Environmental Factors and Cancer, School of Public Health, Fujian Medical University, Fuzhou, P. R. China; Department of Preventive Medicine, School of Public Health, Fujian Medical University, Fuzhou, P. R. China*

Chapter 1

In Vitro Methods for Assessing Nanoparticle Toxicity

Dustin T. Savage, J. Zach Hilt, and Thomas D. Dziubla

Abstract

As a consequence of their increase in annual production and widespread distribution in the environment, nanoparticles potentially pose a significant public health risk. The sought-after catalytic activity granted by their physiochemical properties doubles as a hazard to physiological processes following exposure through inhalation, oral, transdermal, subcutaneous, and intravenous uptake. Upon uptake into the body, their size, morphology, surface charge, coating, and chemical composition augment the response of biological systems to the materials and enhance their toxicity. Identification of each property is necessary to predict the harm imposed by foreign nanomaterials in the body. Assay methods ranging from endotoxin and lactate dehydrogenase (LDH) signaling to apoptosis and oxidative stress detection supply valuable techniques for exposing biomarkers of nanoparticle-induced cellular damage. Spectroscopic investigation of epithelial barrier permeation and distribution within living cells reveals the proclivity of nanoparticles to penetrate the body's natural defensive boundaries and deposit themselves in cytotoxic locations. Combination of the various characterization methodologies and assays is required for every new nanoparticulate system despite preexisting data for similar systems due to the lack of deterministic trends among investigated nanoparticles. The propensity of nanomaterials to denature proteins and oxidize substrates in their local environment generates significant concern for the applicability of several traditional in vitro assays, and the modification of susceptible approaches into novel methods suitable for the evaluation of nanoparticles comprises the focus of future work centered on nanoparticle toxicity analysis.

Key words Nanoparticle toxicity, In vitro assays, Mechanisms of toxicity, Nanoparticle-cell interaction, Nanomaterials, Biocompatibility, Nanoparticle characterization, Reactive oxygen species

1 Introduction

Due to their unique physiochemical properties, nanoparticles have received significant interest over the last several decades as therapeutic agents [1–3], catalysts [4, 5], and commercial material enhancers [6–8]. By combining their small size with individual chemistries, bulk material properties are altered or augmented to grant nanomaterials new features that are otherwise unattainable by their macroscale counterparts. In particular, the characteristic increase in surface area to volume ratio accompanying nanoparticles produces a substantial increase in catalytic activity. The size of

Qunwei Zhang (ed.), *Nanotoxicity: Methods and Protocols*, Methods in Molecular Biology, vol. 1894,
https://doi.org/10.1007/978-1-4939-8916-4_1,

nanomaterials also permits quantum effects to dominate the materials' behavior and bestow fluorescent, magnetic, and electrical capacities that are foreign to their traditional chemistries [9, 10]. These properties have significantly improved the efficacy of everyday consumer products like food, paints, and household cleaners by supplying highly tuned amplification to the goods beyond their stand-alone limits [6, 7, 11, 12]. Albeit useful for improving commodities and the design of highly reactive agents for theranostics or catalysis, the surface reactivity of nanoparticles furthers their potential to interact with biological and environmental substances. In instances where magnified biological interaction is undesired or unforeseen, and even in cases emphasizing specific biological interplay, the materials can present unsought potency toward biosystems that can ultimately lead to adverse physiological consequences.

The frequent use of nanomaterials in everyday consumer products such as sunscreens, cosmetics, and pharmaceutical and food additives accelerates their widespread distribution in the environment [7, 8]. Once deposited therein, bystanders are at risk of exposure through inhalation, oral, or transdermal uptake. This risk can increase even further with intravenous or subcutaneous injection [13]. Inhalation puts the nasopharyngeal, tracheobronchial, and alveolar regions at risk for accumulation in the absence of alveolar–capillary barrier clearance. Oral ingestion of nanoparticles is typically shielded from toxicity by the physiochemical and cellular barriers inhabiting the gastrointestinal tract, but nanoparticles still exhibit size-dependent transition through the digestive system's defenses into the bloodstream [13]. Upon entering the blood, nanoparticles follow the expected absorption, distribution, metabolism, and excretion (ADME) model of pharmacokinetics throughout the body. This model is, however, complicated by potential aggregation and surface absorption of blood plasma proteins which form a "corona" that greatly augments the biological response to these materials [14]. Nonetheless, target organs such as the spleen, kidney, and liver accumulate the nanomaterials for longer periods than traditional pharmaceutical agents with maximal half-lives extending into years. Without clearance, the particles can generate oxidative stress, inflammation, and subsequent cell death in and around the subjected organs and can form agglomerates within vessels that impede blood flow and rupture blockages [13]. As a result, methods for assessing the possible toxicity of newly developed nanoparticles are required to understand the particles' threat to the health of both manufacturers and consumers before their final application.

As new nanomaterials are developed, rapid screening of their biological and health impacts must be performed to assess their potential risk and provide insights into proper handling and care. As part of this screening, in vitro nanoparticle toxicity assessment represents a de facto method of acute hazard identification for potentially dangerous nanoparticles. The methods are not a complete replacement for in vivo evaluation; whereas in vitro analysis records the acute damaging effects of nanoparticles in a specific cellular environment, in vivo animal models track biodistribution and bioaccumulation pathways in a manner that is currently unavailable to in vitro observation. Both methods are needed to fully investigate the toxicity and potential risk of a particular nanomaterial. Often, as a precursor for in vivo studies, in vitro assessment is employed to identify the minimum toxic dose from cell viability protocols. Complementary biomarker analysis is applied thereafter to detect signs of nonnecrotic cellular damage when cell viability is maintained. The absence of terminal markers combined with undisturbed cell viability offers possible categorization of the nanomaterial in question as inert, but the prognosis is moreover a herald for introduction into in vivo trials for confirmation. In vitro studies, moreover, screen for many of the known mechanisms of toxicity that can emerge in in vivo studies and, as a consequence, establish in vitro protocols as a necessary prerequisite. Readers interested in in vivo analysis of nanoparticles are recommended to read the review by Kumar et al. [15] and chapter by Clichici and Filip [16]. The methodology used for in vitro nanoparticle toxicity analysis is the focus of this book and will be discussed herein.

2 Mechanisms of Toxicity

Nanoparticle toxicity stems primarily from the particle's physiochemical properties and individual architecture. Size, shape, surface charge, coating, and chemical constituency all play key roles in determining the particles' uptake and biocompatibility. Established by the National Nanotechnology Initiative, nanoparticles are defined as having characteristic dimensions below 100 nm, but their size is generally recognized to include particles with dimensions of up to 1 μm [17]. In the lower strata of the size regime, particularly below 100 nm [18–20], nanoparticles can take advantage of the enhanced permeation and retention (EPR) effect attributed to highly vascularized tissues such as tumors which makes the size distribution desirable among the pharmacological community [21]. Additionally, as the size of nanoparticles decline, the energy barrier associated with uptake is also reduced, allowing for enhanced transdermal migration and cellular penetration. Decreasing the total surface area exposed to a phagocyte lowers the energy penalty required for energy-dependent endocytosis and raises the probability of phagocytic consumption. The relative increase in particle surface area linked to a reduction in volume also heightens the particle's reactivity and enables further uptake through receptor-mediated endocytosis and nonphagocytic mechanisms.

The shape of nanoparticles plays a significant role in the progression of a material through the body in as much as the particles' size. Morphologies can vary from homogeneous and heterogeneous solid spheres to hollow micellular rods depending on the material in question and the synthesis pathway employed [13, 17]. Spherical nanoparticles are reported to undergo phagocytosis and excretion at faster rates than their high aspect ratio counterparts. The phenomenon is assumed to be due to the minimization of contact area intersecting the cell membrane and the resulting added energy penalty associated with internalization [22]. When the long axis of a cylindrical particle is aligned perpendicular to the membrane surface, the enlarged and unsymmetrical deformation needed to envelope the incident particle is assumed to be energetically unfavorable in comparison to uniform spheres. In another conformation, if the face of the tube first imposes on the cell membrane, phagocytosis may commence without the opportunity for completion. The event can lead to frustrated phagocytosis with eventual cell rupture and localized inflammation as in the case of asbestos. In a countervailing study, however, Gratton et al. [23] identified high aspect ratio nanoparticles as having four-fold increased uptake for HeLa cells in comparison to low aspect ratio particles of similar size and chemistry. The explanation for the difference follows the same reasoning as presented for the rejection hypothesis, but the enlarged surface area affecting high aspect ratio particles is instead theorized to supply beneficial multivalent cationic interactions which promote nonspecific endocytosis. In either case, the morphology of the nanoparticles contributes heavily to their uptake mechanism and represents a major factor in their internalization and clearance potential. Additional shapes such as nonspherical, homogeneous and heterogeneous agglomerates, spherical and tubular micellular capsules, and dendritic structures individually conclude different preferential uptake mechanisms that complicate their ADME profile [13, 17]. Particles that evade phagocytic consumption and remain in circulation for longer periods of time are generally anticipated to possess increased systemic exposure and cytotoxic events, but vast generalizations are inappropriate for nanoparticulate systems due to incongruence among trends in their biocompatibility. Regardless of preexisting information from similar systems, new nanoparticle preparations necessitate in vitro study to verify the biocompatibility of slight morphological or chemical alterations.

Surface charge likewise plays a deterministic role in cellular uptake that rivals the contributions of particle morphology. Both net cationic and anionic charge are correlated with increased toxicity while neutral surfaces are believed to have the greatest biocompatibility [13]. Zwitterionic particles, by contrast, are generally considered benign due to their self-regulated charge balance and have undergone extensive investigation as antimicrobial and

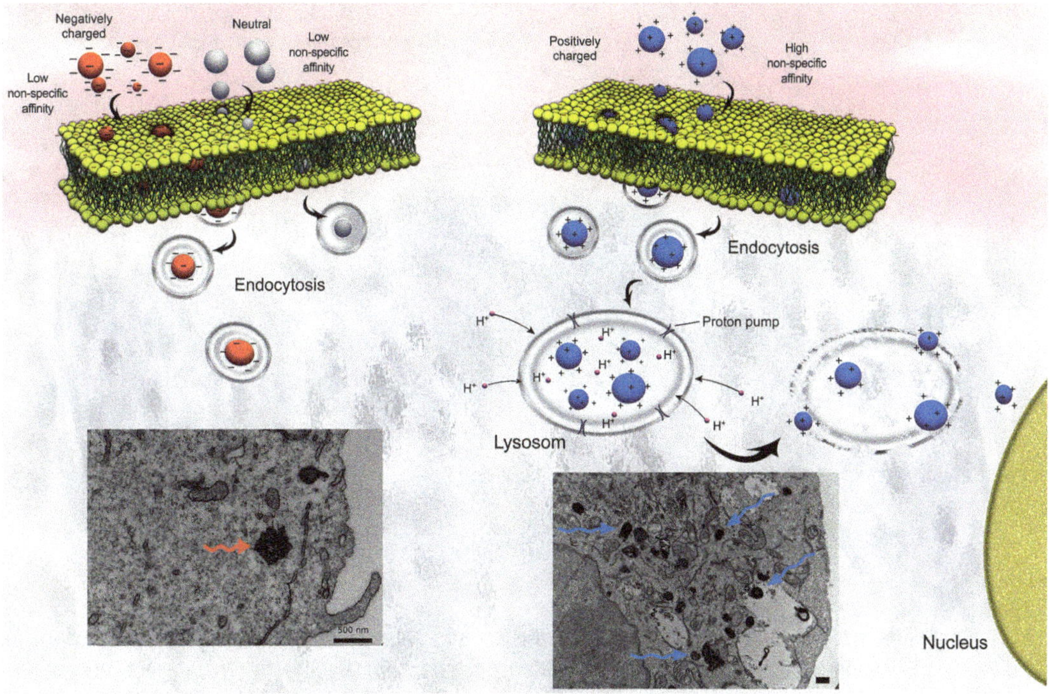

Fig. 1 Schematic displaying endocytosis of anionic (left) and cationic (right) nanoparticles and their resulting cytosolic formations. Cationic nanoparticles show stronger absorption capabilities than their anionic cousins, and, once endocytosed, they act as sponges that pump protons and signal cytotoxic cascades. The lower left transmission electron microscopy (TEM) images show aggregated anionic particles (bottom left) in HeLa cells compared to dispersed cationic particles with heightened uptake (bottom right). Reproduced from ref. 13 with permission from The Royal Society of Chemistry

antifouling agents [24]. Positively charged nanoparticles express affinity toward the negatively charged phospholipid heads populating the lipid bilayer and encourage endocytosis. Once internalized, the cationic surface charge acts as a proton sponge that disrupts normal lysosomal activity and initiates cell death as shown in Fig. 1 [13]. Negatively charged particles, by comparison, display greater potency in breaching the skin barrier via charge density and have the potential to signal coagulation cascades. Under sufficient doses, anionic nanoparticles can induce thrombosis and eventual embolism. In a similar manner, cationic particles assemble platelet aggregates known as "coronas" that disguise their unmasked chemistry and provide an alternative biological identity. Further complicating the functionality of a singular idealized "crown" covering the nanoparticles, protein adhesion to the particle surface operates by competitive affinity which changes the protein mixture surrounding the nanoparticle and modifies its new biological identity over time [14]. Illustrated in Fig. 2, a "hard" corona is initially formed by tightly bound protein aggregates and an exterior "soft" corona constantly exchanges proteins with the surrounding plasma [25].

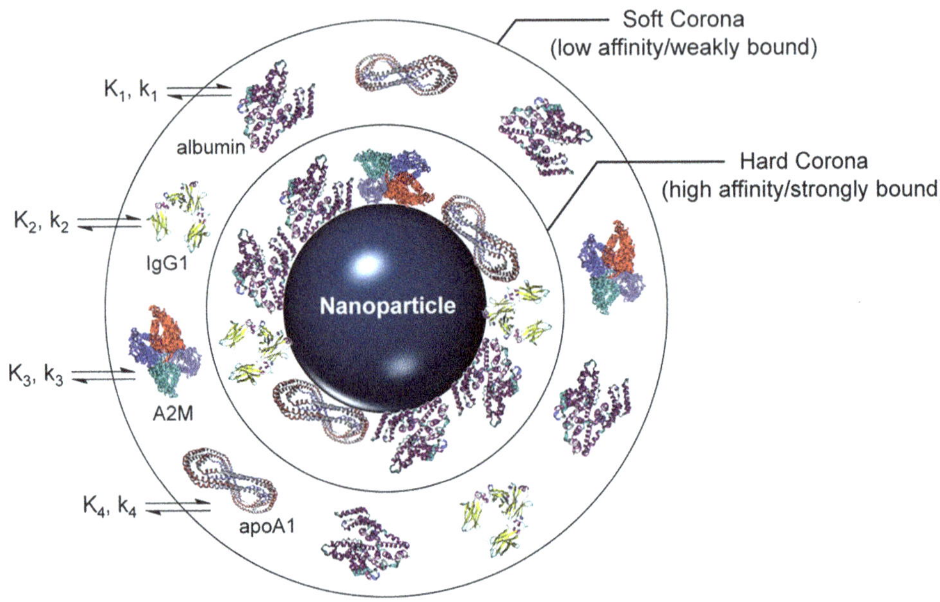

Fig. 2 Representative schematic of a fully developed protein corona surrounding a foreign nanoparticle. Proteins initially adhere to the surface strongly to form a hard corona followed by transient, competitive adsorption in an outer soft corona. Binding in the corona is kinetically (k) and thermodynamically (K) driven by serum proteins (with the common proteins albumin, immunoglobulin G1 (IgG1), alpha-2 macroglobulin (A2M), and apolipoprotein A-1 (apoA1) shown). Reproduced from [25]. Further permissions related to the material excerpted should be directed to the ACS. https:/pubs.acs.org/doi/10.1021/ar500190q

The flux of adsorbed proteins forming the "soft" corona is regulated by a continual state of affinity competition termed the Vroman effect [14, 26]. The presence of a shielding corona can reduce toxicity by preventing the nonspecific cellular internalization of cationic particles and offsetting their membrane disruption and hemolytic capacities or increase toxicity by denaturing attached proteins and generating aberrations that elicit immunogenic and inflammatory responses [14]. Mimicking the myriad of proteins present in biological milieu for in vitro experimentation poses a significant challenge and comprises one of the major sources of disparity between in vitro and in vivo toxicity assessments.

Coating nanoparticles with protein-resistant moieties or agglomeration inhibitors can mitigate the biomodification enveloping bare nanoparticles and counteract their unmodified toxicity. Uncoated nanoparticles often suffer from hydrophobic surfaces, and their preference to aggregate can form blockages that impeded circulation. Polyethylene glycol (PEG) is one of the most commonly employed surface coatings for therapeutic nanoparticles due to its ability to hide the particles from surveillance proteins [27]. The prevention of opsonization using a PEG steric barrier provides the nanoparticles with "stealth" properties that grant elongated circulation [28, 29]. As with shape regulating phagocytotic events, the lengthened biological half-life presents a double-edged sword: as the time in circulation extends, the opportunity for particles to affect both the desired target (e.g., a tumor) and unintended accumulation sites in susceptible tissues simultaneously increases [28]. Although heightened payload delivery to the target region significantly improves drug efficacy, the particles' introduction to otherwise healthy areas can generate deleterious side effects that negate the therapy's benefits. Moieties like chitosan and polylactic acid (PLA) have been combined with PEG to award both "stealth" and therapeutic properties concomitantly, and the modification of coatings to include environmentally responsive degradation cues can prompt even the relatively toxic nanoparticle cores to act as pseudotherapeutic agents. Protection against reactive oxygen species (ROS) generation by bare metallic nanoparticles using antioxidant-infused polymer coatings like poly(trolox ester) with controlled degradation offers a route for the combinatorial suppression of undesired oxidative damage and localized delivery of enzymatically hydrolyzed therapeutic agents while maintaining the core's cytotoxic potential as a secondary mode of treatment [30]. Coatings can also harbor surface charges that selectively take advantage of cationic or anionic behavior without accruing their negative consequences. A cationic nanoparticle neutralized by a negatively charged shell can, for example, exploit extended circulation from a net neutral surface charge and the leaky vascular of tumors to specifically target tumor cells [31]. Shedding brought about by the acidic tumor microenvironment allows the nanocarrier to escape lysosomal destruction and reveal a reactive core. Alternatively, premature coating deterioration can turn an initially inert nanoparticle into a toxic agent by inciting immunogenic or inflammatory responses from its unshielded core prior to reaching its intended destination [13]. The untimely exposure provokes agglomeration, corona formation, and unabated chemical reactivity which potentially results in harmful physiological outcomes.

The chemical composition of nanoparticles governs their interaction with cells and milieu and shapes their capacity for oxidative stress production. Applying comparable size regimes, particles of varying fundamental compositions, especially in the case of metal oxide nanoparticles, display significantly different toxicity profiles due to alterations in their base constituencies [32]. Administered metallic nanoparticles are prone to dislodging toxic metal ions in the presence of fluctuating pH zones throughout the body, and the ions' circulation into accumulation sites such as the liver and kidney present concerns for eventual genotoxic and cytotoxic effects [13]. Iron oxide and copper oxide nanoparticles pose as Fenton or Fenton-like catalysts for radical generation that contribute to lipid peroxidation and deoxyribonucleic acid (DNA) cleavage; gold, highly sought after as photothermal therapy and contrast agents, silver, traditionally used in antimicrobial prophylaxis, and zinc oxide, find use in a variety of applications ranging from filters to food additives, possess dose-dependent cytotoxicity; aluminum oxide and titanium dioxide, both employed in polymer and pharmaceutical industries, were initially considered inert but have since garnered attention as oxidative stress and inflammation promoters [32, 33]. Nanosized silica and carbon-based nanomaterials (e.g., carbon nanotubes, fullerenes, carbon black) constitute over 50% of airborne nanomaterials [34] and have extensive literature characterizing their metabolic resistance and size-dependent cytotoxicity [32, 35]. Polymeric nanoparticles propose additional considerations for their toxicity analysis, namely whether the nanoparticles are liable to degrade within the body and whether their metabolites are biocompatible. Although metallic nanoparticles hold similar concerns for metabolic degradation, therapeutic polymer-based nanoparticles often have the designed caveat of undergoing hydrolysis and breaking into their base monomers or analogs [17]. The feature allows on-demand release of medicinal agents into localized delivery sites to enhance the bioavailable fraction of therapeutics at the site of action while minimizing systemic circulation of drugs with deleterious side effects. Careful engineering is, however, required to ensure toxic degradants are prevented from entering the bloodstream and wreaking havoc downstream of the material's degradation cue. The interplay of balancing the therapeutic and toxic potential of nanoparticles with their metabolites defines a foundational concern for minimizing ROS and inflammation production from therapeutic administration and environmental bioaccumulation, and their evaluation through in vitro testing marks a prerequisite study for any nanoparticle-based treatment.

3 Characterization and Toxicity Analysis

To properly evaluate the safety and impact of a nanomaterial, the fundamental physiochemical properties of the material and its interaction and impact upon living cellular systems must be understood. In this section, the most common methods to characterize nanomaterial properties and a set of in vitro toxicity screenings used to determine material safety are presented. The approaches presented herein do not represent the entirety of all available tools and methods but rather a sufficiently broad initial assessment for the evaluation of a new nanomaterial.

3.1 Size and Surface Charge Evaluation

Numerous analytical techniques are available to characterize the toxicological aspects of nanoparticles, but two methods in particular are regularly used to grant critical quantitative information: dynamic light scattering (DLS) and zeta potential (ZP) analysis. With DLS, the random movements of dilute nanoparticles

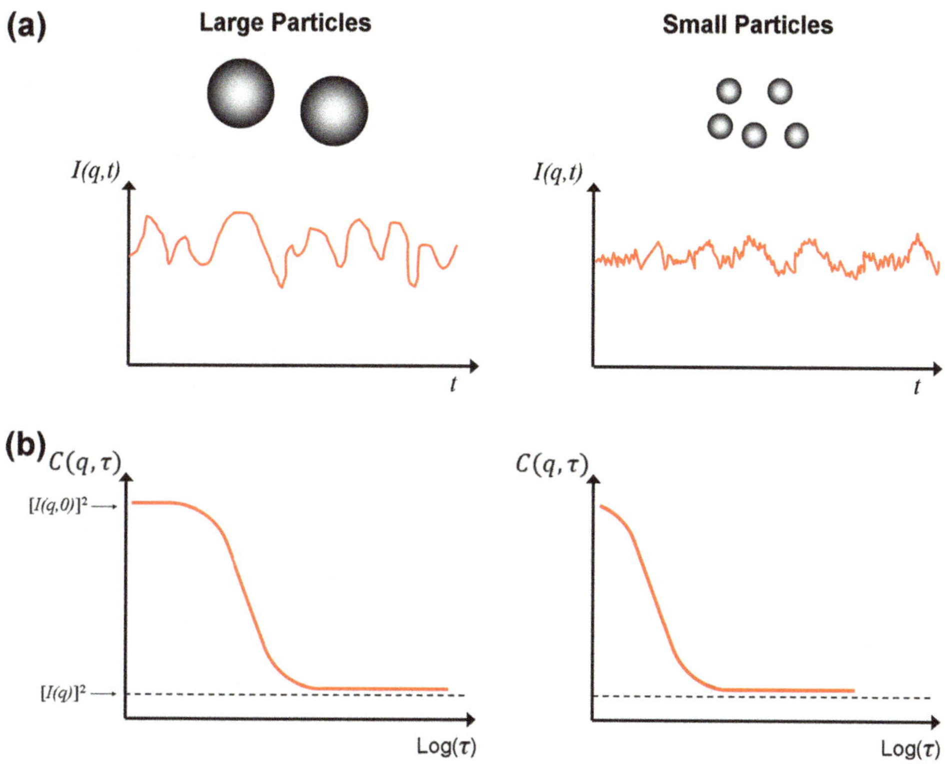

Fig. 3 Schematic scattering intensity as a function of time (**a**) and autocorrelation function variation with delay time (**b**) for large and small particle sizes, respectively. Large particles resist random force fluctuations and maintain smoother intensity plots; smaller particles move rapidly in solution and cause jitter in their intensities. Reproduced in part from [37]

dispersed in solution caused by Brownian motion are detected by monitoring Rayleigh or Mie scattering generated from a monochromatic laser [36]. The intensity fluctuations recorded by the detector are translated into an autocorrelation function which tracks the intensity decay as a function of time. A representative image displaying the translation of scattering intensity into an autocorrelation function is displayed in Fig. 3. In the simplest case, the autocorrelation function is fit to an exponential decay whereby the translational diffusion coefficient is calculated in accordance with the wave vector relating the angle of excitation used by the DLS instrument. The diffusion coefficient is used in conjunction with the Stokes-Einstein equation to estimate the hydrodynamic radius of the particles assuming that the nanoparticles' morphology is confined to a sphere [37]. Averaging the decay rate prior to evaluating the diffusion coefficient yields the ensemble translational diffusion coefficient which is applied to determine the commonly reported z-average nanoparticle diameter. Two primary analytical methods succinctly define the relationship between the autocorrelation function and the sample size distribution: the cumulant and CONTIN algorithms [36]. The cumulant algorithm fits the beginning of the autocorrelation function to a single exponential decay wherein the first cumulant term defines the z-average diameter and the second term indicates the polydispersity index (PDI). The PDI marks the homogeneity of a sample on a zero to one scale; a small PDI (≤ 0.1) is representative of a monodisperse sample while a large PDI (>0.4) designates a highly polydisperse sample [36]. The CONTIN algorithm employs a broader fitting timescale to isolate size distributions for multiple heterogeneous peaks in polydisperse samples. Modern DLS instruments apply both methods to provide the user with the *z*-average diameter, PDI, and heterogeneous peak distributions simultaneously. If the particles lack a spherical geometry and Mie scattering dominates, sample anisotropy will noticeably alter the calculated z-average diameter as a function of the irradiation angle used for the sample analysis. Post-measurement analysis can take advantage of equations derived for estimating the sample's rotational diffusion coefficient together with its translational diffusion coefficient to approximate the aspect ratio of rod-like particles [38, 39].

Zeta potential identifies the apparent surface charge of nanoparticles and is often a complementary capability of DLS systems. Particles dispersed in solution innately attract a closely packed layer of oppositely charged molecules to their surface known as the Stern layer, and the Stern layer is further surrounded by an ionically mixed diffuse layer extending outward toward a hypothetical boundary termed the slipping plane. Together, the Stern layer and slipping plane represent the electric double layer (EDL) enveloping a nanoparticle [40]. As shown in Fig. 4, the electric potential difference between the outermost slipping plane of the EDL and the potential of the dispersant comprises the zeta potential of a colloid. The measured ZP consequently does not signify the surface charge at the nanoparticle–Stern layer interface; the measured potential difference atop the EDL is substantially lower than the potential difference between the surface of the particle and the surrounding medium [41]. The decay of electrostatic force follows Debye's law as an inverse exponential, and the true surface potential, called the Nernst potential, is only attainable through theoretical approximation [36]. The ZP is determined by correlating the speed of particles in transit to the device's anode or cathode to the magnitude of an externally applied electric field. The velocity is assessed by monitoring the Doppler shift, which relates the frequency change between incident light shown onto electrically mobile particles and a reference laser to the velocity of the colloids in the medium [40]. The electrophoretic mobility of the nanoparticles is directly calculated from the experimentally determined particle velocity and electric field strength, and the mobility is thereafter related to the desired ZP with the Helmholtz–Smoluchowski equation for large particles (>100 nm) having relatively

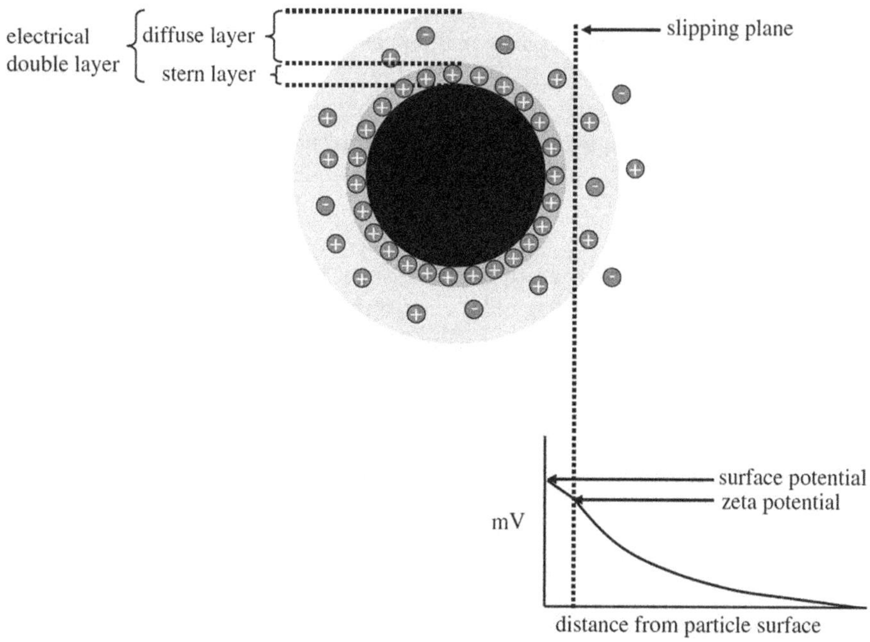

Fig. 4 Schematic representation of the EDL extending from the surface of an anionic nanoparticle into the hypothetical slipping plane. The zeta potential decreases exponentially from the surface outward toward the surrounding medium. Reproduced from [40]

small EDLs with respect to their size or the Hückel equation for small particles ($\leq$100 nm) with comparatively large EDLs [36]. The Helmholtz–Smoluchowski equation is viable for aqueous solutions with high salt concentrations (~10^{-2} M) while the Hückel equation requires minimal salt interference ($<10^{-5}$ M) [36]. The dispersant pH plays a critical role in the stability of nanoparticle solutions by altering the ionic composition of the EDL and modifying the electrostatic repulsive forces between charged particles. As the solution pH approaches the isoelectric point of the nanoparticles, the electrostatic repulsion among particles of like charges diminishes and the van der Waals attractive forces between the floating bodies begins to dominate [42]. The magnitude of the measured ZP, therefore, does not provide a conclusive verification of colloid stability; ZP analyzes only particle surface charge without insight into interparticle attractive forces. Solutions with high ZP ($\pm$30 mV) are often conferred stability while low ZP solutions ($\leq$10 mV) are considered unstable, but the scale of attractive van der Waals forces can (rarely) revoke traditional classifications [43]. The solution ionic strength also contributes to the nanoparticles' stability by compressing the EDL with increasing ionic strength and lowering the measured ZP [41]. As mentioned earlier in this chapter, a particle's calculated ZP and, by extension, surface charge play a significant role in deducing their possible toxicity, advancing integrated DLS-ZP systems as essential instruments for precursor biocompatibility evaluations.

Although DLS and ZP act as the primary characterization techniques for nanoparticles before their introduction to in vitro assays, numerous other techniques are available that offer comparable analyses or additional worthwhile information. Common practices include electron microscopy (e.g., transmission electron microscopy (TEM) and scanning electron microscopy (SEM)), laser diffraction, and atomic force microscopy (AFM) for sizing and geometry, Fourier-transform infrared spectroscopy (FTIR), X-ray diffraction (XRD), surface-enhanced Raman spectroscopy (SERS), and solid-state nuclear magnetic resonance spectroscopy (SSNMR) for composition analysis, and ultraviolet-visible spectroscopy (UV-Vis) and fluorometry for photonic properties [44]. Employing multiple methods in tandem with DLS and ZP analysis help identify some of the more critical parameters composing nanoparticles' toxicity profiles, and their evaluation in concert with in vitro toxicity assessment can reveal the primary mechanisms generating toxicity that require resolution prior to their use.

3.2 Cellular Interaction Assays

An important screen for nanoparticle toxicity is the determination of a nanoparticle's ability to transport across and interact with cellular barriers. Nanoparticle permeation across the cell membrane promoted by cationic surface charges and coatings enticing active transport [45] cultivate interaction between therapeutic or toxic agents and susceptible organelles in the cytoplasm. Assays surveying cellular infiltration desire quantitative analysis of particle positioning within cells and qualitative imaging of the material's destination, but current instrumentation struggles to bridge the gap between the two analytical goals. In conventional procedures, cultivated cells are incubated with nanoparticles for 24 h followed by staining and microscopic analysis [46–48]. Fluorescent methods typically use anterior chemical modification [23, 45] or immunostaining [49] to couple tags such as fluorescein isothiocyanate (FITC), cyanines, and Alexa dyes with fluorescence-activated cell sorting (FACS), confocal laser scanning microscopy (CLSM), and imaging flow cytometry (IFC) for independent quantitative and qualitative identification of nanoparticle internalization following sample incubation. An excellent review by Ostrowski et al. [50] delivers an overview of traditional spectroscopic and microscopic imaging approaches for tissue and cellular internalization studies. Alternatively, methods using inductively coupled plasma mass spectroscopy (ICP-MS) [51], TEM, or transmission X-ray microscopy (TXM) in the case of metallic nanoparticles [52] eliminate the need for fluorophores by applying nonfluorometric instrumentation. None of the individual approaches offers a precise, high-resolution measure for internalization: CLSM and TXM reveal whether nanoparticles are internalized or externally adhered to the surface of cells, but the methods are only semiquantitative; FACS and ICP-MS provide quantitative results without visual resolution; and IFC offers a semiquantitative bridge by sacrificing the throughput of FACS and the resolution of CLSM [53]. Combination of two or more techniques is required to fully characterize the scale of nanoparticle intrusion while maintaining observations of their locality.

Alongside cellular internalization assays evaluating a nanomaterial's proclivity to bypass the cell membrane, quantifying the material's preference to localize in the cytosol or in the nucleus provides further understanding of the nanoparticle's potential routes for therapy and toxicity. After passage into the cytosol, large molecule and particle migration into the nucleus is primarily regulated through active transport mechanisms involving the cytoskeletal motor proteins kinesin and dynein along cellular microtubules [54]. Kinesin-mediated transport exports agents from the centrosome and nucleus while dynein shuttles molecules in the opposite direction, ultimately facing the nuclear pore complex as a gateway into the nucleoplasm. Imaging and quantifying particles that pass the size restrictions of the nuclear envelope ($\leq$40 nm) [54] are typically performed with electron microscopy and fluorometry to visualize nanoparticle populations in the nucleoplasm and surrounding cytosol. Images of Herceptin-loaded gold nanoparticles depositing in both locations depending upon the size of the nanocarrier are presented in Fig. 5. In the case of gold nanoparticles (which have undergone extensive exploration as radiosensitizers), positioning within or outside the nucleus is deduced from TEM while uptake concentrations are determined with ICP-MS [46, 55]. Fluorescent tags for polymeric nanoparticles allow observation of their localization patterns using confocal fluorescence microscopy, epifluorescence microscopy, and CLSM [47, 48]. Beyond transient analysis of internalization behavior, real-time evaluation of nanoparticle transport into cells is available with fluorescence correlation spectroscopy (FCS), raster image correlation spectroscopy (RICS), and time-resolved confocal microscopy [56]. Each method offers insight into the pervasiveness of nanoparticles within the cellular interior and possible explanation for the cytotoxic or biocompatible nature of specific particles.

As a complement to the cellular internalization and distribution schemes offered by microscopic techniques, transcytosis assays identify the proficiency of particles to permeate through epithelial barriers like the lungs, gastrointestinal tract, and blood-brain barrier (BBB). Epithelial cells generally congregate into tight junctions once plated, and measurement of the transepithelial electrical resistance (TEER) across the junction denotes the integrity of the barrier as shown in Fig. 6. If nanoparticles permeate across the barrier and tear the junctions or if construction of the junction is otherwise impaired, the acquired TEER value is typically observed

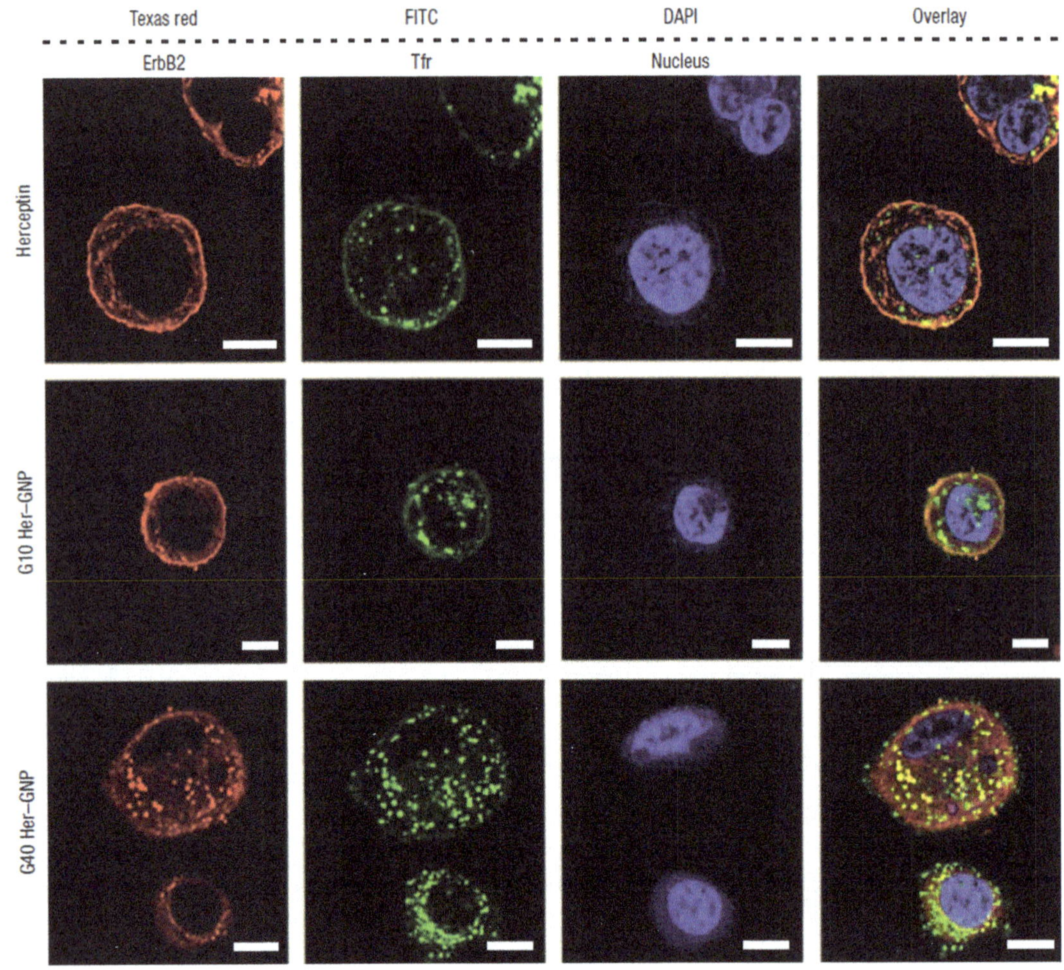

Fig. 5 Herceptin transcytosis into human breast cancer SK-BR-3 cells treated for 3 h promoted by Herceptin-functionalized gold nanoparticles (Her-GNP). Stains from left to right: anti-ErbB2 (Texas red), anti-transferrin receptor (Tfr) antibodies (FITC), and nuclear counterstain (DAPI). Vehicles from top to bottom: free Herceptin, 10 nm Her-GNP, and 40 nm Her-GNP. Each stain was overlaid in the fourth panel. The Her-GNP vehicles display enhanced cytosolic uptake of Herceptin, and the smaller 10 nm Her-GNP carriers demonstrate greater nuclear internalization than their 40 nm counterparts. Scale bars are 10 μm. Reproduced from [20]

to decrease from the range of 500–2000 Ω/cm^2 to less than 500 Ω/cm^2 [57]. Isolating the apical and basolateral compartment concentrations of nanoparticles as a function of time following barrier exposure effectively relates the permeability of the epithelial membrane with respect to the tested nanoparticles [58], and incorporation of the particle translocation tendency with TEER results can decide whether the particles are constructed to innately bypass the junction or whether the transmission occurs as a result of nanoparticle-induced membrane rupture. Basolateral sampling with one of the aforementioned fluorescent stains and fluorometry methods [59] allows direct quantification of the permeated particle

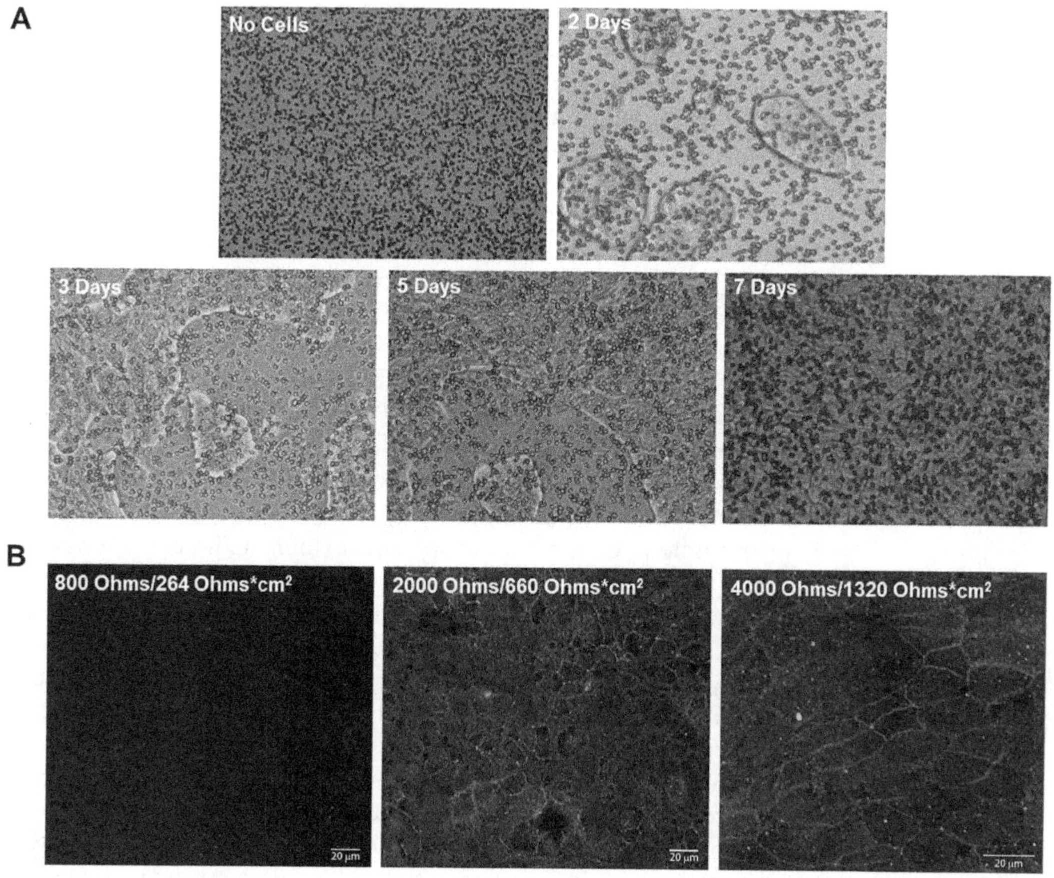

Fig. 6 Human lung epithelial Calu-3 cell confluence over a single week's culture in 10% FBS imaged using an inverted microscope with 10× magnification (**a**). Monolayer formation hides Transwell insert pores throughout the culture duration as seen from the initial image at time zero (top left) to the completion of monolayer formation at the conclusion of a week (bottom right). Confocal microscopy images of ZO-1 (green) and DAPI (blue) stained junctions and nuclei, respectively, display monolayer formation as a function of increased TEER resistance (**b**). Reproduced from [57]. https:/creativecommons.org/licenses/by-nc-nd/4.0/

count and the opportunity for inline characterization. Altogether, data from TEER and migrated nanoparticle populations compose satisfactory reports for the particle's transcytosis performance, and the assay's coupling with other assays describing cellular cytotoxicity details the exposure hazard for both therapeutic and environmental nanoparticles.

3.3 Viability Assays

Lactate dehydrogenase (LDH) is an enzyme produced by living cells to regulate pyruvate and lactate levels through nicotinamide adenine dinucleotide (NAD) oxidation. When cells undergo hemolysis or necrosis, LDH is released into the surrounding extracellular environment while maintaining enzymatic activity. Conversion of pyruvate to lactate follows NADH + Pyruvate $\leftrightarrow$ NAD^+ + Lactate in the presence of LDH where NADH and NAD^+ represent the reduced and oxidized forms of NAD, respectively, and complementary reaction of NADH with tetrazolium salts permits spectroscopic monitoring of LDH enzymatic activity using known initial concentrations of lactate and NAD. The time-dependent change in spectroscopic absorbance of the reduced tetrazolium compound measured by an enzyme-linked immunosorbent assay (ELISA) reader or UV-Vis spectrometer is directly proportional to the sample LDH concentration [60] and, by inference, the extent of cellular trauma. Tetrazolium salts were originally investigated as nonradioactive replacements for the traditional radioactive chromium (^{51}Cr) assay technique [61] and as methods to enhance the sensitivity of detecting NADH absorbance at 340 nm. Common tetrazolium salts include iodonitrotetrazolium (INT), 3-(4,5-dimethylthiazol-2-yl)-2,5-diphenyltetrazolium bromide (MTT), and 3-(4,5-dimethylthiazol-2-yl)-5-(3-carboxymethoxyphenyl)-2-(4-sulfophenyl)-2H-tetrazolium (MTS) which rival the throughput of the ^{51}Cr assay and exhibit a threefold sensitivity increase over ultraviolet NADH assays [62, 63]. Numerous salt-based commercial kits like the Pierce™ LDH Cytotoxicity Assay Kit and CytoTox 96® Non-Radioactive Cytotoxicity Assay are available, and nonsalt fluorometric kits utilizing the reduction of resazurin (nonfluorescent) to resorufin (fluorescent) by NADH offer alternatives to colorimetric assays. Additionally, the luminogenic glycylphenylalanyl-aminofluorocoumarin (GF-AFC) and firefly luciferase ATP assays provide nontoxic and highly sensitive options for assessing cell viability [64]. Regardless of the assay employed, nanoparticles can interfere with viability assay results through several mechanisms: static adsorption of LDH and related proteins to the nanoparticle surface can denature a fixed amount of enzyme prior to surface saturation, dynamic adsorption can continuously inactive LDH throughout the duration of the assay, and ROS generation can prematurely oxidize NADH to skew absorbance values [65]. Careful sample preparation is necessary to minimize perturbations from reactive particles that can severely distort outcomes from in vitro LDH analysis.

3.4 Apoptosis Assays

Acceleration of apoptosis due to nanoparticle exposure can jeopardize cellular regeneration and hasten aging in mammalian hosts. Markers of programmed cell death include two major trackable factors for in vitro analysis: phosphatidylserine (PS) migration to the outer leaflet of the cell membrane and caspase activation into initiator and effector enzymes. Prior to apoptosis initiation, flippases hold PS exclusively on the cytosolic face of the asymmetric cell membrane; during the execution phase of apoptosis, scramblases transport PS from the inner leaflet to the exoplasmic face [66]. The loss of phospholipid asymmetry accompanying PS exchange maintains membrane integrity while signaling for macrophage consumption and platelet aggregation. To prevent rampant blood coagulation occurring from the natural cell cycle, calcium-mediated annexin V binds to exposed PS as a shield from coagulation cascades. Attaching hapten moieties (e.g., FITC) to annexin V permits apoptotic cell labeling, and secondary stains that identify cellular necrosis such as membrane impermeable propidium iodide (PI) combined with fluorescence microscopy or flow cytometry constitute the annexin V-affinity assay, which is capable of quantifying healthy (FITC and PI negative), apoptotic (FITC positive and PI negative), and dead (FITC and PI positive) cells simultaneously [67]. The annexin V assay monitors a seemingly ubiquitous apoptotic event in PS translocation resulting from a number of causal factors [66], establishing the method as a reliable measure for apoptosis signaling. Caspase activation is, however, a precedent to PS transport and a complementary event for verification of premature apoptosis onset. Caspases represent a family of 14 cysteine proteases initially lodged as inactive zymogens (procaspases) within the cellular cytoplasm [68]. Following a host of stimuli-induced signaling pathways, procaspases are oligomerized from encoded prodomains containing large and small subunits through intrinsic or extrinsic pathways. Active caspases offer several assay analysis approaches, including: cleavable substrates with fluorogen and chromogen labels, immunoblotting, immunofluorescence, and affinity assays with attached reporter moieties. Readers are encouraged to refer to the informative review by Kaufmann et al. [69] for detailed explanations and methodologies on each procedure. None of the caspase assays offer definitive evidence for individual quantitative caspase activity, and multiple assays are required for full characterization. The multimodal capability of caspases to cleave their unpreferred substrates hinders isolation with labels; immunoblots are not quantitative and cannot discern non-cleavage-based enzymatic activity; immunofluorescence necessitates specific conformational antibodies with the potential for cross-reactivity; and affinity labels often use expensive reagents that are susceptible to nucleophilic competition [69]. Nonetheless, the caspase assays provide a useful technique for identifying cellular apoptosis signals preceding PS translocation.

3.5 Oxidative Stress/ Inflammation Assays

The enhanced reactivity of nanoparticles imposed by their high surface area to volume ratio boosts cellular oxidative stress and promotes intracellular damage. Detection of oxidation events through direct measurement of ROS, indicators of oxidative damage such as protein carbonyl content and genotoxicity, and inflammatory markers reveals the in vitro potential of nanoparticles to produce detrimental cellular oxidants. Generation of ROS within the cytoplasm beyond natural levels is quantifiable via introduction of ROS sensitive dyes such as the nonionic, nonpolar, membrane-permeable fluorophore 2′,7′-dichlorofluorescein diacetate (DCFH-DA) as described by Keston and Brandt [70]. Upon cellular internalization of nonfluorescent DCFH-DA, the fluorophore is enzymatically hydrolyzed by cytosolic esterases into its nonfluorescent polar analog dichlorofluorescein (DCFH), whereby the analog becomes trapped within the cytosol. Hydroxyl radicals and comparable cellular ROS oxidize DCFH into highly fluorescent dichlorofluorescein (DCF) which is monitored using fluorescence microscopy or flow cytometry [71]. Albeit relatively easy to implement and quantitative, the DCFH-DA method for evaluating ROS content is susceptible to inaccuracy due to nonspecific enzymatic oxidation and photooxidation [71, 72]. Catalase offers possible inhibition for enzymatic oxidation, but the results from DCF assays must, nevertheless, be interpreted with caution to avoid overestimating nanoparticles' ROS generation capability. In a comparable method for analyzing mitochondrial respiration, commercial Seahorse Extracellular Flux (XF) Analyzers measure the oxygen consumption rate (OCR) and energy production potential of cells subjected to chemical inhibitors as markers of mitochondrial oxidative stress. Checking the OCR following incubation with antioxidants and subsequent oxidizers tracks oxidation-induced mitochondrial damage inhibition capacity, and the offset in OCR decline observed by the introduction of a therapeutic agent can signify the efficacy of a treatment [73]. Post-analysis treatment with cell viability kits can verify ROS mitigation and the inherent safety of proposed treatments as in the case of curcumin versus curcumin nanogels displayed in Fig. 7.

The carbonyl content of proteins increases in response to oxidation from ROS and provides a general indicator of oxidative damage. Several approaches are available for measuring protein carbonyl levels, but two are particularly notable: tritiated borohydride and 2,4-dinitrophenylhydrazine (DNPH). Borohydride reduces protein carbonyls to alcohols with stable tritium labels detectable by spectrophotometric absorbance at 340 nm [74]. As with other carbonyl reagents, extraneous nucleic acids necessitate removal prior to labeling; streptomycin treatment is typically recommended as a pretreatment to precipitate nucleic acids [75]. Employing DNPH as the carbonyl reagent offers a nonradiochemical labeling method, but larger quantities of sampled protein are required for successful analysis. Reaction of the protein carbonyl group with DNPH generates a stable 2,4-dinitrophenyl (DNP) hydrazone product that is detected from its maximum absorbance between 360 and 390 nm and translated to a carbonyl content value using a molar absorption coefficient of 22,000 M^{-1} cm^{-1} [74]. Both assays produce identical values for the evaluated carbonyl content assuming protein-bound chromophores with absorbances in the range of the applied reagent are subtracted via a blank. The sensitivity and specificity of the DNPH assay is further improved while eliminating the expenditure of excess sample by applying high-performance liquid chromatography (HPLC) or

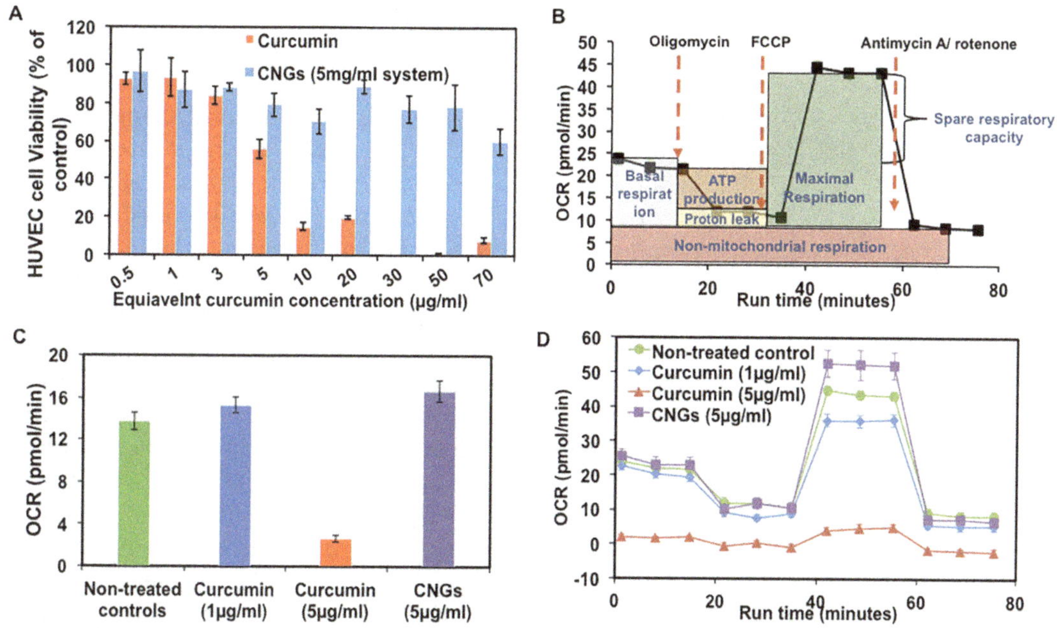

Fig. 7 Cytotoxicity of curcumin and curcumin nanogels (CNGs) for human umbilical vein endothelial cells (HUVECs) following 24 h of treatment at specified concentrations. (**a**) Cell viability results using calcein AM red-orange live cell tracer assay. (**b**) Seahorse XF96 calculated OCR for untreated cells undergoing a typical mitochondrial stress assay under the conditions shown. (**c**) Endpoint basal OCR rates for select samples from **a**. (**d**) Mitochondrial stress assay profiles for curcumin and CNG treatments following inhibitor additions as described in **b**. Reproduced from [73]

Western blotting with a sodium dodecyl sulfate polyacrylamide gel electrophoresis (SDS-PAGE) system [76]. Immunoassays in the form of ELISA and slot blotting can likewise be applied as highly sensitive techniques for analyzing carbonyl content, but the approaches are less common than the standard DNPH and borohydride methods [75].

Genotoxicity assays survey DNA and chromosomal damage and gene mutations occurring as a consequence of toxin-induced oxidative stress. The comet, micronucleus, Ames, and chromosome aberration assays are comprehensively reviewed by Golbamaki et al. [77] for metal oxide and silica nanomaterials and will be related for their general use herein. The single-cell gel electrophoresis, or comet, assay is a routine method for quantifying DNA breaks using fluorescence microscopy. Under alkaline electrophoresis conditions, supercoiled loops of DNA straighten into tails resembling comets, and the comet's head-to-tail distance reveals the number of DNA breaks in the sample. The Olive tail moment (OTM), first described by Olive et al. [78], relates the amount of damage in a standard format by reporting the comet tail's length multiplied by its DNA encapsulation percentage. Micronucleus (MN) assays regularly utilize cytochalasin B under the direction of the Organisation for Economic Co-operation and Development (OECD) Test Guideline no. 487 to test chromosomal breakage by preventing daughter cell separation following mitosis [79]. Visualization of binucleate cells using fluorescent stains like acridine orange permits quantification of micronucleus frequency among treated mitotic cell populations [80]. The Ames test uses *Salmonella* (*S. typhimurium*) and *Escherichia coli* (*E. coli*) bacterial strains to test for amino acid production among genetically defunct bacteria as prescribed by OECD Test Guideline no. 471 [81]. In the test, mutated bacteria that are incapable of producing an essential amino acid are incubated with the tested substance and the growth of revertant bacteria that regain the ability to synthesize the amino acid is observed. Implementation is rapid and facile but often considered inappropriate for nanoparticles due to the materials' meager uptake by bacterial cells [77]. The chromosome aberration test monitors chromosomal repair process malfunctions by halting mammalian cell cycles using a metaphase-arresting substance as per OECD Test Guideline no. 473 and registering metaphase chromosome aberrations microscopically [82]. The test is limited to clastogen identification and is, therefore, considered inferior to MN assays that also allow for aneugen detection [83].

Lipid peroxidation presents another quantifiable effect of ROS overproduction through evaluation of two major secondary peroxidation products in malondialdehyde (MDA) and 4-hydroxyl-2-nonenal (4-HNE). The more mutagenic of the products, MDA, arises from the decomposition of large polyunsaturated fatty acids (PUFAs) and the metabolism of arachidonic acid (AA) during thromboxane A_2 synthesis [84]. Reaction of the by-product with thiobarbituric acid (TBA) at pH 3.5 forms a MDA-TBA adduct that is detected fluorescently at 553 nm with an excitation of 515 nm or spectrophotometrically at 532 nm as part of the thiobarbituric acid reactive substances (TBARS) assay [85]. The assay has received intense scrutiny for its lack of specificity; TBA reacts with a number of substances other than MDA ranging from oxidized lipids to urea, altogether producing drastic overestimations of ROS lipid peroxidation. Efforts to raise the specificity of the assay include using HPLC to isolate the desired MDA-TBA adduct and eliminate background signals from conflicting reactive species [86]. The more cytotoxic lipid peroxidation product, 4-HNE, occurs as a by-product of AA decomposition and enzymatic and nonenzymatic PUFA peroxidation. The compound's high reactivity toward primary amines to form Schiff bases and thiol or amino compounds to make Michael adducts [87] enables detection using HNE-protein adduct ELISA assays [88]. In samples containing both MDA and 4-HNE, the TBA assay approach described for MDA analysis normally assembles fluorescent adducts for both peroxidation markers due to the assay's nonspecific nature, but substitution of TBA with 1-methyl-2-phenylindole in a hydrochloric acid reaction medium has been shown to promote MDA adduct yields over 4-HNE [89]. Despite its misgivings, the TBARS assay remains the predominant method for determining toxin lipid peroxidation and a viable approach for nanoparticles' peroxidation proclivity.

Inflammatory response markers include numerous families of cytokines activated by the immune system to combat hazardous invaders like reactive nanoparticles. One family in particular, interleukins, hosts 43 cytokines expressed by proinflammatory and anti-inflammatory macrophages that promote T-helper type 1 (Th1) and T-helper type 2 (Th2) cell responses, respectively [90]. Activity by Th1 and Th2 cells delivers tumor necrosis factor alpha (TNF-α) and interleukin-10 (IL-10) into the extracellular milieu whereby the concentrations are readily measured using ELISA [90] to gauge inflammatory responses occurring from treating macrophages with nanoparticles. As a precursor to interleukin upregulation, nuclear factor kappa-light-chain-enhancer of activated B cells (NF-κB) activity controls the cytokine production pathway and presents a foundational inflammation test using electrophoretic mobility shift assays (EMSAs). Binding of NF-κB to DNA response elements forms a bulky complex which, when exposed to an electrophoretic gel, inhibits migration and provides a gap between complexes that is frequently visualized with ^{32}P radiolabeling [91, 92]. Confirmation of NF-κB activity offers a qualitative or, at best, semiquantitative signal of proinflammation. As a quantitative alternative, firefly-derived luciferase assays, which use expression vectors cloned upstream of the *Photinus pyralis* luciferase gene, encode enzymes capable of measuring the genetic expression of inflammatory response markers such as the nuclear factor for interleukin-6 (NF-IL6) [93]. Following conjugation of clones containing the regulatory region of the inflammatory marker with the interleukin gene-of-interest during cell incubation, the produced luciferase reporter enzymes transiently oxidize injected luciferin into oxyluciferin which is quantified using a luminometer. Adding coenzyme A to the post-incubation luciferin spike greatly enhances the assay's sensitivity by augmenting and sustaining the emitted luminescence [94]. Applying quantitative luciferase assays in combination with inflammatory response and ROS assays contributes vital information for characterizing the oxidative and inflammatory potential of any nanoparticle species.

3.6 Endotoxin Assays

A common challenge for nanoparticles arises from their ability to absorb ambient contaminants to their surface, which can result in an enhanced inflammatory response over what would be expected if the absorbed chemicals were simply free in solution. This is most commonly seen in the case of endotoxins that cause acute inflammatory responses in humans. Endotoxins, or lipopolysaccharides (LPS), are environmentally prevalent pyrogens found in the outer cell wall of gram-negative bacteria that elicit inflammatory cytokines following activation of the coagulation signaling cascade in mammalian systems. The particular cascade sequence discovered for the analogous Atlantic horseshoe crab (*Limulus polyphemus*) by Bang [95] capitalizes upon the crabs' lethal intravascular coagulation when exposed to *Vibrio* endotoxin, and the reaction was developed into a routine series of in vitro assay procedures identified under the umbrella of the *Limulus* amebocyte lysate (LAL) assay using the blood cells (amebocytes) of the *Limulus polyphemus* or the homologous Japanese horseshoe crab (*Tachypleus tridentatus*). Three main assays stem from the LAL approach: the gel clot assay, the coagulogen-based (turbidity) assay, and the chromogenic assay [96]. The gel clot method employs endotoxin-activated enzymatic coagulogen cleavage by combining a portion of LAL solution with the endotoxin sample solution and checking for clotting following sufficient incubation. The technique is somewhat subjective due to confirmation arising from a simple positive or negative tube inversion to visualize clot formation, and quantitation requires inference from serial dilutions. Coagulogen-based assays vary in their quantitation by examining either changes in turbidity, coagulogen reduction during clotting, or peptide fragmentation [96]. Chromogenic approaches substitute chromogens for coagulogen that release chromophores when cleaved. Traditionally, *para*-nitroaniline is attached to an amino acid sequence resembling the clotting enzyme cleavage site in LAL and colors the solution upon liberation. Absorbance at 405 nm indicates the available concentration of clotting enzyme, which, in turn, reveals the concentration of endotoxin [96, 97]. Chromogenic LAL assays are included in commercial kits such as the Endosafe®-PTS (Portable Test System) for routine endotoxin analysis. In an alternative approach to using the blood of horseshoe crabs for assays, recombinant Factor C (rFC), the priming agent for coagulation, has developed into a standard reagent for endotoxin detection as a method for improving the sensitivity of LAL assays and sparing horseshoe crabs from endangerment [98]. Isolation and implementation of endotoxin-sensitive rFC eliminates possible false-positive reads from β-glucan contamination in LAL assays by eliminating glucan-reactive factor G that acts as a secondary clotting cascade pathway [99]. Additional methodologies have explored using immunoassays and rabbit pyrogen as alternatives to the popular LAL and rFC assays, but insensitivity and difficulty quantifying biological activity have curtailed their use in comparison to bioassays. Notably, evidence has demonstrated that nanoparticles can perturb LAL assay approaches and disrupt their accuracy [97], which has generated interest in identifying alternative routes for endotoxin detection to accommodate nanoparticles. Advances include using toll-like receptor 4 (TLR4) as a reporter protein, and the technology has made its way into commercial kits like the HEK-Blue™ detection system [97].

Table 1
Summary of toxins or injuries surveyed by each in vitro assay, their corresponding biomarkers, and select references applying the assays

Toxin/injury	Assays	Biomarkers	References
Barrier degradation	Cellular internalization, cytosol/ nuclear localization, TEER	Epithelial barrier damage, pervasive nanoparticle cellular internalization	[23, 45–49, 51–53, 55–57, 59]
Hemolysis or necrosis	INT, MTT, resazurin, NADH, GF-AFC, firefly luciferase ATP	Extracellular LDH	[60, 62–65]
Apoptosis	Annexin V, fluorogenic and chromogenic caspase, caspase immunoblotting, caspase immunofluorescence, caspase affinity	PS transport across to the outer leaflet of the cell membrane, procaspase oligomerization	[67, 69]
Hydroxyl radicals (ROS)	DCF, Seahorse XF Analyzers	Heightened intracellular ROS	[70–73]
	Tritiated borohydride, DNPH	Heightened protein carbonyl content	[74, 76]
	Comet, micronucleus, Ames, chromosome aberration	DNA/chromosome damage, gene mutations	[78–83]
Lipid peroxidation	TBARS, HNE-protein ELISA	MDA, 4-HNE	[85, 86, 88, 89]
Inflammation	ELISA, EMSA luciferase	Interleukin and nuclear factor release	[90–94]
Endotoxin/ LPS	Gel clot LAL, coagulogen-based LAL, chromogenic LAL, rFC, rabbit pyrogen, TLR4	Release of inflammatory cytokines IL-1β, TNF-α, and IL-6 following CD14 binding and MD2/TLR4 association	[96, 97, 99]

From the assays reviewed in the previous sections, the toxins and biomarkers corresponding to each assay are summarized in Table 1.

4 Conclusions/Outlook

Despite similarities in size, nanoparticles threaten multimodal forms of toxicity to unfortunate hosts through numerous mechanisms. Nanomaterial toxicity occurs due to the physicochemical properties of the material determining its proclivity to interact with the various proteins and cells comprising the biological milieu. Catalyzing ROS generation forms one of the most potent contributors to nanoparticles' toxicological components and sparks cascades of oxidative stress and inflammatory signals that ultimately lead to necrosis, expedited apoptosis, or carcinogenesis. The roots of the disastrous cascades are uncovered by observing the interplay between the particles' size and morphology and their chemical composition and apparent surface charge. Evaluation of each property is required to fully understand the toxicity profile of the queried material, and, even with exhaustive characterization, causes for toxicity can be shrouded by the complexity of biological systems. No individual gold standard exists for foreshadowing the toxicity of a unique nanomaterial; rather, combinations of several techniques are necessary to adequately describe the material's toxicological profile. Albeit ubiquitous, sizing from DLS does not provide an insurmountable threshold to bar cellular infiltration and epithelial barrier penetration, and ZP relates only the particle's apparent surface charge. Deduction of cellular uptake, protein corona formation, catalysis potential, and protein denaturation proficiency from routine nanoparticle analysis is, at best, inferential and necessitates in vitro study for verification.

Akin to the limitations plaguing characterization of physiochemical properties, in vitro assays also lack a one-size-fits-all method for exposing evidence regarding the toxicity or biocompatibility of tested nanoparticles. The myriad of cell types and assays impose a formidable array of tests for identifying individual markers of toxicity, but none of the studies provides an ideal pass-or-fail qualification. Multiple cell types should ideally be screened to replicate the heterogeneity of in vivo conditions, and singular signs of apparent inertness do not exclude alternative toxicological mechanisms from remaining in play. Combinations of multiple assays are, therefore, needed to sufficiently elucidate physiological responses to the nanoparticle system in question. Issues still persist for several of the established in vitro assays, namely: a method for the parallel high-resolution imaging and precise quantification of nanoparticle internalization beyond the sacrifices present for IFC has yet to be drawn into a standalone instrument; protein-based catalysis assays frequently assume a risk of cross-reactivity with secondary analytes that can mar data from the assays; and the enhanced reactivity of nanoparticles can preemptively oxidize analytical reagents or denature proteins that constitute the basis of numerous in vitro approaches. Resolution to the analytical and application-based problems involved with in vitro assays, particularly those associated with nanoparticulate systems, embodies the focus of future endeavors into nanoparticle toxicity analysis.

References

1. Salata OV (2004) Applications of nanoparticles in biology and medicine. J Nanobiotechnol 2:3–3. https://doi.org/10.1186/1477-3155-2-3
2. Eifler AC, Thaxton CS (2011) Nanoparticle Therapeutics: FDA Approval, Clinical Trials, Regulatory Pathways, and Case Study. In: Hurst SJ (ed) Biomedical Nanotechnology: Methods and Protocols. Humana, Totowa, NJ, pp 325–338. https://doi.org/10.1007/978-1-61779-052-2_21

3. Priyadarsini S, Mukherjee S, Mishra M (2018) Nanoparticles used in dentistry: a review. J Oral Biol Craniofac Res 8(1):58–67. https://doi.org/10.1016/j.jobcr.2017.12.004
4. Copéret C, Héroguel F (2017) Recent advances in surface organometallic chemistry. In: Cornils B, Herrmann WA, Beller M, Paciello R (eds) Applied homogeneous catalysis with organometallic compounds. Wiley-VCH Verlag GmbH & Co, Weinheim, pp 1069–1084. https://doi.org/10.1002/9783527651733.ch15
5. Yan N, Xiao C, Kou Y (2010) Transition metal nanoparticle catalysis in green solvents. Coord Chem Rev 254(9):1179–1218. https://doi.org/10.1016/j.ccr.2010.02.015
6. Weiss J, Takhistov P, McClements DJ (2006) Functional materials in food nanotechnology. J Food Sci 71(9):R107–R116. https://doi.org/10.1111/j.1750-3841.2006.00195.x
7. Contado C (2015) Nanomaterials in consumer products: a challenging analytical problem. Front Chem 3:48. https://doi.org/10.3389/fchem.2015.00048
8. Raj S, Jose S, Sumod US, Sabitha M (2012) Nanotechnology in cosmetics: opportunities and challenges. J Pharm Bioallied Sci 4 (3):186–193. https://doi.org/10.4103/0975-7406.99016
9. Boxberg F, Tulkki J (2004) Quantum dots: phenomenology, photonic and electronic properties, modeling and technology. the handbook of nanotechnology. Nanometer structures: theory, modeling, and simulation. SPIE Press, Bellingham. https://doi.org/10.1117/3.537698.ch4
10. Akbarzadeh A, Samiei M, Davaran S (2012) Magnetic nanoparticles: preparation, physical properties, and applications in biomedicine. Nanoscale Res Lett 7(1):144–144. https://doi.org/10.1186/1556-276X-7-144
11. Smulders S, Luyts K, Brabants G, Landuyt KV, Kirschhock C, Smolders E, Golanski L, Vanoirbeek J, Hoet PHM (2014) Toxicity of nanoparticles embedded in paints compared with pristine nanoparticles in mice. Toxicol Sci 141(1):132–140. https://doi.org/10.1093/toxsci/kfu112
12. Rai M, Yadav A, Gade A (2009) Silver nanoparticles as a new generation of antimicrobials. Biotechnol Adv 27(1):76–83. https://doi.org/10.1016/j.biotechadv.2008.09.002
13. Sharifi S, Behzadi S, Laurent S, Forrest ML, Stroeve P, Mahmoudi M (2012) Toxicity of nanomaterials. Chem Soc Rev 41 (6):2323–2343. https://doi.org/10.1039/c1cs15188f
14. Corbo C, Molinaro R, Parodi A, Furman NET, Salvatore F, Tasciotti E (2016) The impact of nanoparticle protein corona on cytotoxicity, immunotoxicity and target drug delivery. Nanomedicine 11(1):81–100. https://doi.org/10.2217/nnm.15.188
15. Kumar V, Sharma N, Maitra SS (2017) In vitro and in vivo toxicity assessment of nanoparticles. Int Nano Lett 7(4):243–256. https://doi.org/10.1007/s40089-017-0221-3
16. Clichici S, Filip A (2015) In vivo assessment of nanomaterials toxicity. Nanomaters toxicity and risk assessment. https://doi.org/10.5772/60707
17. Vasilakes AL, Dziubla TD, Wattamwar PP (2013) Polymeric nanoparticles. In: Bader RA (ed) Engineering polymer systems for improved drug delivery. John Wiley & Sons, Inc., pp 117–161. https://doi.org/10.1002/9781118747896.ch5
18. Cabral H, Matsumoto Y, Mizuno K, Chen Q, Murakami M, Kimura M, Terada Y, Kano MR, Miyazono K, Uesaka M, Nishiyama N, Kataoka K (2011) Accumulation of sub-100 nm polymeric micelles in poorly permeable tumours depends on size. Nat Nanotechnol 6:815. https://doi.org/10.1038/nnano.2011.166 https://www.nature.com/articles/nnano.2011.166#supplementary-information
19. Perrault SD, Walkey C, Jennings T, Fischer HC, Chan WCW (2009) Mediating tumor targeting efficiency of nanoparticles through design. Nano Lett 9(5):1909–1915. https://doi.org/10.1021/nl900031y
20. Jiang W, Kim BYS, Rutka JT, Chan WCW (2008) Nanoparticle-mediated cellular response is size-dependent. Nat Nanotechnol 3:145. https://doi.org/10.1038/nnano.2008.30 https://www.nature.com/articles/nnano.2008.30#supplementary-information
21. Jain RK, Stylianopoulos T (2010) Delivering nanomedicine to solid tumors. Nat Rev Clin Oncol 7:653. https://doi.org/10.1038/nrclinonc.2010.139
22. Caldorera-Moore M, Guimard N, Shi L, Roy K (2010) Designer nanoparticles: incorporating size, shape and triggered release into nanoscale drug carriers. Expert Opin Drug Deliv 7 (4):479–495. https://doi.org/10.1517/17425240903579971
23. Gratton SEA, Ropp PA, Pohlhaus PD, Luft JC, Madden VJ, Napier ME, DeSimone JM (2008) The effect of particle design on cellular internalization pathways. Proc Natl Acad Sci 105 (33):11613–11618. https://doi.org/10.1073/pnas.0801763105

24. Huo S, Jiang Y, Gupta A, Jiang Z, Landis RF, Hou S, Liang XJ, Rotello VM (2016) Fully zwitterionic nanoparticle antimicrobial agents through tuning of core size and ligand structure. ACS Nano 10(9):8732–8737. https://doi.org/10.1021/acsnano.6b04207
25. Fleischer CC, Payne CK (2014) Nanoparticle–cell interactions: molecular structure of the protein corona and cellular outcomes. Acc Chem Res 47(8):2651–2659. https://doi.org/10.1021/ar500190q
26. Vroman L, Adams AL (1969) Identification of rapid changes at plasma–solid interfaces. J Biomed Mater Res 3(1):43–67. https://doi.org/10.1002/jbm.820030106
27. Owens DE, Peppas NA (2006) Opsonization, biodistribution, and pharmacokinetics of polymeric nanoparticles. Int J Pharm 307(1):93–102. https://doi.org/10.1016/j.ijpharm.2005.10.010
28. Li S-D, Huang L (2010) Stealth nanoparticles: high density but sheddable PEG is a key for tumor targeting. J Control Release 145(3):178–181. https://doi.org/10.1016/j.jconrel.2010.03.016
29. Perry JL, Reuter KG, Kai MP, Herlihy KP, Jones SW, Luft JC, Napier M, Bear JE, DeSimone JM (2012) PEGylated PRINT nanoparticles: the impact of peg density on protein binding, macrophage association, biodistribution, and pharmacokinetics. Nano Lett 12(10):5304–5310. https://doi.org/10.1021/nl302638g
30. Cochran DB, Wattamwar PP, Wydra R, Hilt JZ, Anderson KW, Eitel RE, Dziubla TD (2013) Suppressing iron oxide nanoparticle toxicity by vascular targeted antioxidant polymer nanoparticles. Biomaterials 34(37):9615–9622. https://doi.org/10.1016/j.biomaterials.2013.08.025
31. Fan M, Zeng Y, Ruan H, Zhang Z, Gong T, Sun X (2017) Ternary nanoparticles with a sheddable shell efficiently deliver microRNA-34a against CD44-positive melanoma. Mol Pharm 14(9):3152–3163. https://doi.org/10.1021/acs.molpharmaceut.7b00377
32. Bahadar H, Maqbool F, Niaz K, Abdollahi M (2016) Toxicity of nanoparticles and an overview of current experimental models. Iran Biomed J 20(1):1–11. https://doi.org/10.7508/ibj.2016.01.001
33. Han SG, Newsome B, Hennig B (2013) Titanium dioxide nanoparticles increase inflammatory responses in vascular endothelial cells. Toxicology 306:1–8. https://doi.org/10.1016/j.tox.2013.01.014
34. Donaldson K, Stone V (2003) Current hypotheses on the mechanisms of toxicity of ultrafine particles. Ann Ist Super Sanita 39(3):405–410
35. Napierska D, Thomassen LC, Lison D, Martens JA, Hoet PH (2010) The nanosilica hazard: another variable entity. Part Fibre Toxicol 7(1):39. https://doi.org/10.1186/1743-8977-7-39
36. Bhattacharjee S (2016) DLS and zeta potential – what they are and what they are not? J Control Release 235:337–351. https://doi.org/10.1016/j.jconrel.2016.06.017
37. Lim J, Yeap SP, Che HX, Low SC (2013) Characterization of magnetic nanoparticle by dynamic light scattering. Nanoscale Res Lett 8(1):381–381. https://doi.org/10.1186/1556-276X-8-381
38. Pecora R (1968) Spectrum of light scattered from optically anisotropic macromolecules. J Chem Phys 49(3):1036–1043. https://doi.org/10.1063/1.1670189
39. Rodríguez-Fernández J, Pérez-Juste J, Liz--Marzán LM, Lang PR (2007) Dynamic light scattering of short Au rods with low aspect ratios. J Phys Chem C 111(13):5020–5025. https://doi.org/10.1021/jp067049x
40. Kaszuba M, Corbett J, Watson FM, Jones A (2010) High-concentration zeta potential measurements using light-scattering techniques. Philos Transact A Math Phys Eng Sci 368(1927):4439–4451. https://doi.org/10.1098/rsta.2010.0175
41. Brown MA, Goel A, Abbas Z (2016) Effect of electrolyte concentration on the stern layer thickness at a charged interface. Angew Chem Int Ed 55(11):3790–3794. https://doi.org/10.1002/anie.201512025
42. Pfeiffer C, Rehbock C, Hühn D, Carrillo-Carrion C, de Aberasturi DJ, Merk V, Barcikowski S, Parak WJ (2014) Interaction of colloidal nanoparticles with their local environment: the (ionic) nanoenvironment around nanoparticles is different from bulk and determines the physico-chemical properties of the nanoparticles. J R Soc Interface 11(96):20130931. https://doi.org/10.1098/rsif.2013.0931
43. Clogston JD, Patri AK (2011) Zeta potential measurement. In: McNeil SE (ed) Characterization of nanoparticles intended for drug delivery. Humana Press, Totowa, NJ, pp 63–70. https://doi.org/10.1007/978-1-60327-198-1_6
44. Lin P-C, Lin S, Wang PC, Sridhar R (2014) Techniques for physicochemical characterization of nanomaterials. Biotechnol Adv 32

(4):711–726. https://doi.org/10.1016/j.biotechadv.2013.11.006

45. Muro S, Garnacho C, Champion JA, Leferovich J, Gajewski C, Schuchman EH, Mitragotri S, Muzykantov VR (2008) Control of endothelial targeting and intracellular delivery of therapeutic enzymes by modulating the size and shape of ICAM-1-targeted carriers. Mol Ther 16(8):1450–1458. https://doi.org/10.1038/mt.2008.127
46. Lechtman E, Pignol JP (2017) Interplay between the gold nanoparticle sub-cellular localization, size, and the photon energy for radiosensitization. Sci Rep 7(1):13268. https://doi.org/10.1038/s41598-017-13736-y
47. Singh L, Parboosing R, Kruger HG, Maguire GEM, Govender T (2016) Intracellular localization of gold nanoparticles with targeted delivery in MT-4 lymphocytes. Adv Nat Sci Nanosci Nanotechnol 7(4). https://doi.org/10.1088/2043-6262/7/4/045013
48. Tammam SN, Azzazy HM, Breitinger HG, Lamprecht A (2015) Chitosan nanoparticles for nuclear targeting: the effect of nanoparticle size and nuclear localization sequence density. Mol Pharm 12(12):4277–4289. https://doi.org/10.1021/acs.molpharmaceut.5b00478
49. Hewitt RE, Vis B, Pele LC, Faria N, Powell JJ (2017) Imaging flow cytometry assays for quantifying pigment grade titanium dioxide particle internalization and interactions with immune cells in whole blood. Cytometry A 91(10):1009–1020. https://doi.org/10.1002/cyto.a.23245
50. Ostrowski A, Nordmeyer D, Boreham A, Holzhausen C, Mundhenk L, Graf C, Meinke MC, Vogt A, Hadam S, Lademann J, Ruhl E, Alexiev U, Gruber AD (2015) Overview about the localization of nanoparticles in tissue and cellular context by different imaging techniques. Beilstein J Nanotechnol 6:263–280. https://doi.org/10.3762/bjnano.6.25
51. Bao D, Oh ZG, Chen Z (2016) Characterization of silver nanoparticles internalized by Arabidopsis plants using single particle ICP-MS analysis. Front Plant Sci 7:32. https://doi.org/10.3389/fpls.2016.00032
52. Chen H-H, Chien C-C, Petibois C, Wang C-L, Chu YS, Lai S-F, Hua T-E, Chen Y-Y, Cai X, Kempson IM, Hwu Y, Margaritondo G (2011) Quantitative analysis of nanoparticle internalization in mammalian cells by high resolution X-ray microscopy. J Nanobiotechnol 9(1):14. https://doi.org/10.1186/1477-3155-9-14
53. Gottstein C, Wu G, Wong BJ, Zasadzinski JA (2013) Precise quantification of nanoparticle internalization. ACS Nano 7(6):4933–4945. https://doi.org/10.1021/nn400243d
54. Cohen O, Granek R (2014) Nucleus-targeted drug delivery: theoretical optimization of nanoparticles decoration for enhanced intracellular active transport. Nano Lett 14 (5):2515–2521. https://doi.org/10.1021/nl500248q
55. McNamara AL, Kam WW, Scales N, McMahon SJ, Bennett JW, Byrne HL, Schuemann J, Paganetti H, Banati R, Kuncic Z (2016) Dose enhancement effects to the nucleus and mitochondria from gold nanoparticles in the cytosol. Phys Med Biol 61(16):5993–6010. https://doi.org/10.1088/0031-9155/61/16/5993
56. Hemmerich PH, von Mikecz AH (2013) Defining the subcellular interface of nanoparticles by live-cell imaging. PLoS One 8(4): e62018. https://doi.org/10.1371/journal.pone.0062018
57. Derk R, Davidson DC, Manke A, Stueckle TA, Rojanasakul Y, Wang L (2015) Potential in vitro model for testing the effect of exposure to nanoparticles on the lung alveolar epithelial barrier. Sens Biosensing Res 3:38–45. https://doi.org/10.1016/j.sbsr.2014.12.002
58. Srinivasan B, Kolli AR, Esch MB, Abaci HE, Shuler ML, Hickman JJ (2015) TEER measurement techniques for in vitro barrier model systems. J Lab Autom 20(2):107–126. https://doi.org/10.1177/2211068214561025
59. Bannunah AM, Vllasaliu D, Lord J, Stolnik S (2014) Mechanisms of nanoparticle internalization and transport across an intestinal epithelial cell model: effect of size and surface charge. Mol Pharm 11(12):4363–4373. https://doi.org/10.1021/mp500439c
60. Ponsoda X, Jover R, Castell JV, Gómez-Lechón MJ (1991) Measurement of intracellular LDH activity in 96-well cultures: a rapid and automated assay for cytotoxicity studies. J Tissue Cult Methods 13(1):21–24. https://doi.org/10.1007/bf02388199
61. Brunner KT, Mauel J, Cerottini JC, Chapuis B (1968) Quantitative assay of the lytic action of immune lymphoid cells of (51)Cr-labelled allogeneic target cells in vitro; inhibition by isoantibody and by drugs. Immunology 14 (2):181–196
62. Babson AL, Babson SR (1973) Kinetic colorimetric measurement of serum lactate dehydrogenase activity. Clin Chem 19(7):766
63. Mosmann T (1983) Rapid colorimetric assay for cellular growth and survival: application to proliferation and cytotoxicity assays. J

Immunol Methods 65(1):55–63. https://doi.org/10.1016/0022-1759(83)90303-4

64. Riss T, Moravec R, Niles A, Duellman S, Benink H, Worzella T, Minor L (2013, Updated 1 Jul 2016) Cell viability assays. [Internet]
65. Han X, Gelein R, Corson N, Wade-Mercer P, Jiang J, Biswas P, Finkelstein JN, Elder A, Oberdorster G (2011) Validation of an LDH assay for assessing nanoparticle toxicity. Toxicology 287(1–3):99–104. https://doi.org/10.1016/j.tox.2011.06.011
66. van Engeland M, Nieland LJW, Ramaekers FCS, Schutte B, Reutelingsperger CPM (1998) Annexin V-affinity assay: a review on an apoptosis detection system based on phosphatidylserine exposure. Cytometry 31(1):1–9. https://doi.org/10.1002/(SICI)1097-0320(19980101)31:1<1::AID-CYTO1>3.0.CO;2-R
67. Koopman G, Reutelingsperger C, Kuijten G, Keehnen R, Pals S, van Oers M (1994) Annexin V for flow cytometric detection of phosphatidylserine expression on B cells undergoing apoptosis. Blood 84(5):1415–1420
68. Fan T-J, Han L-H, Cong R-S, Liang J (2005) Caspase family proteases and apoptosis. Acta Biochim Biophys Sin 37(11):719–727. https://doi.org/10.1111/j.1745-7270.2005.00108.x
69. Kaufmann SH, Lee SH, Meng XW, Loegering DA, Kottke TJ, Henzing AJ, Ruchaud S, Samejima K, Earnshaw WC (2008) Apoptosis-associated caspase activation assays. Methods 44(3):262–272. https://doi.org/10.1016/j.ymeth.2007.11.005
70. Keston AS, Brandt R (1965) The fluorometric analysis of ultramicro quantities of hydrogen peroxide. Anal Biochem 11(1):1–5. https://doi.org/10.1016/0003-2697(65)90034-5
71. Bass DA, Parce JW, Dechatelet LR, Szejda P, Seeds MC, Thomas M (1983) Flow cytometric studies of oxidative product formation by neutrophils: a graded response to membrane stimulation. J Immunol 130(4):1910–1917
72. Wang H, Joseph JA (1999) Quantifying cellular oxidative stress by dichlorofluorescein assay using microplate reader11Mention of a trade name, proprietary product, or specific equipment does not constitute a guarantee by the United States Department of Agriculture and does not imply its approval to the exclusion of other products that may be suitable. Free Radic Biol Med 27(5):612–616. https://doi.org/10.1016/S0891-5849(99)00107-0
73. Gupta P, Jordan CT, Mitov MI, Butterfield DA, Hilt JZ, Dziubla TD (2016) Controlled curcumin release via conjugation into PBAE nanogels enhances mitochondrial protection against oxidative stress. Int J Pharm 511(2):1012–1021. https://doi.org/10.1016/j.ijpharm.2016.07.071
74. Levine RL, Garland D, Oliver CN, Amici A, Climent I, Lenz A-G, Ahn B-W, Shaltiel S, Stadtman ER (1990) Determination of carbonyl content in oxidatively modified proteins. In: Abelson JN (ed) Methods in enzymology, vol 186. Academic, Cambridge, MA, pp 464–478. https://doi.org/10.1016/0076-6879(90)86141-H
75. Dalle-Donne I, Rossi R, Giustarini D, Milzani A, Colombo R (2003) Protein carbonyl groups as biomarkers of oxidative stress. Clin Chim Acta 329(1–2):23–38. https://doi.org/10.1016/s0009-8981(03)00003-2
76. Levine RL, Williams JA, Stadtman EP, Shacter E (1994) Carbonyl assays for determination of oxidatively modified proteins. In: Abelson JN (ed) Methods in enzymology, vol 233. Academic, Cambridge, MA, pp 346–357. https://doi.org/10.1016/S0076-6879(94)33040-9
77. Golbamaki N, Rasulev B, Cassano A, Marchese Robinson RL, Benfenati E, Leszczynski J, Cronin MT (2015) Genotoxicity of metal oxide nanomaterials: review of recent data and discussion of possible mechanisms. Nanoscale 7(6):2154–2198. https://doi.org/10.1039/c4nr06670g
78. Olive PL, Banath JP, Durand RE (2012) Heterogeneity in radiation-induced DNA damage and repair in tumor and normal cells measured using the "comet" assay. 1990. Radiat Res 178(2):AV35–AV42
79. OECD. Test no. 487: in vitro mammalian cell micronucleus test. OECD, Paris
80. Ellard S, Parry EM (1993) A modified protocol for the cytochalasin B in vitro micronucleus assay using whole human blood or separated lymphocyte cultures. Mutagenesis 8(4):317–320. https://doi.org/10.1093/mutage/8.4.317
81. OECD. Test no. 471: bacterial reverse mutation test. OECD, Paris
82. OECD. Test no. 473: in vitro mammalian chromosome aberration test. OECD, Paris
83. Doak SH, Manshian B, Jenkins GJ, Singh N (2012) In vitro genotoxicity testing strategy for nanomaterials and the adaptation of current OECD guidelines. Mutat Res 745(1–2):104–111. https://doi.org/10.1016/j.mrgentox.2011.09.013
84. Ayala A, Munoz MF, Arguelles S (2014) Lipid peroxidation: production, metabolism, and signaling mechanisms of malondialdehyde and

4-hydroxy-2-nonenal. Oxidative Med Cell Longev 2014:360438. https://doi.org/10.1155/2014/360438

85. Ohkawa H, Ohishi N, Yagi K (1979) Assay for lipid peroxides in animal tissues by thiobarbituric acid reaction. Anal Biochem 95 (2):351–358. https://doi.org/10.1016/0003-2697(79)90738-3
86. Moselhy HF, Reid RG, Yousef S, Boyle SP (2013) A specific, accurate, and sensitive measure of total plasma malondialdehyde by HPLC. J Lipid Res 54(3):852–858. https://doi.org/10.1194/jlr.D032698
87. Esterbauer H, Schaur RJ, Zollner H (1991) Chemistry and biochemistry of 4-hydroxynonenal, malonaldehyde and related aldehydes. Free Radic Biol Med 11(1):81–128. https://doi.org/10.1016/0891-5849(91)90192-6
88. Weber D, Milkovic L, Bennett SJ, Griffiths HR, Zarkovic N, Grune T (2013) Measurement of HNE-protein adducts in human plasma and serum by ELISA-Comparison of two primary antibodies. Redox Biol 1:226–233. https://doi.org/10.1016/j.redox.2013.01.012
89. Gérard-Monnier D, Erdelmeier I, Régnard K, Moze-Henry N, Yadan J-C, Chaudière J (1998) Reactions of 1-methyl-2-phenylindole with malondialdehyde and 4-hydroxyalkenals. Analytical applications to a colorimetric assay of lipid peroxidation. Chem Res Toxicol 11 (10):1176–1183. https://doi.org/10.1021/tx9701790
90. Bartosh TJ, Ylostalo JH (2014) Macrophage inflammatory assay. Bio Protoc 4(14):e1180
91. Fujita T, Nolan GP, Ghosh S, Baltimore D (1992) Independent modes of transcriptional activation by the p50 and p65 subunits of NF-kappa B. Genes Dev 6(5):775–787. https://doi.org/10.1101/gad.6.5.775
92. L-f C, Fischle W, Verdin E, Greene WC (2001) Duration of nuclear NF-κB action regulated by reversible acetylation. Science 293 (5535):1653–1657. https://doi.org/10.1126/science.1062374
93. Kinoshita S, Akira S, Kishimoto T (1992) A member of the C/EBP family, NF-IL6 beta, forms a heterodimer and transcriptionally synergizes with NF-IL6. Proc Natl Acad Sci 89(4):1473–1476
94. Smale ST (2010) Luciferase assay. Cold Spring Harb Protoc 2010(5):pdb prot5421. https://doi.org/10.1101/pdb.prot5421
95. Bang FB (1956) A bacterial disease of Limulus polyphemus. Bull Johns Hopkins Hosp 98 (5):325–351
96. Hurley JC (1995) Endotoxemia: methods of detection and clinical correlates. Clin Microbiol Rev 8(2):268–292
97. Smulders S, Kaiser JP, Zuin S, Van Landuyt KL, Golanski L, Vanoirbeek J, Wick P, Hoet PH (2012) Contamination of nanoparticles by endotoxin: evaluation of different test methods. Part Fibre Toxicol 9:41. https://doi.org/10.1186/1743-8977-9-41
98. Ding JL, Ho B (2010) Endotoxin detection – from limulus amebocyte lysate to recombinant factor C. In: Wang X, Quinn PJ (eds) Endotoxins: structure, function and recognition. Springer, Dordrecht, pp 187–208. https://doi.org/10.1007/978-90-481-9078-2_9
99. Alwis KU, Milton DK (2006) Recombinant factor C assay for measuring endotoxin in house dust: comparison with LAL, and (1 → 3)-β-D-glucans. Am J Ind Med 49 (4):296–300. https://doi.org/10.1002/ajim.20264

Chapter 2

Methods for Assessing Mast Cell Responses to Engineered Nanomaterial Exposure

Nasser B. Alsaleh and Jared M. Brown

Abstract

Mast cells are key effector cells in inflammatory and allergic immune responses such as asthma, rhinitis, and atopic dermatitis. Activation of mast cells leads to immediate release of preformed mediators such as histamine and proteases, which can regulate vascular permeability and the function of a number of immune and nonimmune cells. Engineered nanomaterials (ENM) have been utilized for a wide range of applications and introduced into a number of consumer products; yet the consequent increase in human exposure and any potential adverse effects have not been fully evaluated. Modulation of the immune system function has been shown to be a major toxicological consequence of ENM exposure. The implication of mast cells in ENM-mediated toxicity, including the most widely utilized carbon and metal-based ENMs, has been previously demonstrated; and therefore, understanding direct ENM interaction with mast cells at the cellular and molecular level is of critical importance for the safe implementation of ENMs into consumer products.

Key words Mast cell, Degranulation, Engineered nanomaterials, Nanoparticles, Nanotoxicity, Immunotoxicity

1 Introduction

Mast cells are an innate immune effector cell type primarily known for their role in allergic disease. They are long-lived tissue resident cells that are found in greater numbers within host–environment interfaces (e.g., skin, respiratory tract, and GI mucosa), and hence they play key roles in host defense through regulation of innate and adaptive immune responses [1]. Importantly, mast cells contribute significantly to allergic and Th2 immune responses, which typically developed following an initial exposure to an allergen (pollen, animal dander, etc.) that consequently leads to B cell-mediated production of immunoglobulin type E (IgE) [2]. Subsequently, IgE binds to the high-affinity IgE receptor (FcεR1) on the membrane of mast cells and a second exposure to the same allergen (epitope) will trigger cross-linking of FcεR1 of resident mast cells

Qunwei Zhang (ed.), *Nanotoxicity: Methods and Protocols*, Methods in Molecular Biology, vol. 1894,
https://doi.org/10.1007/978-1-4939-8916-4_2,

leading to a rapid release of preformed granular content including vasoactive mediators such as histamine, serotonin, cytokines, and a number of proteases, a process known as degranulation. Mast cell degranulation ranges from mild allergic reactions to severe anaphylaxis. Importantly, the underlying mechanism of IgE-mediated mast cell degranulation is fairly characterized; however, non-IgE mediated mechanisms of mast cell degranulation, for instance by neuropeptides, compound 48/80, metals, and engineered nanomaterials, are poorly understood [3].

Engineered nanomaterials (ENM) are any materials with at least one dimension at the size of 1–100 nm. At such a small scale, ENMs possess unique physicochemical properties and behave differently from their bulk counterparts [4]; hence, ENMs have been utilized for numerous applications (electronics, biotechnology, pharmaceuticals, etc.) and introduced into many consumer products. Over the past few years, the use of ENMs in consumer products has increased significantly, yet we lack a thorough understanding of ENM associated health and environmental adverse effects [5]. Therefore, it is crucial to investigate any adverse effects associated with acute and chronic ENM exposure at both the cellular and systemic levels.

Assessing the immune system function is key in the evaluation of ENM toxicity. Recent literature demonstrates a critical role for the immune system in dictating ENM-induced toxicity [6–8]. Mast cells regulate the immune system through regulating the function of other innate and adaptive immune cells as well as nonimmune cells and their activation can be of critical consequences [1]. Importantly, non-IgE mediated mast cell activation has been demonstrated in response to various types of ENMs [9–12]. For instance, it has been demonstrated that instillation of cerium oxide nanoparticles in the lungs of C57BL/6 mice resulted in pulmonary inflammation that was absent in mast cell deficient mice [12]. However, the underlying molecular mechanisms of ENM-induced mast cell activation are poorly understood but it has recently been shown that in vitro exposure to silver nanoparticles resulted in robust mast cell degranulation by potentially a membrane-mediated activation of signal transduction pathways involved in calcium signaling [13]. Recently, administration of ferumoxytol (Feraheme®), an iron oxide nanoparticle based medication for iron deficiency, resulted in severe anaphylaxis in patients of which 18 were fatal [14]. Serum histamine levels were elevated in ferumoxytol-administered patients suggesting the potential involvement of mast cells. It is worth noting that exposure to ENMs has been shown to activate the complement system and lead to the release of anaphylatoxins [15]. This could indirectly result in mast cell activation leading to allergic-like responses. Taken together, mast cells represent an important cell model in the assessment of ENM associated allergic- and allergic-like responses and hypersensitivity reactions.

Mast cells are derived from CD34⁺ hematopoietic stem cells, which become fully differentiated after reaching peripheral tissues under the influence of the tissue microenvironment. Mast cells are heterogeneous in nature and based on the microenvironment (cytokines and growth factors), they can differentiate into a number of phenotypes that vary in their functional properties and content of their secretory granules [16]. For instance, in rodents, stem cell factor (SCF) give rise to connective tissue type mast cells (CTMC) whereas IL-3 gives rise to mucosal-type mast cells (MMC). Similarly, in humans there are two major populations of mast cells, which are differentiated based on their protease content: *tryptase* mast cells (MC_T), which are commonly found in the mucosa and *tryptase/chymase* mast cells (MC_{TC}), which are commonly found in connective tissues [16]. While specific roles of mast cell heterogeneity are largely undetermined, it is generally thought that based on their tissue location, such heterogeneity could be important for optimal mast cell responses in the regulation of immune and non-immune cells depending on the physiological (e.g., neuron-mediated mast cell activation) or pathological (e.g., host defense) context [17]. In the laboratory, a number of primary and immortalized cell lines of murine and human origin have been employed to study mast cells. Primary murine mast cells are typically differentiated from $CD34^+$ cells obtained from the bone marrow (i.e., bone marrow-derived mast cell, BMMCs) into mucosal-type (in the presence of recombinant murine IL-3) or connective tissue type (in the presence of IL-3 and SCF). Differentiated (mature, connective tissue type) mast cells can be obtained from lavaging the rodent peritoneal cavity while the yield is much lower compared to generation of BMMCs. Primary human mast cells are typically differentiated from $CD34^+$ cells obtained from peripheral blood (can also be obtained from cord blood and bone marrow) in the presence of recombinant human SCF, IL-3 and IL-6 [18]. On the other hand, a number of immortalized mast cell lines have also been developed and widely utilized to understand the biology and function of mast cells. For instance, rat basophilic leukemia (RBL) cells have been widely used to study mast cell signaling through the IgE receptor and cell secretory function [19]. Other common cell lines of human origin include HMC-1 and LAD2. It is important to note that both murine and human primary mast cell models are the most closely representative of in situ mast cells. Other mast cell lines have some limitations such as lack of phenotype (e.g., lack of an IgE receptor in the HMC cell line), alerted phenotype (e.g., mutated stem cell factor receptor (cKIT) in RBL cell line), ease and cost of growth and maintenance (e.g., LAD2 and LUVA cell lines). Thus, it is of critical importance to address phenotypical differences among these cell lines and confirm findings using primary mast cells before drawing any major conclusions. This chapter describes methods used to culture primary mouse mast cells and focuses on key end points of in vitro mast cell activation such as degranulation and cytokine release. It also describes in vivo models of mast cell activation such as passive cutaneous anaphylaxis. These methods are key in the assessment of ENM-induced modulation of mast cell function and toxicity.

2 Materials

All solutions are made using ultrapure grade water (ddH_2O). All cell culture procedures are carried out using standard aseptic techniques. Animal work is approved by Institutional Animal Use guidelines.

2.1 Isolation of Mouse BMMCs and Assessment of Cell Maturity

1. 60 mm cell culture dishes.
2. T-75 cell culture flasks.
3. Cell culture incubator (37 °C/5% CO_2).
4. Laminar flow cell culture hood.
5. 15- and 50-ml sterile conical centrifuge tubes.
6. Centrifuge for 15- and 50-ml tubes (Eppendorf 5810 R).
7. Sterile tweezers and two sets of scissors.
8. Sterile 1.5 ml eppendorf tubes.
9. 75% ethanol sprayer.
10. Complete mast cell media (see recipe below).
11. 0.22 μM filtration system (Autofil™ laboratory filtration system, catalogue No. 1103-RLS, Nova-Tech International, Inc., Kingwood, TX).
12. Sterile 1 ml syringe.
13. Sterile 25-G needle.
14. PBS, pH 7.4.
15. Microcentrifuge (Eppendorf 5424 R).
16. Flow cytometer (Accuri C6, BD Biosciences).
17. FcεR1 (PE) and cKIT (APC) antibodies (eBioscience Inc., San Diego, CA).
18. Staining buffer (BD Biosciences, Franklin Lakes, NJ).

2.2 Mast Cell Degranulation and Cell Viability

1. HEPES buffer, pH 7.4.
2. IgE anti-dinitrophenyl-human serum albumin (Sigma-Aldrich, St. Louis, MO).
3. Dinitrophenyl-human serum albumin (Sigma-Aldrich, St. Louis, MO).
4. Propidium iodide (Molecular Probes, Waltham, MA).

5. Annexin V-APC antibody (BD Biosciences, Franklin Lakes, NJ).
6. 15- and 50-ml sterile conical centrifuge tubes.
7. Centrifuge for 15- and 50-ml tubes and 96-well plate (Eppendorf 5810 R).
8. Cell culture 96-well plates.
9. Flat bottom 96-well clear nonsterile plates.
10. Microplate spectrophotometer (BioTek Synergy HT).
11. Multichannel pipette.
12. 25-ml sterile reservoirs.
13. Microbalance (Mettler Toledo XP6).
14. Ultrasonic processor.
15. Flow cytometer (Accuri C6, BD Biosciences).

2.3 Media, Buffers, and Solutions

1. Complete mast cell media: RPMI 1640 without L-glutamine (Corning, Manassas, VA), 10% heat-inactivated fetal bovine serum (FBS), 4 mM L-glutamine (Life Technologies, Carlsbad, CA), 100 U/ml penicillin/100 μg/ml streptomycin, 100 μg/ml primocin, 25 mM HEPES (Corning, Manassas, VA), 1.0 mM sodium pyruvate (Sigma-Aldrich, St. Louis, MO), 1.0 mM nonessential amino acids (Sigma-Aldrich, St. Louis, MO), 30 ng/ml recombinant murine IL-3 (Peprotech, Rocky Hill, NJ), 50 mM 2-mercaptoethanol (Sigma-Aldrich, St. Louis, MO). Filter-sterilize (0.22 μm).
2. HEPES buffer for degranulation assay: 10 mM HEPES, 137 mM NaCl, 2.7 mM KCl, 0.4 mM Na_2HPO_4, 5.6 mM Glucose. pH to 7.4 with 1 M NaOH, then add: 1.8 mM $CaCl_2$, 1.3 mM $MgSO_4$. Filter-sterilize (0.22 μm).
3. Citrate solution: 40 mM citric acid, 20 mM Na_2HPO_4. pH to 4.5 with 1 M NaOH. Filter-sterilize (0.22 μm).
4. p-nitrophenyl *N*-acetyle-B-D-glucosaminide (PNAG) solution: PNAG stock is prepared by dissolving powder (3.5 mg/ml) into citrate buffer (70 mg per 20 ml buffer is enough for 2 full 96-well plates). Brief sonicate the solution to dissolve PNAG.
5. Binding buffer: 10 mM HEPES, 140 mM NaCl. pH to 7.4 with 1 M NaOH and then add 2.5 mM $CaCl_2$.

3 Methods

3.1 Growing Mouse BMMCs

1. Euthanize a C57BL/6 mouse by CO_2 asphyxiation or other approved method following Institutional Animal Use guidelines. Use a secondary method of euthanasia (e.g., cervical dislocation).

2. Use sterile tweezers and two sets of scissors. Spray the mouse fur with 70% ethanol.
3. To collect femurs, with the first set of scissors, make an incision then a complete circle cut around the ankle and then perpendicular cut through the legs. Peal the skin, spray the leg with 70% ethanol.
4. With the second set of scissors, cut away muscles from the knee up and around the femur bone.
5. Using the second set of scissors, cut the femur bone at the knee joint, hold the femur with tweezers and make another cut at the other end of femur bone (near the hip-joint).
6. Place the femur in 1.5 ml sterile eppendorf tube-containing complete BMMC media.
7. Repeat **steps 3–6** for the mouse other femur.
8. Fill a 60 mm cell culture petri dish with complete BMMC media.
9. Using sterile 1 ml syringe and 25-G needle, flush each bone to collect the marrow into BMMC media-containing petri dish.
10. Repeat **step 9** several times for each end of the femur bone to ensure complete collection of bone marrow cells (femur bone turns white after a complete flushing of bone marrow cells).
11. For a total of four femur marrows (two mice), transfer the 10 ml of bone marrow cell-containing media to a T-75 flask and add 30 ml of complete media.
12. Change media and flasks (to get rid of adherent cells) every 3–4 days for 4–6 weeks.
13. Check cell maturity by measuring the surface expression of FcεR1 and cKIT (see details below).

3.2 Mast Cell Maturity: Surface Expression of FcεR1 and cKIT (CD117)

1. Plate 2×10^5 cells per sample (at 1×10^6 cell per ml).
2. Centrifuge cells at $600 \times g$ for 5 min and resuspend cells into 100 μl of 1:100 FcεR1 (PE) and cKIT (APC) antibody-containing staining buffer and incubate for at least 30 min at room temperature protected from direct light. Use PE- and APC-conjugated IgG isotype for nonspecific binding control.
3. Wash two times with cold PBS.
4. Determine surface expression using a flow cytometer (typical mast cell purity is about 95–99%).
   (a) PE (Ex-Max 496 nm/Em-Max 578 nm).
   (b) APC (Ex-Max 650 nm/Em-Max 660 nm).

3.3 Mast Cell Degranulation Assay and Cell Viability

3.3.1 Mast Cell Degranulation Assay

Resting (mature) mast cells contain a large number of preformed mature granules, which contain mediators such as histamine, serotonin, cytokines, and a number of proteases. Mature mast cells can immediately degranulate upon exposure to an appropriate stimulus and released mediators influence several different cell types resulting in quick biological response including vascular dilatation, tissue remodeling and recruitment of effector immune cells [1, 2]. Therefore, measuring such a key event (i.e., mast cell degranulation) following exposure to ENM is of great importance in the assessment of ENM-induced allergic reactions. In this protocol, mast cell degranulation is measured based on the release of β-hexosaminidase, a protease found in mast cell granules (Fig. 1):

1. *Preincubation step for IgE-mediated degranulation*: Coat mature mast cells with IgE anti-dinitrophenyl-human serum albumin (IgE anti-DNP-HSA) (0.1 μg/ml) overnight in complete mast cell media.
2. Wash cells two times and plate 5×10^4 cells per well (96-well plate) at a total volume of 90 μl per well.
3. Prepare DNP-HSA stock at a concentration of 10 mg/ml in sterile ultrapure water (ddH_2O) (can be used for up to 2 weeks, to be stored at 4 °C).
4. Make a DNP-HSA working solution (in HEPES buffer) with a concentration of 1000 ng/ml and then add 10 μl (to give a

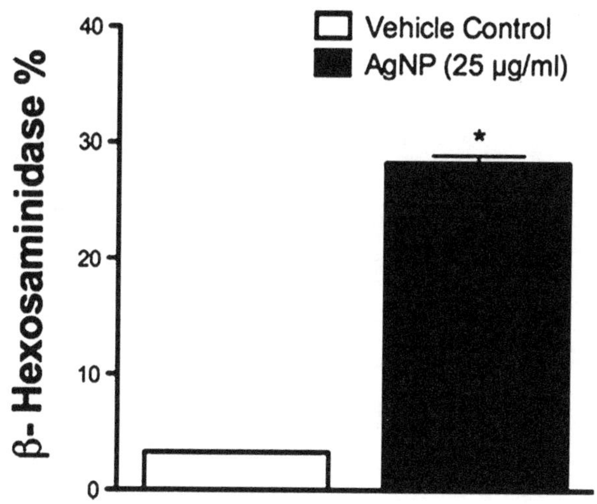

Fig. 1 Mast cell degranulation following exposure to silver nanoparticles based on the release of β-hexosaminidase. BMMCs were exposed to vehicle control or silver nanoparticles (25 μg/ml) for 1 h and percentage of β-hexosaminidase release was measured in supernatant relative to cellular content. Values are expression as mean ± SEM of three independent experiments. *Indicates significant difference from control group ($p \leq 0.05$)

final concentration of 100 ng/ml) to DNP-treated group in triplicates and incubate for 30 min at cell culture incubator. Add 10 μl of HEPES buffer to control group.

5. For a DNP dose-response, the following concentrations are suggested: 0.01, 0.1, 1, 10, 100, and 1000 ng/ml. To make original working stocks: Add 5 μl of original DNP stock (10 mg/ml) to 5 ml of HEPES to give a final stock concentration of 10,000 ng/ml and then perform serial dilutions: 0.5 ml into 4.5 ml of HEPES.
6. For ENM exposure: Add ENMs at the desired concentration (s) in a total volume of 10 μl (HEPES buffer) (*see* **Notes 1–4**) and incubate for the desired time point(s) in a cell culture incubator (37 °C/5% CO_2). Suggested ENM concentrations: 0.01, 0.1, 1, 10, 100 μg/ml or 1.56, 3.12, 6.25, 12.5, 25, 50, 100 μg/ml. Suggested ENM incubation time points: 5, 10, 20, 30, 60 min (*see* **Notes 5** and **6**).
7. Centrifuge plate at 300 × *g* for 5 min and collect 50 μl per well of supernatant into a new 96-well nonsterile clear plate (plate 1).
8. Add 150 μl per well of 0.1% Triton X-100 to remaining cells and pipette up/down five times to lyse cells.
9. Collect 50 μl per well of lysed cells into a new 96-well nonsterile clear plate (plate 2).
10. Add 100 μl per well of p-nitrophenyl N-acetyle-B-D-glucosaminide (PNAG) to plate 1 and 2 and incubate for 90 min at 37 °C.
11. Add 100 μl per well of 0.4 M glycine (pH 10.7) to stop the reaction.
12. Read absorbance by a spectrophotometer at 405 nm (*see* **Notes 7** and **8**).
13. To obtain % β-hexosaminidase apply the following formula:

$$\%\beta\text{-hexosaminidase} = [(\text{supernatant} \times 2)/(\text{lysis} \times 4)] \times 100.$$

3.3.2 Mast Cell Viability Based on Propidium Iodide/Annexin V Staining

1. Plate 2×10^5 cells per well (at 1×10^6 cells per ml).
2. Following exposure to ENMs for the desired concentrations and time points, collect cells into 1.5 ml eppendorf tubes, wash two times with cold binding buffer.
3. Resuspend cells in 100 μl of propidium iodide-containing binding buffer at a final concentration of 3 μM).
4. Add 2.5 μl of annexin V-APC antibody per sample.
5. Incubate samples for 15 min at room temperature protected from direct light.

6. Read on a flow cytometer using two channels:
   (a) Propidium iodide (Ex-Max 533 nm/Em-Max 617 nm).
   (b) APC (Ex-Max 650 nm/Em-Max 660 nm).
7. Use a positive control, for example:
   (a) 20 μM Camptothecin, 6 h for early apoptosis.
   (b) 10 mM H_2O_2, 1 h for late apoptosis/necrosis.
8. Plot the two channels (i.e., for PI and APC-Annexin V) and calculate the percentage of each cell population as follows:
   (a) Q1 (lower left): Live cells.
   (b) Q2 (lower right): Early apoptosis.
   (c) Q3 (upper right): Late apoptosis.
   (d) Q4 (upper left): Necrosis.

3.4 Mast Cell Cytokine Release (Late-Phase Activation)

Mast cells can be activated through two phases, that is, an *early* phase (also known as degranulation), which typically occurs in a short time (~minutes), and a *late* phase (synthesis and release of arachidonic acid metabolites and cytokines/chemokines), which takes a longer time (~minutes to hours). Late phase activation could contribute to the late phase of allergic responses and has been shown to play an important role in the pathophysiology of allergic disease [20].

1. Plate 1×10^6 cells per well (24-well plate, 1 ml of total media per well) (*see* **Notes 9** and **10**).
2. Expose cells to the desired concentrations of ENMs. Include DNP-HSA (100 ng/ml) with prior IgE anti-DNP-HSA sensitization step as a positive control as demonstrated above in the degranulation assay protocol.
3. For ENM exposure: Suggested ENM concentrations: 0.01, 0.1, 1, 10, 100 μg/ml or 1.56, 3.12, 6.25, 12.5, 25, 50, 100 μg/ml. Suggested ENM incubation time points: 4, 6, 12, 24, and 48 h (*see* **Notes 1–4**).
4. Centrifuge cells for 200 × *g* for 5 min at 4 °C and collect supernatants.
5. Process supernatant following standard ELISA protocol or store at −80 °C until use.

3.5 Peritoneal Mast Cell Degranulation Assay

This assay is designed to assess mast cell degranulation in vivo by measuring the release of β-hexosaminidase in the mouse peritoneal cavity. It involves passively sensitizing the mice with IgE anti-DNP-HSA overnight followed by antigen challenging (mast cell activation) by DNP-HSA (positive control).

1. Inject 1 μg monoclonal IgE anti-DNP in 100 μl PBS intraperitoneally to sensitize peritoneal mast cells overnight.

2. In one set of mice, inject DNP-HSA (100 ng/ml in 100 μl PBS) intraperitoneally for 1 h (positive control).
3. In another set of mice, inject ENMs (in 100 μl PBS or appropriate vehicle) intraperitoneally for 1 h (*see* **Notes 1–4** and **11**).
4. Irrigate the peritoneal cavity with PBS (2–3 ml).
5. Measure β-hexosaminidase content in the collected fluid (i.e., from irrigated peritoneal cavity) as described above in the degranulation assay. Briefly, add 100 μl of PNAG per 50 μl of collected fluid (in triplicate) and incubate for 90 min at 37 °C. Stop reaction with 0.4 M glycine and read optical density (O.D.) by a spectrophotometer at 405 nm (Fig. 3).

3.6 Passive Cutaneous Anaphylaxis (PCA)

Mast cell activation involves release of preformed vasoactive mediators such as histamine. The PCA method described below assesses in vivo mast cell degranulation by measuring mast cell-induced vasodilatation based on the extravasation of administered Evans blue dye.

1. In one set of mice (BALB/c mice are often used due to ease of visualizing Evan's blue dye in white mice, but any rodent model can be applied), inject 1 μg IgE anti-DNP in 25 μl PBS intradermally in the right ear overnight. For control, inject 25 μl of PBS in the left ear.
2. In the following day, in another set of mice apply ENMs dermally (with DMSO) or inject intradermally at the desired dose (can be in the range of μg/ml to mg/ml based on utilized ENMs and study design) in 25 μl PBS in the right ear. For control, inject 25 μl of PBS in the left ear.
3. Thirty minutes to several hours following ENM exposure (determined empirically) (including a 30 min of DNP treatment, *see* **step 4**), inject 100 μl of 0.5 mg/ml DNP-HSA in 1% Evan's blue in saline intravenously into the tail vein (positive control group) or 1% Evan's blue in saline (ENM and vehicle control groups) (*see* **Notes 1–4**).
4. Euthanize mice by CO_2 asphyxiation 30 min after antigen challenge, excise the ears and incubate in 200 μl formamide at 55 °C for 24 h (to extract the Evan's blue dye).
5. Remove ears and read color absorbance by a spectrophotometer at 620 nm.
6. Subtract background using vehicle control from treated samples for comparison across groups.

4 Notes

This is an overview and important considerations during ENM preparation and characterization.

1. ENM preparation for cell culture (in vitro) and animal administration (in vivo) can vary largely depending on ENM physicochemical properties and the desired vehicle of exposure in vitro (PBS, HEPES, unsupplemented vs. supplemented media, etc.) and route of administration in vivo (inhalation, instillation, oral gavage, etc.). The ultimate goal is to deliver ENMs at the desired dose and in the desired form.
2. ENMs have very high surface-to-volume ratio and they possess an active surface area. Biological media often contain buffering systems and nutrients such as sugars, amino acids, and growth factors. Introducing ENMs into biological fluids often leads to ENM aggregation and agglomeration. This issue has undeniably resulted in false interpretation of nanotoxicological outcomes. Therefore, it is very important to choose the appropriate method for ENM preparation before exposure to biological systems. Furthermore, thorough characterization of ENMs into biological media particularly over time in studies with long exposure times is also of great importance for accurate data interpretation.
3. *ENM dispersion methods*: Ensuring that ENMs are consistently suspended (i.e., ENM dispersity) in aqueous media is important for toxicity testing. ENM dispersion methods for toxicity testing include use of dispersants, ultrasonication, stirring, and shaking [21]. Importantly, several specific protocols have been established for dispersion of ENMs in aqueous media. Readers can refer to the review by Hartmann et al. for more details about this topic [22].
4. *ENM dosimetry*: Another important consideration is ENM dosimetry. ENM aggregation, agglomeration, and poor dispersity can drastically influence ENM dosimetry. Due to their large and active surface area, ENM can agglomerate and aggregate and thus eventually sediment due to the effect of gravity. Indeed, Wittmaack demonstrated that toxic consequences of ENMs at high exposure concentrations in in vitro settings can be a result of mechanical overload of insoluble matter and a consequent interference with cellular functions without necessarily being an inherent ENM toxicity [23]. Measuring cellular or tissue uptake of ENMs has been suggested as a solution to this concern; however, other issues arise from such an approach including: (a) technical difficulty of measuring intracellular ENM concentration; (b) intracellular degradation of ENM

over time; and (c) it does not account for cell membrane-mediated ENM interaction.

5. It is important to note when testing for mast cell degranulation that ENMs are to be suspended in HEPES buffer and therefore characterization of ENMs in HEPES should be included.
6. Another important consideration is dosimetry as BMMCs are suspension cells, which means a larger surface area of cells is exposed to ENM (versus adherent cells).
7. *ENM interference with toxicological assays*: An important consideration in designing nanotoxicological studies is interference of ENMs with classical colorimetric and fluorometric assays such as tetrazolium compound [3-(4,5-dimethylthiazol-2-yl)-5-(3-carboxymethoxyphenyl)-2-(4-sulfophenyl)-2H-tetrazolium (MTS) and lactate dehydrogenase (LDH) colorimetric assays. For instance, metal ENMs, depending on their physicochemical properties, can absorb light at a wide range of UV-Visible spectrum. Several publications have discussed this topic in detail including ENM interference with biological/toxicological assays and provided alternative methods [24–26]. Thus, it is important to consider such interferences during the process of experimental design including the use of appropriate controls and secondary methods to confirm results.
8. ENMs used for the first time should always be tested for interference with the degranulation assay (visible spectrum). This can be done by including "ENMs only" control or using a secondary method to confirm the obtained results such as histamine or protease release from mast cells using commercial ELISA kits. Another alternative method is measuring surface expression of lysosome-associated membrane protein 2 (reflecting mast cell degranulation, i.e., fusion of granular membranes with cell membrane) by fluorescent microscopy (Fig. 2) or flow cytometry.
9. When exposing cells in supplemented with serum vs. unsupplemented media, it is important to consider the formation of biocorona and potential subsequent consequences.
10. *ENM characterization methods*: Factors such as pH, ionic strength and surface charge are known to influence ENM stability in aqueous solutions [27]. Therefore, thorough characterization of ENMs in relevant aqueous solutions and biological media is of critical importance for nanotoxicological studies. Common methods used to characterize ENMs include (but are not limited to) [28]: *ENM size*: Transmission electron microscopy (TEM), atomic force microscopy (AFM) and dynamic light scattering (DLS); *ENM shape*: TEM and AFM; *ENM aggregation/agglomeration*: DLS and UV-Vis; *ENM*

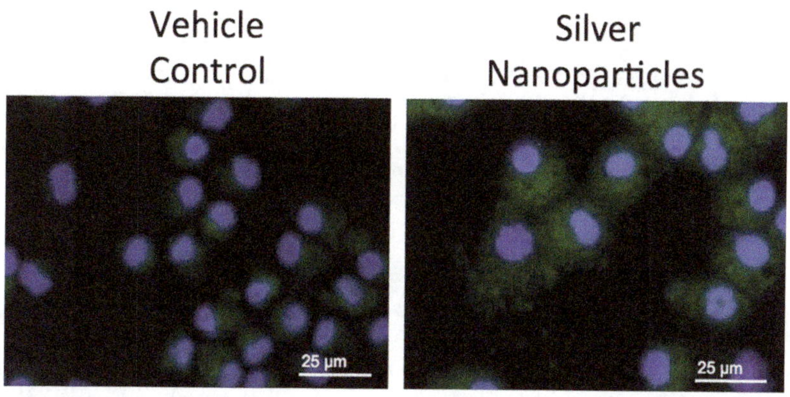

Fig. 2 Mast cell degranulation following exposure to silver nanoparticles based on the surface expression of lysosome-associated membrane protein 2 (Lamp-2). Representative immunofluorescent images showing the surface expression of Lamp-2 (green) on BMMCs that were exposed to vehicle control (left image) or silver nanoparticles (25 μg/ml) for 15 min (right image). DAPI (blue) visualizes nucleus (Images generated and provided by Abdullah A. Aldossari)

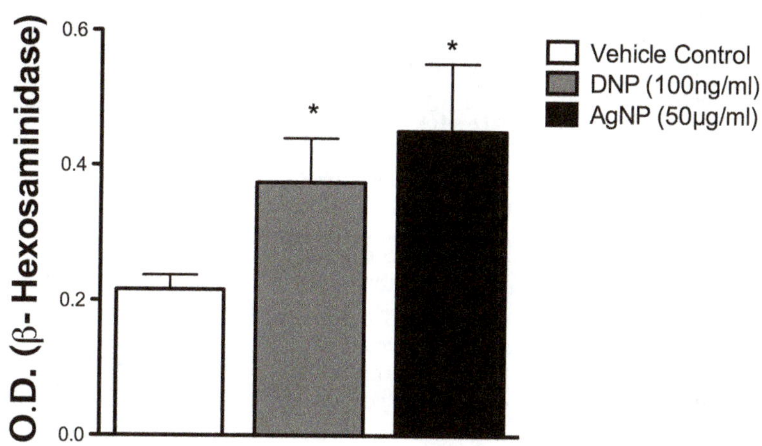

Fig. 3 Peritoneal mast cell degranulation following exposure to DNP-HSA or silver nanoparticles based on the release of β-hexosaminidase. Vehicle control, DNP-HSA (100 ng/ml) (with prior IgE anti-DNP-HSA sensitization step) or silver nanoparticles (50 μg/ml) were injected intraperitoneally for 1 h and percentage of β-hexosaminidase release was measured in the collected fluid from peritoneal irrigation. Values are expression as mean ± SEM of three independent experiments. *Asterisk* indicates significant difference from control group ($p \leq 0.05$)

surface charge: ζ-potential; *ENM dissolution*: Inductively coupled plasma mass spectrometry (ICP-MS); *ENM cellular uptake*: ICP-MS, TEM and flow cytometry.

11. In peritoneal mast cell degranulation assay, ENM doses can be in the range of μg/ml to mg/ml based on the utilized ENMs and study design.

References

1. Abraham SN, St John AL (2010) Mast cell-orchestrated immunity to pathogens. Nat Rev Immunol 10(6):440–452. https://doi.org/10.1038/nri2782
2. Galli SJ, Nakae S, Tsai M (2005) Mast cells in the development of adaptive immune responses. Nat Immunol 6(2):135–142. https://doi.org/10.1038/ni1158
3. Gilfillan AM, Tkaczyk C (2006) Integrated signalling pathways for mast-cell activation. Nat Rev Immunol 6(3):218–230. https://doi.org/10.1038/nri1782
4. Buzea C, Pacheco II, Robbie K (2007) Nanomaterials and nanoparticles: sources and toxicity. Biointerphases 2(4):MR17–MR71
5. Vance ME, Kuiken T, Vejerano EP, McGinnis SP, Hochella MF Jr, Rejeski D, Hull MS (2015) Nanotechnology in the real world: redeveloping the nanomaterial consumer products inventory. Beilstein J Nanotechnol 6:1769–1780. https://doi.org/10.3762/bjnano.6.181
6. Dobrovolskaia MA, McNeil SE (2007) Immunological properties of engineered nanomaterials. Nat Nanotechnol 2(8):469–478. https://doi.org/10.1038/nnano.2007.223
7. Dobrovolskaia MA, Shurin M, Shvedova AA (2016) Current understanding of interactions between nanoparticles and the immune system. Toxicol Appl Pharmacol 299:78–89. https://doi.org/10.1016/j.taap.2015.12.022
8. Alsaleh NB, Brown JM (2017) Immune responses to engineered nanomaterials: current understanding and challenges. Curr Opin Toxicol. https://doi.org/10.1016/j.cotox.2017.11.011
9. Aldossari AA, Shannahan JH, Podila R, Brown JM (2015) Influence of physicochemical properties of silver nanoparticles on mast cell activation and degranulation. Toxicol In Vitro 29(1):195–203. https://doi.org/10.1016/j.tiv.2014.10.008
10. Chen EY, Garnica M, Wang YC, Mintz AJ, Chen CS, Chin WC (2012) A mixture of anatase and rutile TiO(2) nanoparticles induces histamine secretion in mast cells. Part Fibre Toxicol 9:2. https://doi.org/10.1186/1743-8977-9-2
11. Katwa P, Wang X, Urankar RN, Podila R, Hilderbrand SC, Fick RB, Rao AM, Ke PC, Wingard CJ, Brown JM (2012) A carbon nanotube toxicity paradigm driven by mast cells and the IL-(3)(3)/ST(2) axis. Small 8(18):2904–2912. https://doi.org/10.1002/smll.201200873
12. Wingard CJ, Walters DM, Cathey BL, Hilderbrand SC, Katwa P, Lin S, Ke PC, Podila R, Rao A, Lust RM, Brown JM (2011) Mast cells contribute to altered vascular reactivity and ischemia-reperfusion injury following cerium oxide nanoparticle instillation. Nanotoxicology 5(4):531–545. https://doi.org/10.3109/17435390.2010.530004
13. Alsaleh NB, Persaud I, Brown JM (2016) Silver nanoparticle-directed mast cell degranulation is mediated through calcium and PI3K signaling independent of the high affinity IgE receptor. PLoS One 11(12):e0167366. https://doi.org/10.1371/journal.pone.0167366
14. U.S. Food and Drug Administration (2015) FDA strengthens warnings and changes prescribing instructions to decrease the risk of serious allergic reactions with anemia drug Feraheme (ferumoxytol). https://www.fda.gov/Drugs/DrugSafety/ucm440138.htm
15. Szebeni J (2005) Complement activation-related pseudoallergy: a new class of drug-induced acute immune toxicity. Toxicology 216(2–3):106–121. https://doi.org/10.1016/j.tox.2005.07.023
16. Marshall JS (2004) Mast-cell responses to pathogens. Nat Rev Immunol 4(10):787–799. https://doi.org/10.1038/nri1460
17. Schwartz LB (1994) Mast cells: function and contents. Curr Opin Immunol 6(1):91–97
18. Yin Y, Bai Y, Olivera A, Desai A, Metcalfe DD (2017) An optimized protocol for the generation and functional analysis of human mast cells from CD34+ enriched cell populations. J Immunol Methods 448:105–111. https://doi.org/10.1016/j.jim.2017.06.003
19. Maeyama K, Hohman RJ, Metzger H, Beaven MA (1986) Quantitative relationships between aggregation of IgE receptors, generation of intracellular signals, and histamine secretion in rat basophilic leukemia (2H3) cells. Enhanced responses with heavy water. J Biol Chem 261(6):2583–2592
20. Galli SJ, Tsai M, Piliponsky AM (2008) The development of allergic inflammation. Nature 454(7203):445–454. https://doi.org/10.1038/nature07204
21. Farre M, Gajda-Schrantz K, Kantiani L, Barcelo D (2009) Ecotoxicity and analysis of nanomaterials in the aquatic environment. Anal Bioanal Chem 393(1):81–95. https://doi.org/10.1007/s00216-008-2458-1
22. Hartmann NB, Jensen KA, Baun A, Rasmussen K, Rauscher H, Tantra R, Cupi D,

Gilliland D, Pianella F, Riego Sintes JM (2015) Techniques and protocols for dispersing nanoparticle powders in aqueous media-is there a rationale for harmonization? J Toxicol Environ Health B Crit Rev 18(6):299–326. https://doi.org/10.1080/10937404.2015.1074969

23. Wittmaack K (2011) Excessive delivery of nanostructured matter to submersed cells caused by rapid gravitational settling. ACS Nano 5(5):3766–3778. https://doi.org/10.1021/nn200112u
24. Kroll A, Pillukat MH, Hahn D, Schnekenburger J (2012) Interference of engineered nanoparticles with in vitro toxicity assays. Arch Toxicol 86(7):1123–1136. https://doi.org/10.1007/s00204-012-0837-z
25. Monteiro-Riviere NA, Inman AO, Zhang LW (2009) Limitations and relative utility of screening assays to assess engineered nanoparticle toxicity in a human cell line. Toxicol Appl Pharmacol 234(2):222–235. https://doi.org/10.1016/j.taap.2008.09.030
26. Ong KJ, MacCormack TJ, Clark RJ, Ede JD, Ortega VA, Felix LC, Dang MK, Ma G, Fenniri H, Veinot JG, Goss GG (2014) Widespread nanoparticle-assay interference: implications for nanotoxicity testing. PLoS One 9(3): e90650. https://doi.org/10.1371/journal.pone.0090650
27. Jingkun Jiang GO, Biswas P (2009) Characterization of size, surface charge, and agglomeration state of nanoparticle dispersions for toxicological studies. J Nanopart Res 11 (1):77–89
28. Love SA, Maurer-Jones MA, Thompson JW, Lin YS, Haynes CL (2012) Assessing nanoparticle toxicity. Annu Rev Anal Chem 5:181–205. https://doi.org/10.1146/annurev-anchem-062011-143134

Chapter 3

Preparation and Utilization of a 3D Human Liver Microtissue Model for Nanotoxicological Assessment

Ali Kermanizadeh

Abstract

The liver is the principal detoxification center of the body, removing xenobiotics and waste products which could potentially include some nanomaterials (NM). With the ever increasing public and occupational exposure associated with accumulative production of nanomaterials, there is an urgent need to consider the possibility of harmful health consequences of engineered NM exposure. It is understood that following exposure via inhalation, ingestion, or direct intravenous injection a fraction of NMs reach the liver. Traditional in vitro or ex vivo hepatic nanotoxicology models are often limiting and/or troublesome (i.e., reduced metabolism enzymes, lacking important cell populations, unstable with very high variability, etc.). This chapter highlights a methodology for the preparation of a physiologically relevant 3D human liver microtissue model which addresses most of the negative issues associated with the models used in traditional in vitro hepatic toxicological investigations. The spheroids are a very promising model for the assessment of the toxicological effects associated with engineered NM exposure.

Key words Liver, 3D microtissue spheroid, Hepatocytes, Kupffer cells, Nanomaterials, Nanotoxicology

1 Introduction

The rapid expansion of technological and commercial uses of molecular scale materials has led to an escalating interest in the fields of nanoscience, nanotechnology, and nanomedicine [1]. As a negative however, the same unique chemical and physical characteristics which make NMs so desirable might also contribute to their potential adverse effects, which raises concerns that some NMs could be hazardous for people living and working with said materials [2, 3]. As the potential for public and occupational exposure is likely to rise with increasing production of nanomaterials (NM), there is an urgent need to consider the possibility of detrimental health consequences of engineered NMs.

The lungs and the gastrointestinal tract are in constant contact with the external environment, and hence these systems are the primary exposure sites for NMs [4]. However, it has been

Qunwei Zhang (ed.), *Nanotoxicity: Methods and Protocols*, Methods in Molecular Biology, vol. 1894,
https://doi.org/10.1007/978-1-4939-8916-4_3, © Springer Science+Business Media, LLC, part of Springer Nature 2019

demonstrated that some NMs can translocate from these primary exposure sites [5, 6]. As a secondary exposure tissue, the liver is extremely important, as it has been shown to accumulate NMs at much higher concentrations compared to other organs [6, 7]. In addition, the prominent advances in nanomedicine will result in an increase in direct entry of NMs into the circulatory system. The presence of NMs in the blood will result in the materials reaching the liver faster and in large quantities and will cause the induction of an immune response from the organ. The liver is characterized by its distinct populations of cells, each with their own unique morphology amongst which the hepatocytes and the resident macrophage population (Kupffer cells—KCs) being of utmost importance due to their numbers, location within a healthy liver and the wide arrays of functions that are crucial in overall liver activity [8–12].

It is widely argued that in vitro hepatocyte systems (including cell lines and systems without optimal artificial extracellular matrices) might not be ideal for functional and metabolic studies as the cells lose key liver specific functions especially their cytochrome P450 (CYP450) activity [13, 14]. Hence, the cells used in such experiments are not representative of "real" hepatocytes in vivo. In addition, most hepatic studies of the effects of nanomaterials are undertaken on hepatocyte cell lines or primary cultures lacking any nonparenchymal cells (namely KCs). However, these cells are extremely important as they are components of the reticuloendothelial system and are involved in the clearance of particles from blood as well as being crucial in the initiation of an immune response to foreign material challenge. Finally, in typical in vitro or ex vivo systems cells have a very limited life span, and therefore the opportunity for repeated exposure is not usually possible. To address all above issues will highlight a detailed protocol for the preparation and utilization of a 3D human liver microtissue model using GravityPLUS™ microtissue production plate in a 96 well format in order to investigate the adverse effects of a panel of engineered NMs as a model of the human liver. Following isolation or sourcing of primary hepatic cell the formation of the 3D microtissue is relatively simple. In principle, the cell suspension is delivered to individual inlet funnels. At the outlets under the plate, the hanging drops will form and the cells will aggregate into microtissues by gravity-enforced assembly within 4 days. The use of more physiologically relevant models such as the 3D spheroid tissue is an excellent candidate for the replacement of traditional in vitro single cell hepatic models and a valuable tool in further progression of liver nanotoxicology.

2 Materials

1. The GravityPLUS™ plate assembly (Fig. 1) consists of the following components:

   Bottom plate with reservoir.

   GravityPLUS™ plate (raster plate) with 12 × 8-well strips.

   Lid.

   Hanging drop 8-well strips.

   Humidifier pads.

2. Hepatic cells—either cell lines or primary cells (*see* **Note 1**).
3. GravityTRAP™ plate.
4. Cell culture medium—formulation will vary depending on the cell types being utilized (*see* **Note 2**).
5. Sterile phosphate buffered saline (PBS).
6. Inverted microscope.
7. Cell counter.
8. Multichannel pipette (10–200 μl).
9. Sterile medium reservoir for multichannel pipettes.
10. Sterile reservoir large enough to fit 96-well plate.
11. Microplate centrifuge.
12. Humidified CO_2 incubator.
13. Level 1 biosafety cabinet.
14. Water or bead heating bath (37 °C).
15. Sterile tweezers.

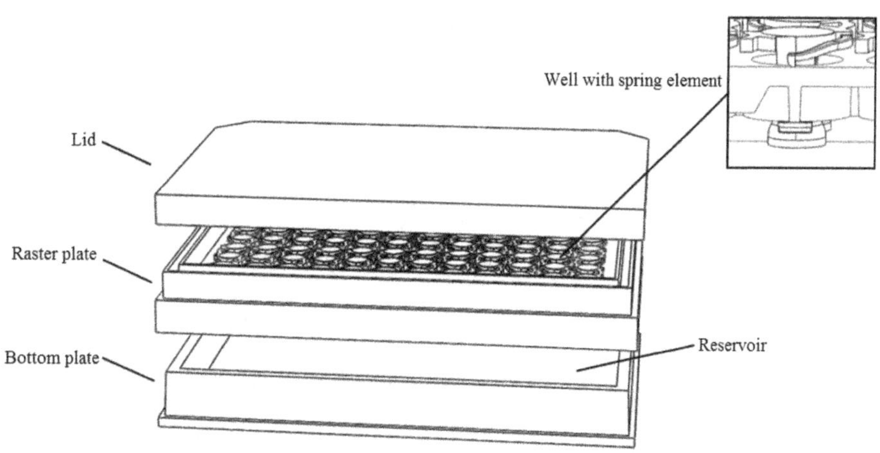

Fig. 1 GravityPlus™ plate components (modified and reproduced from [15])

16. Additional consumables and reagents for cell culture, characterization of microtissue and subsequent toxicological testing, i.e., 4% PFA (Sigma Aldrich, UK) or hemotoxylin and eosin stain (Sigma-Aldrich, UK).

3 Methods

3.1 Formation of the Hepatic Microtissues

1. Open the bag containing the GravityPLUS™ Plate assembly under sterile conditions.
2. Prepare a sterile reservoir with 20 ml of PBS.
3. Using the tweezers, remove one humidifier pad and place in sterile PBS for 5 min.
4. Place the soaked humidifier pad in the bottom plate of the GravityPLUS™ plate.
5. Prepare hepatic cells (*see* **Note 1**).
6. Count the cells.
7. Gently deliver 40 μl of cell suspension into each well (*see* **Note 2**) of the GravityPLUS™ plate. Ensure tight contact between the pipette tip and the well inlet by applying slight pressure to form the SureDrop™ seal (Fig. 2). (Use of 1000–2000 proliferating cells is recommended. If using nonproliferating cells, a minimum of 2000–5000 cells per drop are required.).
8. Close the lid on the plate and place assembly in a humidified CO_2 incubator at 37 °C for 4 days (*see* **Note 3**).
9. After 4 days in culture hepatic cells should reaggregate and form a 3D spheroid.

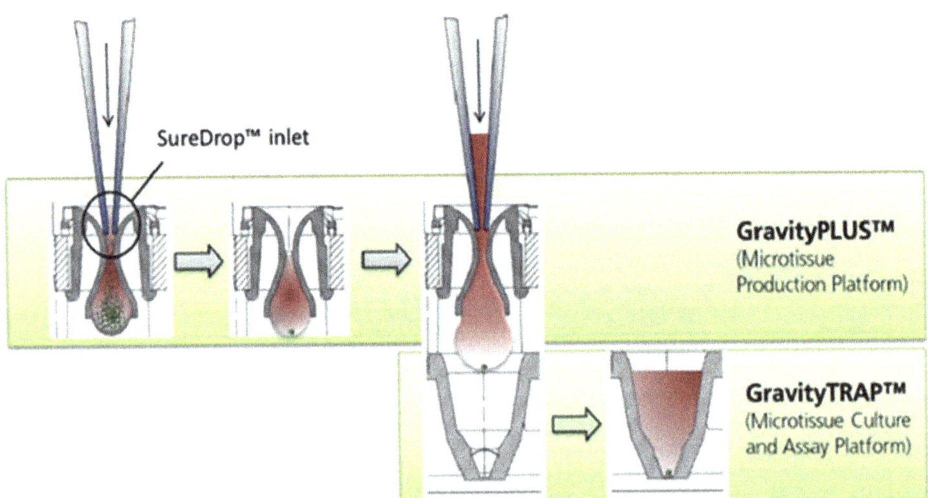

Fig. 2 SureDrop™ inlet/GravityPlus™ and GravityTRAP™ platforms (reproduced from [16])

3.2 Transfer of Microtissue to GravityTRAP™ Plate (See Note 4)

1. Preheat the medium required for microtissue culture and maintenance to 37 °C.
2. Under sterile conditions open the bag containing the GravityTRAP™ plate.
3. Add 40 μl of cell culture to each well by placing the tip deep into the wells (avoid touching the well bottom) (*see* **Note 5**).
4. Place the raster plate of the GravityPLUS™ plate onto the GravityTRAP™ plate by positioning the three pins into the corresponding holes on the top surface of the GravityTRAP™ plate. Using this step should ensure that the drops are aligned perfectly with the wells of the GravityTRAP™ plate underneath.
5. Very slowly add 70 μl of cell culture medium through the inlet of the GravityPLUS™ plate wells. It is important that the pipette tips should be in direct contact with the well inlets. The drops containing the microtissues will fall into the wells in the GravityTRAP™ plate.
6. Check the transfer of the microtissues using an inverted microscope.
7. OPTIONAL STEP—spin the plates at 250 RCF for 2 min to ensure successful transfer of all tissues and removal of trapped air bubbles in the GravityTRAP™ plate wells.
8. OPTIONAL STEP—to ensure accurate medium volumes in each wells aspirate and replace the cell culture medium with 70 μl of fresh medium. Remove medium by placing the tip at the ledge of the upper cavity of the well (Fig. 3). Remove the medium at low pipetting speed. Add 70 μl of fresh medium by placing the pipette tip at the ledge.

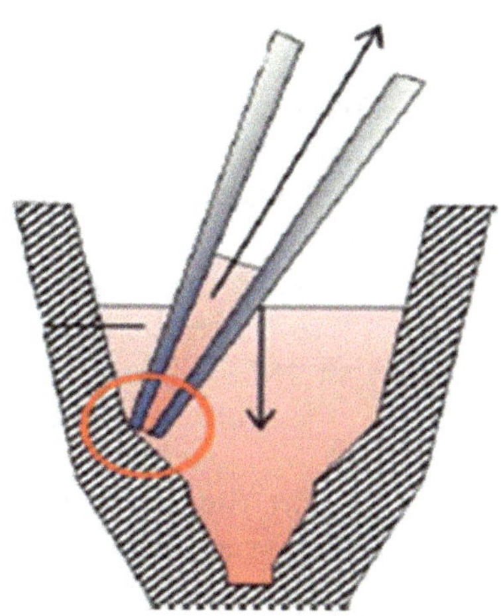

Fig. 3 The removal of medium from GravityTRAP™ well (modified and reproduced from [15]). (*See* **Note 6**)

9. The cell culture medium should be exchanged every 48 h. The human hepatic 3D microtissue maintenance and viability has been checked for up to 28 days using the above protocol (*see* **Note 1**).

3.3 Harvest of Microtissue from the GravityTRAP™ Plate

1. Place the tip of a 1000 μl pipette tip in a vertical position to cover the center of the lower cavity of the well. The tip orifice is positioned directly above the microtissue at the bottom of the well. The utilization of a 1 ml tip size prevents the disruption of the microtissue by being squeezed inadvertently at the tip of the pipette.
2. Very carefully collect the microtissues by aspirating 50 μl of the medium. It is important to avoid aspiration of air bubbles which may cause the break-up of the microtissue.
3. Transfer the microtissue to the required vessel or plate for subsequent testing.

3.4 Microtissue Characterization (Hepatocyte and KC 3D Microtissue)

1. For characterization purposes the microtissues should be harvested at around day 7.
2. Transfer the microtissue into 1.5 ml tubes.
3. Wash with 1 ml PBS before fixing with 4% PFA for 2 h at room temperature.
4. The specimens are covered with agarose and further processed for paraffin embedding and histological staining.
5. Stain paraffin sections with H&E (using standard protocols).
6. OPTIONAL STEP—immunohistochemistry staining for KCs can be performed with a CD68 antibody (Fig. 4).

As an example of the utilization of technology for toxicological assessment of NMs; the loss of cell membrane integrity was evaluated utilizing a ToxiLight™ bioassay kit (Lonza, USA) in primary human hepatic microtissue (hepatocytes and Kupffer cells) (Fig. 5). Following NM treatment single or repeated NM treatment over a period of 360 h, 20 μl of cell supernatant was transferred to a luminescence compatible plate before the addition of 80 μl of adenylate kinase detection buffer. The plates were incubated for 5 min at room temperature before the luminescence was measured. These experiments included the appropriate controls which included tissue treated with medium or lysis reagent.

See **Notes** 7 and **8**.

3.5 Limitations and Considerations

Despite the numerous advantages of the generated human liver microtissue using the above methodology, there are also some limitations which need to be considered in the design of any toxicological experiment. The wells contain limited volumes of supernatant which means there are some restrictions to the biochemical and toxicological end-points which can be examined (although it is

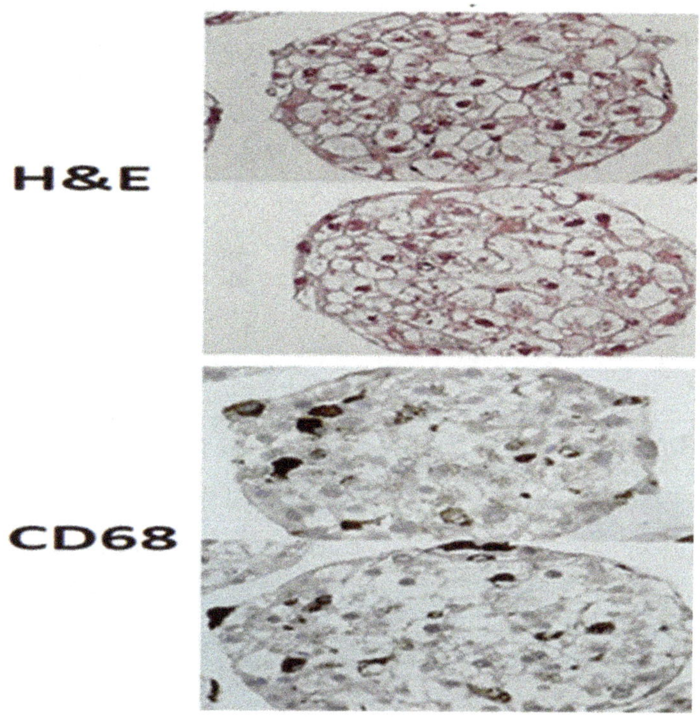

Fig. 4 Morphological characterization of intact 3D human liver microtissue. H&E staining and CD68 immunohistochemistry of formalin fixed microtissue after day 7 in culture (modified and reproduced from [17])

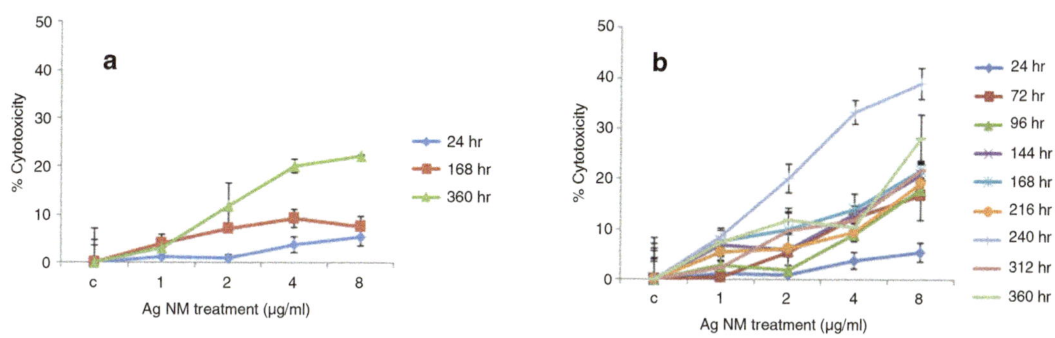

c **Single exposure**

Treatment 1 - 0 hr(day 0)
Medium change - 24 hr (day 1)
Medium change - 72 hr (day 3)
Medium change - 168 hr (day 7)
Medium change - 216 hr (day 9)
Medium change - 264 hr (day 11)
Medium change - 336 hr (day 14)
Medium change - 360 hr (day 15)

Fig. 5 Cytotoxicity in human liver microtissue following a single (**a**) or repeated (**b**) exposures to Ag NMs. The microtissue were exposed to cell medium (**c**)/or Ag NMs over a period of 360 h as measured by adenylate kinase release cytotoxicity assay. Values represent mean $\pm$ SEM ($n = 3$). Microtissue maintenance and NM treatment in the singular and repeated exposure experiments over a period of 15 days (figure reproduced from [17])

possible to pool the supernatants from wells with the same treatment). On the same note, for subsequent assays which require individual cells (i.e., the comet assay used to investigate DNA damage) an efficient homogenization method is required due to small cell numbers in each individual microtissue. Finally, the consideration size of the microtissue is very important in any study design. Due to lack of blood flow and 3D spheroid structure of the tissue the inner cells will not receive enough nutrients if the spheroid is too large. From a toxicological prospective the inner cells might also not encounter NMs (in particular nonsoluble materials) in the larger spheres which might result in false findings.

4 Notes

1. The above protocol has been used successfully with cocultures of primary human hepatocytes and cryopreserved Kupffer cells (Thermo Fischer Scientific, UK) (4:1 ratio), HepRG (Thermo Fischer Scientific, UK) and cryopreserved Kupffer cells (Thermo Fischer Scientific, UK) (4:1 ratio), as well as monocultures utilizing HepG2 (Sigma-Aldrich, UK) and HepRG hepatocytes.
2. For the homogeneity of the forming microtissues it is essential to assure a homogeneous distribution of the cells by gently pipetting up and down prior to the seeding.
3. Assess the progress of microtissue formation at least every 24 h. The formation of the microtissue can be observed using inverted microscopy.
4. For long-term cultivation and subsequent toxicological analysis using the hepatic cells the transfer of microtissues from the GravityPLUS™ plate to the GravityTRAP™ plate is required.
5. All attempts should be made to avoid air bubbles in the pre-wetting steps to ensure better positioning of the microtissue in the center region of wells.
6. It is impossible to remove all medium from the wells with a volume of around 10 μl of medium will remain in the well using the above protocol.
7. The 3D hepatic microtissue spheroids (both cell line and primary cells) generated using the above protocol have been previously exposed to a wide range of NMs including silica, TiO_2, silver, zinc oxide and multiwalled carbon nanotubes either via a single treatment or repeated dosing regiments for up to 15 days.
8. Previous tested biochemical analysis and nanotoxicological end-points using the generated hepatic 3D microtissue have included but not limited to cell viability (adenylate kinase assay), inflammatory response (cytokine secretion), DNA

damage (comet assay), hepatic function (albumin production), cytochrome P450 metabolic activity, and fluorescent and confocal microscopy.

References

1. Nel A, Xia T, Meng H, Wang X, Lin S, Ji Z, Zhang H (2013) Nanomaterial toxicity testing in the 21st century: use of a predicvtive toxicological approach and high-throughput screening. Acc Chem Res 46:607–621
2. Johnston H, Brown D, Kermanizadeh A, Gubbins E, Stone V (2012) Investigating the relationship between nanomaterial hazard and physicochemical properties: informing the exploitation of nanomaterials with therapeutic and diagnosis applications. J Control Release 164:307–313
3. Kermanizadeh A, Gosens I, MacCalman L, Johnston H, Danielsen PH, Jacobsen NR, Lenz AG, Fernandes T, Schins RPF, Cassee FR, Wallin H, Kreyling W, Stoeger T, Loft S, Møller P, Tran L, Stone V (2016) A multilaboratory toxicological assessment of a panel of ten engineered nanomaterials to human health—ENPRA project—the highlights, limitations and the current and future challenges. J Toxicol Environ Health B Crit Rev 19:1–28
4. Bakand S, Hayes A, Dechsakulthorn F (2012) Nanoparticles: a review of particle toxicology following inhalation exposure. Inhal Toxicol 24:125–135
5. Semmler-Behnke M, Kreyling W, Lipka J, Fertsch S, Wenk A, Takeneka S, Schmid G, Brandau W (2008) Bio-distribution of 1.4 and 18 nm gold particles in rats. Small 4 (12):2108–2111
6. Kermanizadeh A, Balharry D, Wallin H, Loft S, Møller P (2015) Nanomaterial translocation—the biokinetics, tissue accumulation, toxicity and fate of materials in secondary organs—a review. Crit Rev Toxicol 45:837–872
7. Sadauskas E, Jacobson NR, Danscher G, Soltenberg M, Larsen A, Kreyling W, Wallin H (2009) Bio-disruption of gold nanoparticles in mouse lung following intratracheal instillation. Chem Cent J 3:16–23
8. Kermanizadeh A, Brown DM, Hutchison G, Stone V (2013) Engineered nanomaterial impact in the liver following exposure via an intravenous route—the role of polymorphonuclear leukocytes and gene expression in the organ. Nanomed Nanotechnol 4:157
9. Kermanizadeh A, Chauché C, Balharry D, Brown DM, Kanase N, Boczkowski J, Lanone S, Stone V (2014) The role of Kupffer cells in the hepatic response to silver nanoparticles. Nanotoxicology 8:149–154
10. Kmiec Z (2001) Co-operation of liver cells in health and disease. Adv Anat Embryol Cell Biol 161:1–151
11. Godoy P, Hewitt NJ, Albrecht U, Andersen ME, Ansari N, Bhattacharya S, Bode JH, Bolleyn J, Borner C, Bottger J et al (2014) Recent advances in 2D and 3D in vitro Systems using primary hepatocytes, alternative hepatocyte sources and nonparenchymal liver cells and their use in investigating mechanisms of hepatotoxicity, cell signalling and ADME. Arch Toxicol 87:1315–1530
12. Teigs G, Lohse AW (2009) Immune tolerance: what is unique about the liver. J Autoimmun 34:1–6
13. Mingoia RT, Nabb DL, Yang CH, Han X (2007) Primary culture of rat hepatocytes in 96 well plates: effects of extracellular matrix configuration on cytochrome P450 enzyme activity and inducibility and its application *in vitro* cytotoxicity screening. Toxicol In Vitro 21:165–173
14. Messner S, Agarkova I, Moritz W, Kelm JM (2013) Multi-cell human liver microtissues for hepatotoxicity testing. Arch Toxicol 87:209–213
15. PerkinElmer website. 14 Oct 2017. http://www.perkinelmer.com/
16. Khetani SR, Berger DR, Ballinger KR, Davidson MD, Lin C, Ware BR (2015) Microengineered liver tissue for drug testing. J Lab Autom 20:216–250
17. Kermanizadeh A, Løhr M, Roursgaard M, Messner S, Gunness P, Kelm JM, Møller P, Stone V, Loft S (2014) Hepatic toxicology following single and multiple exposure of engineered nanomaterials utilising a novel primary human 3D liver microtissue model. Part Fibre Toxicol 11:56

Chapter 4

Deriving Neural Cells from Pluripotent Stem Cells for Nanotoxicity Testing

Yiling Hong, Nymph Chan, and Aynun N. Begum

Abstract

Stem cells are undifferentiated biological cells that can differentiate into all lineages under defined control condition. Stem cell neuronal differentiation can faithfully recapitulate stages of neural development and generate neuronal progenitors, mature neurons, and glial cells. Stem cell technology will largely allow for the replacement of animal studies and reduce costs, and will provide a new paradigm for in toxic genomics, bioinformatics, systems biology, and epigenetics studies. Here, we describe a nonadherent neuronal differentiation methodology developed in our laboratory, which can rapidly derive neurons and astrocytes from human embryonic stem cells (hESCs) and induced pluripotent stem cell (hiPSC) and use of this platform for nanoparticle neurotoxicity study.

Key words Human embryonic stem cells, Induced pluripotent stem cells neuronal differentiation, Neurotoxicity, Neuronal progenitors, Neurons and astrocyte, Silver nanoparticles

1 Introduction

Human embryonic stem cells (hESCs) were first derived by Thomson's group in 2001 [1]. Induced pluripotent stem cells (iPSCs) are a type of pluripotent stem cell that can be generated directly from adult cells. The iPSC technology was pioneered by Shinya Yamanaka's lab in 2006 [2]. The ability to derive stem cells into neuron/astrocyte network and cerebral organoids that recapitulate corticogenesis provided a powerful model to identify the human neuronal disease pathogenic mechanism [3, 4] and for toxicity studies [5]. Stem cell neuronal differentiation can be derived by the adherent or nonadherent culturing conditions [6]. In the adherent method, hESCs/iPSCs are grown in a monolayer called neuroectoderm, whereas in the nonadherent method, cells are initially grown as nonadhering neurospheres. We have demonstrated that the nonadherent method formed larger neural tube type rosette (NTTR) structure and expressed high level of PAX6, SOX2, and NESTIN neuroprogenitor genes compared with neuroectoderm-

Qunwei Zhang (ed.), *Nanotoxicity: Methods and Protocols*, Methods in Molecular Biology, vol. 1894,
https://doi.org/10.1007/978-1-4939-8916-4_4,

derived neuroprogenitors. Furthermore, most of the functional subtype neurons can be generated around 27–40 days, which is faster than traditional neurodifferentiation protocols (42–60 days) [7].

In our laboratory, we initiated neuronal differentiation by culturing hESCs/iPSCs in knockout serum replacement medium (SKSRM) supplemented with bFGF, ROCK inhibitor, EGF, LIF, and heparin and incubating in a 37 °C incubator with 10% CO_2 for 3 days. Using this method, the expression of neural progenitor cell markers is higher than that of cells incubated in 5% CO_2. Afterwards, neurospheres were broken down into smaller fragments mechanically by a step called AdSTEP, and then plated onto Matrigel-coated plates to generate a monolayer called neurospheederm. Differentiation with AdSTEP increased the expression of PAX6 and FOXG1 and facilitated the production of neurons and astrocytes. When neurospheres were transplanted into mouse brains, they differentiated into neural stem cells as well as neurons and astrocytes efficiently. These suggest that our nonadherent method enhances the neurodifferentiation capacity of stem cells both in vitro and in vivo [7] (Fig. 1).

Deriving neural cells of all lineages from hESCs/iPSCs not only allows us to study neural development, it can also serve an analytical purpose. Utilizing the hESCs neurodevelopment model, we can test the toxicity of various agents elicited at any stage of the development of the brain. In our laboratory, we employed this neurodifferentiation process to produce mature glutamatergic neurons for testing the neurotoxicity of nanoparticles. Silver nanoparticles (AgNPs) have already entered consumer market, having been

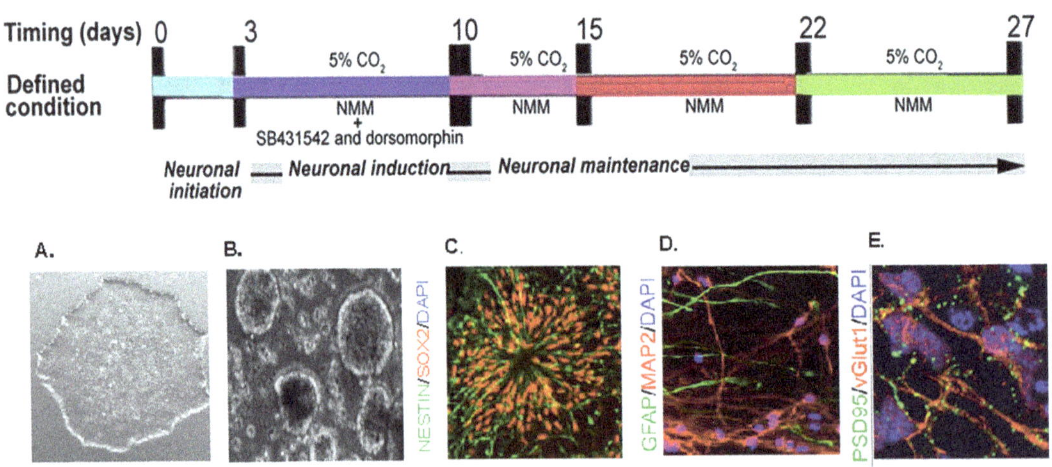

Fig. 1 Diagram the time course of derivation of neuronal progenitors, mature neurons and astrocytes from hESCs. (**a**) Human embryonic stem cells (hESCs). (**b**) Neurospheres derived from hESCs (**c**) Rosette-forming neuroepithelial expressed Nestin and Sox2. (**d**) Neurons and astrocytes expressed Map2 (red) and GFAP (green). (**e**) Synapses expressed PSD95 and vGlut1 synaptic [7]

applied in therapy and everyday household items such as textiles, cosmetic and plastics. We tested two types of AgNPs, 20 nm electrostatically stabilized citrated-coated AgNPs (AgSCs) and 20 nm sterically stabilized polyvinylpyrrolidone-coated AgNPs (AgSPs). The results showed that both types of AgNPs negatively affected neuritic growth and cell viability, with AgSCs exhibiting higher neurotoxicity. AgNPs also induced reactive oxygen species (ROS) production and calcium ion influx into the glutamatergic neurons, as well as the phosphorylation of GSK3β and Tau, suggesting that AgNP exposure may stimulate the initiation and progression of neurodegeneration (Fig. 2). Our work provided a template for using hESCs/iPSCs-derived neurodevelopment to mimic human brain development and for testing neurotoxicity [8].

2 Materials

2.1 Culturing H9 Human Embryonic Stem Cells and Induced Pluripotent Stem Cells

1. Human embryonic stem cells (H9 lines, National Stem Cell Bank code WA09) were ordered from Wicell and maintained in mTeSR1 medium (STEMCELL Technologies). Induced pluripotent stem cells (iPSC) was derived as descripted in Begum et al. [7]. The colonies were maintained in an undifferentiated state in Matrigel-coated (BD Biosciences) T25 flasks.
2. mTeSR medium: Add 100 mL of thawed 5× mTeSR supplements to 400 mL of filtered mTeSR Basal Medium and mix by swirling thoroughly. Aliquot this mTeSR media into 40 mL portions into sterile 50 mL tubes and store at −20 °C. This medium can be frozen up to 6 months (*see* **Note 1**).
3. ReLeSR enzyme-free hESC and hiPSC selection and passaging reagent.
4. mFreSR defined cryopreservation medium for human embryonic stem cells.
5. Matrigel coating solution: Add 500 μL of knockout DMEM/F12 medium to 300 μL of Matrigel hESC-qualified matrix, LDEV-free, and mix thoroughly by pipetting up and down with a cold 5 mL pipet. Transfer this mixture to 25 mL of knockout DMEM/F12 medium and mix thoroughly with a cold 25 mL pipette (*see* **Note 2**).
6. Dulbecco's phosphate-buffered saline, no calcium, no magnesium.
7. Knockout DMEM/F12 medium.
8. Washing medium: 50% PBS and 50% DMEM.

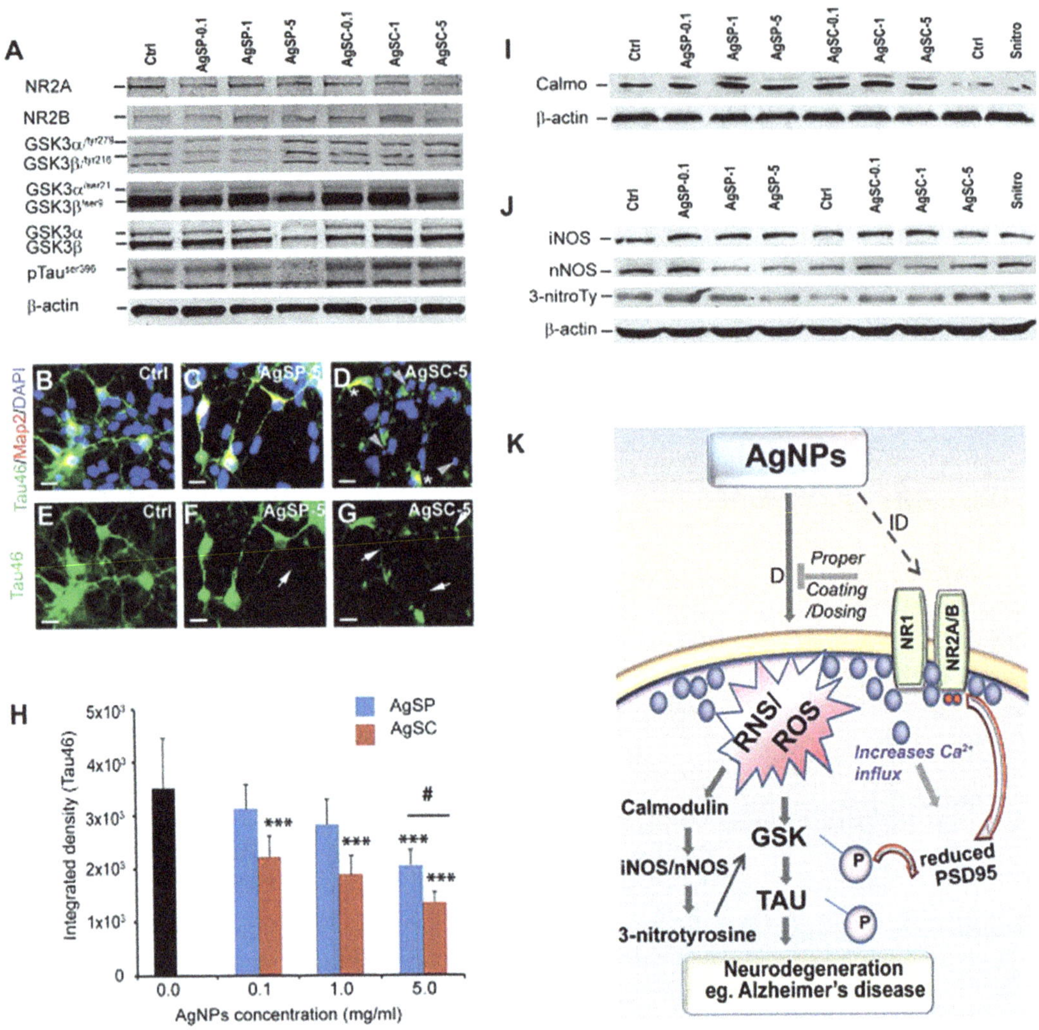

Fig. 2 AgNPs induced the phosphorylation of GSK-3β and Tau and the impairment of the microtubule dynamics protein Tau46. (**a**) Immunoblotting of NR2A, NR2B, phosphorylated GSK-3α/β at serine and tyrosine and Tau after exposure to three different concentrations (0.1, 1, and 5 μg/mL) of AgNPs for 72 h. β-Actin was used as the loading control. Immunostaining was performed with a Tau46/Map2 antibody to examine the effect of AgNP on microtubule dynamics by staining the axons and dendrites. (**b**, **e**) The untreated sample (Ctrl) showed no changes in either the axons or dendrites, whereas (**c**, **f**) AgSP exposure slightly damaged the axons and dendrites. (**d**, **g**) AgSC (5 μg/mL) caused a significant loss of dendrites and substantial damage of the axonal network (white arrow). AgSCs also caused fragmented nuclei. (**d**) The grey arrowhead represents apoptotic neurons, but (**b**) the control and (**c**) AgSP treatments did not result in neuronal apoptosis. The nuclei are stained with DAPI. Scale bars, 25 μm. (**h**) Image J quantification confirmed the dose-dependent effect of AgNPs on microtubule dynamics through observing the reduction in the Tau46 integrated density. Data are presented as the means ± SD, $N = 4$. $^{*}p < 0.05$ or $^{\#}p < 0.05$ represent significant differences. (**i**) The proposed mechanism underlying AgNP-induced neurotoxicity could follow two pathways. The first is the direct pathway (D), where the production of ROS causes excessive Ca^{2+} influx into neurons and affects the phosphorylation status and activity of GSK-3β and Tau. Ultimately, axonal networks are disrupted through the reduction or loss of Tau46, leading to an AD-like pathology as shown in this study. The second mechanism is the indirect mechanism (ID), which is a change in the expression of NR2A/B and other NMDA receptor proteins. These proteins are important for maintaining ion channel-mediated synaptic signaling and their loss can induce the phosphorylation of GSK and Tau

2.2 Neuronal Differentiation

1. Collagenase: Prepare a 20 mg/mL Collagenase IV solution by dissolving Collagenase IV in knockout DMEM/F12 medium. Aliquot this collagenase solution into 1 mL portions and freeze at −20 °C. For the working stock, dilute 1 mL of the 20 mg/mL collagenase solution in 20 mL of knockout DMEM/F12 medium.
2. 0.5% (V/V) FBS: Dilute FBS in PBS to a concentration of 1% (v/v) and freeze at −20 °C. For the working stock, dilute the 1% (v/v) FBS 1:1 with PBS to make 0.5% (v/v) FBS.
3. KSRM medium (SR basal): Add 5 mL of 100× nonessential amino acids solution, 2.5 mL of 100× GlutaMAX supplement, 3.5 μL of β-mercaptoethanol, 100 mL of KnockOut™ serum replacement, and 5 mL of 10,000 U/mL penicillin/streptomycin into 500 mL of DMEM/F12 (1:1) medium.
4. SKSRM medium (SR+): Add 40 μL of 10 ng/mL bFGF, 40 μL of 500 ng/mL EGF, 40 μL of ROCK inhibitor Y-27632, 8 μL of 1 μg/mL heparin, and 4 μL of 10^7 units ESGRO Leukemia Inhibitory Factor (LIF) into 40 mL of KSRM medium (SR basal).
5. SR+ medium without ROCK inhibitor: Add 40 μL of 10 ng/mL bFGF, 40 μL of 500 ng/mL EGF, 8 μL of 1 μg/mL of heparin, and 4 μL of 10^7 units ESGRO Leukemia Inhibitory Factor (LIF) into 40 mL of KSRM medium (SR basal).
6. N2 medium: Add 5 mL of 100× MEM nonessential amino acids solution, 5 mL of 100× GlutaMAX™ supplement, 5.5 mL of 10,000 U/mL penicillin-streptomycin, 3.5 μL of β-mercaptoethanol, 250 μL of 10 mg/mL of insulin, and 5 mL of 100× N-2 supplement into 500 mL of DMEM/F12 medium (*see* **Note 3**).
7. B27 medium: Add 5.5 mL of 100× GlutaMAX™ supplement, 5.5 mL of 10,000 U/mL of penicillin-streptomycin, and 10 mL of 50× B-27® supplement into 500 mL of Neurobasal®-A medium, minus phenol red.
8. NMM medium: 50% N2 medium and 50% B27 medium.
9. Gentle cell dissociation reagent.
10. Neurosphere induction medium (Day 5): Add 1 μM of dorsomorphin and 10 μM of SB421542 into 70% SR basal medium and 30% NMM medium.
11. Neurosphere induction medium (Day 7): Add 1 μM of dorsomorphin and 10 μM of SB421542 into 50% SR basal medium and 50% NMM medium.
12. Neurosphere induction medium (Day 9): Add 1 μM of dorsomorphin and 10 μM of SB421542 into 30% SR basal medium and 70% NMM medium.

13. Neurosphere induction medium (Day 11): Add 1 μM of dorsomorphin and 10 μM of SB421542 into 100% NMM medium.
14. Low adhesion suspension 6-well culture plates.

2.3 Exposing Glutamatergic Neurons (hGNs) to Silver Nanoparticles

The 20 nm citrate-stabilized colloidal silver nanoparticles (AgSCs) and the polyvinlypyrrolidone (PVP)-stabilized colloidal silver nanoparticles (AgSPs) were generous gifts from the National Institute of Environment and Health Sciences (NIEHS). The average primary particle size and the size distribution were determined using high-resolution transmission electron microscopy (TEM). The silver concentration was determined by inductively coupled plasma mass spectrometry (ICPMS). Both samples had the same silver concentration (1.1 mg/g). The physical and chemical characterization data of these nanoparticles can be found in the booklet provided by NIEHS (NCL-NIEHS201305A). The particles of AgNPs were supplied in water at a concentration of 1 mg/mL. The dosing solutions were prepared in cell culture media (NMM) for the treatments.

2.4 Determining Morphology, Toxicity, and Induction of Reactive Oxygen Species

1. Neurite outgrowth cell kit.
2. Phosphate-buffered saline (PBS).
3. LDH cytotoxicity assay kit.
4. CellROX Deep Red Reagent.
5. Microplate fluorescence reader.
6. EVOS fluorescence microscope.

2.5 Intracellular Calcium Staining

1. Neuro basal medium (low Ca^{2+} and Mg^{2+}).
2. PBS without Ca^{2+} and Mg^{2+}.
3. Fluo-4 Ca^{2+} AM ester solution: Dilute the DMSO stock to 5 μM in PBS containing 0.001% Pluronic F-127.
4. Microplate fluorescence reader.

2.6 Immuno-cytochemistry

1. Coverslips.
2. PBS.
3. 4% Paraformaldehyde: Dilute 16% paraformaldehyde stock by mixing 4 mL of the stock with 12 mL of PBS.
4. 0.1% Triton X-100: Dilute 16 μL of 100% Triton X-100 in 16 mL of PBS.
5. Blocking buffer: Add 2.5 mL of 10% normal goat serum (NGS) into 22.25 mL of PBS, and then dissolve 1.25 g of bovine serum albumin (BSA) into the NGS in PBS.
6. Primary antibody solution: Dilute monoclonal mouse anti-MAP2 antibody, polyclonal rabbit anti-vGLUT1 antibody, monoclonal mouse anti-PSD95 antibody, or monoclonal mouse anti-Tau46 antibody in blocking buffer.

7. Washing buffer: Add 500 μL of 10% normal goat serum and 250 μL of 10% Tween 20 to 50 mL of PBS.
8. Secondary antibody solution: Dilute goat anti-rabbit IgG-Alexa Fluor 546 or goat anti-mouse IgG-Alexa Fluor 488 conjugates in washing buffer.
9. DAPI Fluoromount-G.
10. EVOS fluorescence microscope.

2.7 Western Blotting

1. RIPA buffer: Dissolve 0.88 g of sodium chloride, 0.05 g of sodium deoxycholate, 1 g of SDS and 0.61 g of Tris base in 80 mL of water and add 1 mL of NP-40. Adjust pH with 6 N HCl to pH 8.0, then add water to 100 mL.
2. Protease inhibitors.
3. 1.5 M Tris–HCl, pH 8.8: Dissolve 181.5 g of Tris base in 800 mL of water and adjust pH with 6 N HCl to pH 8.8, then add water to 1 L.
4. 0.5 M Tris–HCl, pH 6.8: Dissolve 60 g of Tris base in 800 mL of water and adjust pH with 6 N HCl to pH 6.8, then add water to 1 L.
5. 10% SDS: Dissolve 10 g of SDS in 90 mL of water, and then add water to 100 mL.
6. 10% ammonium persulfate: Dissolve 0.1 g of ammonium persulfate in 1 mL of water (*see* **Note 4**)
7. 30% acrylamide–bis solution, 29:1.
8. TEMED.
9. SDS PAGE sample buffer.
10. Running buffer: Dissolve 3.03 g of Tris base, 14.41 g of glycine, and 1 g of SDS in 800 mL of water, and then add water to 1 L.
11. Polyvinylidene difluoride (PVDF) membranes.
12. Transfer buffer: Dissolve 3.03 g of Tris base and 14.41 g of glycine in 800 mL of water and 200 mL of methanol.
13. Odyssey blocking buffer in PBS: Mix Odyssey blocking buffer with PBS at a 1:1 ratio.
14. Primary antibody solution: Dilute antibodies targeting PSD95, vGLUT1, NR2A, NR2B, pGSK3$^{tyr216/279}$, pGSK3^{Ser9}, GSK3, pTau, calmodulin, iNOS, nNOS, 3-nitrotyrosine, and β-actin in blocking buffer according to manufacturers' recommendation.
15. PBS with Tween 20: Add 1 mL of Tween 20 to 1 L of PBS.
16. Odyssey infrared-conjugated secondary antibodies.
17. Odyssey infrared imager.

3 Methods

3.1 Coating Flasks/Plates with Matrigel

1. Transfer 4 or 2 mL of Matrigel coating solution per T25 flask and per well of a 6-well plate, respectively.
2. Immediately rock the flask or plate back and forth until the coating solution is distributed evenly on the surface of the flask or plate.
3. Incubate the flask or plate with the coating solution for 1–2 h at room temperature. Alternatively, seal the side of the plate with Parafilm, and store the flask or plate horizontally at 4 °C (*see* **Note 5**).

3.2 Plating Cryopreserved H9 Cells

1. Before using the Matrigel-coated plate or flask that had been stored at 4 °C, incubate them for 2 h at room temperature.
2. Thaw and warm frozen mTeSR medium in the 37 °C water bath for 2 h.
3. Mix prewarmed mTeSR medium by pipetting up and down.
4. Remove excess Matrigel coating solution by aspiration and wash the plate or flask with PBS for complete removal of Matrigel.
5. Transfer 1.5 or 3 mL of mTeSR medium per well of a 6-well plate or per T25 flask, respectively.
6. Transfer a vial of cryopreserved cells from the liquid nitrogen storage tank onto ice.
7. Thaw the vial of cryopreserved cells in a 37 °C water bath with continuous shaking.
8. Once the cells are thawed, transfer 1 mL of the thawed cells into a 15 mL tube using 1 mL pipette tips.
9. Immediately add 9 mL of mTeSR medium to the thawed cells in the 15 mL tube (*see* **Note 6**).
10. After mixing the cells with mTeSR medium, centrifuge at 300 × *g* for 5 min.
11. Carefully aspirate the supernatant and leave 50–60 μL of the mTeSR medium above the cell pellet.
12. Resuspend the cells with 2 mL of mTeSR medium.
13. Transfer 0.5 mL of the cell suspension drop-wise and equally distribute it into each coated well or flask.
14. Rock the plate or flask back and forth and then place them into a 37 °C incubator.
15. Wash the cells 1 day after plating. Remove the existing medium by aspiration, then wash the cells using 1.5 mL or 2 mL of Knockout DMEM/F12 per well or per flask, respectively. Rock the plate back and forth. Aspirate the Knockout DMEM/F12

and transfer 2 or 3 mL of mTeSR medium per well or flask, respectively.

16. Change medium with fresh mTeSR medium every other day.
17. Incubate the cells at 37 °C, 5% CO_2.

3.3 Passaging H9 Cells with ReLeSR

1. Coat plates or flasks with Matrigel coating solution as described above, or take out coated plates or flasks from 4 °C and incubate at room temperature for 2 h.
2. Wash cells with washing medium.
3. Aspirate the washing medium, then transfer 2 or 4 mL of ReLeSR per T25 flask or per T75 flask, respectively.
4. Incubate at 37 °C, 5% CO_2 for 1–3 min.
5. Transfer 3 or 6 mL of mTeSR medium to a T25 flask or T75 flask, respectively, and then tab and shake the flask to detach the cells.
6. Transfer 100–200 μL of cell suspension to a new coated flask containing mTeSR medium.
7. Incubate the cells at 37 °C, 5% CO_2.
8. Wash the cells and replace with fresh mTeSR medium one day after passaging, and change medium every other day.

3.4 Picking Colonies

1. Coat plates or flasks with Matrigel as described above, or retrieve coated plates or flasks from 4 °C and incubate at room temperature for 2 h.
2. Aspirate existing medium, and wash the cells with washing medium.
3. Transfer 4 or 8 mL of mTeSR medium per T25 flask or per T75 flask, respectively.
4. Search for a well-formed colony using a microscope inside a biosafety cabinet, then using a P-200 pipette with sterile tips, gently scrape off cells from the colony and immediately suck up the detached cells. Transfer the cells to the flask containing mTeSR medium.
5. Pick and transfer 5–7 colonies per flask, and incubate the cells at 37 °C, 5% CO_2.
6. Wash the cells and replace with fresh mTeSR medium 1 day after passaging, and change medium every other day.

3.5 Cryopreserving H9 Cells

1. Wash cells with washing medium, and then transfer 4 mL of mTeSR medium to the flasks.
2. Using a sterile cell scraper, scrape cells off the flask and then transfer the cell suspension into a 15 mL tube.
3. Centrifuge at 400 × g for 5 min, and then aspirate the supernatant.

4. Resuspend the cells in mFreSR.
5. Aliquot 1 mL of the cell suspension per cryovial.
6. Place the cells in the cryovials into a Mister Frosty and store at −80 °C overnight. On the next day, transfer the cells into a liquid nitrogen storage tank.

3.6 Neuronal Differentiation

Day 0 (Neuronal Initiation—10% CO_2, 37 °C incubator)

1. Wash H9 cells with 2 mL of washing medium.
2. Transfer 2 mL of collagenase onto the cells and incubate the cells at 37 °C for 20 min until the edges of the colonies become folded.
3. Neutralize the activity of the collagenase with 0.5% FBS, using double the volume of collagenase used.
4. Detach cells by scraping using sterile cell scrapers.
5. Transfer the cell suspension to a 15 mL tube and centrifuge at 400 × *g* for 4 min, and then remove the supernatant.
6. Resuspend cells with SR+ medium by pipetting up and down for 5–10 min.
7. Wash a low adhesion suspension 6-well culture plate with PBS.
8. Distribute the cells evenly into each well, and fill each well with up to 2 mL of SR+ medium. Incubate the cells under 10% CO_2, 37 °C culture condition.

Day 1

9. Add 2 mL of SR+ medium without ROCK inhibitor per well.

Day 3

10. Remove 2 mL of the existing medium from the surface of the medium so as not to disturb the neurosphere, and then transfer 2 mL of SR+ medium without ROCK inhibitor per well.

Day 5 (Neuronal Induction—5% CO_2)

11. Remove 2 mL of the existing medium from the surface of the medium so as not to disturb the neurosphere.
12. Flush the neurospheres to resuspend them with a 1 mL pipette by pipetting up and down 3–4 times.
13. Add 2 mL of the neurosphere induction medium (Day 5).

Day 7

14. Remove 2 mL of the existing medium from the surface of the medium so as not to disturb the neurosphere.
15. Flush the neurospheres to resuspend them with a 1 mL pipette by pipetting up and down 3–4 times.
16. Add 3 mL of the neurosphere induction medium (Day 7).

Day 9

17. Remove 2 mL of the existing medium from the surface of the medium so as not to disturb the neurosphere.
18. Flush the neurospheres to resuspend them with a 1 mL pipette by pipetting up and down 3–4 times.
19. Add 2 mL of the neurosphere induction medium (Day 9).

Day 11

20. Remove 2 mL of the existing medium from the surface of the medium so as not to disturb the neurosphere.
21. Flush the neurospheres to resuspend them with a 1 mL pipette by pipetting up and down 3–4 times.
22. Add 2 mL of the neurosphere induction medium (Day 11).

Day 13—Neurosphederm—AdStep—5% CO_2, 37 °C incubation

23. Coat 6-well plates with Matrigel coating solution for 2 h at room temperature.
24. After coating, remove the coating solution, wash the plates with PBS, transfer 2 mL of NMM medium per well, and then incubate in the 5% CO_2, 37 °C incubator.
25. Retrieve culture plates containing the neurospheres from the incubator, and transfer all cells to a 15 mL tube.
26. Centrifuge at 400 × *g* for 5 min and then remove the supernatant.
27. Wash the cells with PBS (do not resuspend the cells).
28. Centrifuge at 400 × *g* for 5 min and then remove the supernatant.
29. Add 300 μL of NMM media to each 15 mL tube.
30. AdSTEP: using a serological pipette, mechanically break down the neurospheres by striking them (*see* **Note 7**).
31. Retrieve the Matrigel-coated plates containing NMM media from the incubator, and plate the resuspended cells with 2 mL of NMM media per well.

Day 14

32. Remove existing medium.
33. Wash each well with 1 mL of PBS.
34. Transfer 2 mL of fresh NMM medium per well.

Day 16

35. Remove existing medium.
36. Transfer 2 mL of fresh NMM medium per well.

Day 18

37. Remove existing medium.
38. Transfer 2 mL of fresh NMM medium per well.

Day 20 (replate neuronal progenitors)

39. Coat plates or flasks with the Matrigel coating solution for 2 h at room temperature, and then wash once with PBS.
40. Transfer NMM medium to the plates: use 500 μL per well for 12- or 24-well plates, and 1 mL per well for 6-well plates. Place the plates in the incubator.
41. Retrieve the plates containing neurosphederm from the incubator and wash the cells with PBS.
42. Transfer 500 μL or 1 mL of Gentle Cell Dissociation Reagent per well in a 12-/24-well plate or 6-well plate, respectively.
43. Incubate at 37 °C for 7 min.
44. Remove the Gentle Cell Dissociation Reagent, and transfer 500 μL or 1 mL of NMM medium per well in a 12-/24-well plate or 6-well plate, respectively.
45. Scrape cells using sterile cell scrapers.
46. Transfer 500 μL or 1 mL of NMM medium per well in a 12-/24-well plate or 6-well plate, respectively, and resuspend the cells.
47. Plate the resuspended cells in the Matrigel-coated plates (0.2 million/mL).

Day 21

48. Remove the existing medium.
49. Wash each well with PBS.
50. Transfer 500 μL or 1 mL of NMM medium per well in a 12-/24-well or 6-well plate, respectively.

Day 22

51. Refresh the medium every other day until mature neurons and astrocytes form.

3.7 hGNs Differentiation

Differentiate hESCs into neurons as described above in Subheading 3.6 and keep cells in NMM medium for 1–3 weeks until hGNs are observed and functional synapses are generated.

3.8 Exposing hGNs to AgNPs

1. Dilute 20 nm AgSCs or AgSPs supplied in water at a concentration of 1 mg/mL with NMM medium to desired concentrations.

2. Sonicate the diluted NPs twice for 1 min at 40 W, room temperature to prevent agglomeration.
3. Add the sonicated NPs to hGNs at 0, 0.1, 1.0, or 1.5 μg/mL and incubate at 37 °C for 72 h.

3.9 Determining the Change in Morphology and Cell Viability in NP-Exposed hGNs

1. Culture hGNs in 24-well or 96-well plates using NMM medium.
2. After exposing hGNs to the NPs, wash the cells once with PBS.
3. Using the neurite outgrowth cell kit, incubate the cells with 1× working stain solution containing the cell membrane stain and cell viability indicator and incubate at 25 °C for 20 min.
4. Remove the stain solution and wash the cells once with PBS.
5. Add 1× background suppression dye and capture the images from the 24-well plate using the EVOS fluorescence microscope at an excitation wavelength of 555 nm and an emission wavelength of 565 nm.
6. The 96-well plate was read with a microplate fluorescence reader at an excitation wavelength of 495 nm and emission wavelength of 515 nm.
7. All the data were normalized using the blank.

3.10 Determining Cytotoxicity in NP-Exposed hGNs

1. After exposing hGNs to NPs, transfer 50 μL of culture medium from each treatment condition into each well of a 96-well plate.
2. Using a LDH cytotoxicity assay kit, add 50 μL of reaction mixture per well. Mix the medium and reaction mixture well and then incubate at room temperature for 30 min.
3. Add 50 μL of stop solution per well and mix well.
4. Read the plate with a colorimetric microplate reader at the excitation wavelength of 490 nm. Perform the experiment in triplicates.

3.11 Determining the Induction of ROS Production in NP-Exposed hGNs

1. After exposing hGNs to NPs, incubate the cells with 5 μM CellROX Deep Red Reagent for 30 min at 37 °C with 5% CO_2.
2. Wash the cells three times with PBS.
3. Capture the red fluorescent images using the EVOS fluorescence microscope.

3.12 Determining ROS Induced by NPs Causes Ca^{2+} Influx

1. To examine the neurotoxicity of the NPs by measuring the amount of Ca^{2+} influx into the cells, after exposing hGNs to NPs at 0, 0.1, 1.0, or 5.0 μg/mL for 24, 72 or 144 h, wash the cells twice with NMM medium (low Ca^{2+} and Mg^{2+}) and then wash the cells once with PBS (without Ca^{2+} and Mg^{2+}).
2. Incubate the cells with a 5 μM Fluo-4 Ca^{2+} AM ester solution for 1 h at 37 °C with 5% CO_2, in the dark.

3. Remove the Fluo-4 solution and wash the cells twice with PBS.
4. Read the plate with a microplate fluorescence reader at an excitation wavelength of 485 nm and an emission wavelength of 520 nm.
5. Calculate the intraneuronal Ca^{2+} $[Ca^{2+}]_i$ using the equation: $[Ca^{2+}]_i = K_d \times (F - F_{min})/(F_{max} - F)$.
6. To determine whether the Ca^{2+} influx is caused by ROS, after exposing hGNs to NPs at 0, 0.1, 1.0, or 5.0 μg/mL for 72 h, cells were lyzed in RIPA buffer containing protease inhibitors and 5–10 μg of protein per treatment condition was resolved on a 10% SDS-polyacrylamide gel and then transferred onto a PVDF membrane.
7. The membrane was blocked in Odyssey blocking buffer in PBS for 1 h at 25 °C.
8. The membrane was incubated with anti-calmodulin, anti-iNOS, anti-nNOS, or anti-3-nitrotyrosine in blocking buffer overnight at 4 °C.
9. The membrane was washed three times with PBST, and then incubated with Odyssey infrared-conjugated secondary antibodies for 1 h at 25 °C.
10. The membrane was washed three times with PBST, and then scanned with the Odyssey infrared imager.

3.13 Assessing the Excitatory Synaptotoxicity and Neurotoxicity in NP-Exposed hGNs

1. After exposure of hGNs grown on Matrigel-coated coverslips to NPs, fix the cells with 4% paraformaldehyde on ice for 30 min.
2. Wash once with PBS, and permeabilize the cells with 0.1% Triton X-100 for 5 min at 25 °C.
3. Wash once with PBS, and block the cells with blocking buffer for 1 h at 25 °C.
4. Coincubate the cells either with anti-MAP2 (cytoskeletal protein in neurons particularly in dendrites) and anti-vGLUT1 (excitatory synaptic-associated protein) antibodies, or anti-vGLUT1 and anti-PSD95 (excitatory synaptic-associated protein) antibodies that are diluted in blocking buffer at 4 °C overnight.
5. Wash the cells three times with washing buffer for 10 min each, and then incubate with secondary antibodies diluted with washing buffer for 3 h at 25 °C.
6. Wash the cells three times with washing buffer for 10 min each, and mount the coverslips containing the cells onto glass slides with DAPI Fluoromount-G.
7. To further examine the effect of the NPs on the expression of vGLUT1 and PSD95, perform Western blotting on

NP-exposed hGNs as described in Subheading 3.12, but instead probe the membrane with anti-vGLUT1 or anti-PSD95 to demonstrate whether the NPs dose-dependently affect the expression of these two proteins.

3.14 Investigating the Effect of NPs on Neurodegeneration

1. Perform Western blotting on NPs-exposed hGNs as described in Subheading 3.12, but instead incubate the membrane with anti-NR2A, anti-NR2B (postsynaptic receptor proteins), anti-pGSK3$^{tyr216/279}$ (increase of which may lead to Tau phosphorylation), anti-pGSK3^{Ser9} (associated with neural apoptosis in many neurodegeneration disorder), anti-GSK3, and anti-pTau.
2. Perform immunocytochemistry as described in Subheading 3.13, but instead incubate the cells with anti-Tau46 or coincubate with anti-MAP2 and anti-Tau46 (stabilizes microtubules particularly in axons).

4 Notes

1. Making 40 mL aliquots in 50 mL tubes avoids the tubes bursting open after freezing.
2. Thaw Matrigel on ice and store all flasks and plates to be coated and pipettes to be used for coating at 4 °C overnight to avoid gel formation.
3. When preparing the various media for neuronal differentiation, always add the supplements fresh and dilute the collagenase right before use. For N2 medium, warm up and add all the other supplements first, and then take from the fridge and add insulin. Put the insulin immediately back into the fridge afterwards as it is heat-sensitive.
4. Always make small volume of ammonium persulfate solution because its activity starts decreasing after 1 month of storage at 4 °C.
5. Matrigel-coated plates or flasks can be kept at 4 C for 7–10 days.
6. When thawing cryopreserved stem cells, after transferring the 1 mL of thawed cells to a 15 mL tube, add the first mL of the 9 mL of mTeSR medium dropwise to avoid sudden shock to the cells.
7. When performing AdSTEP, use a 5 mL serological pipette and strike the neurospheres suspension 100 times to break them down.

References

1. Abbondanzo SJ, Gadi I, Stewart CL (1993) Derivation of embryonic stem cells. Methods Enzymol 225:803–823
2. Takahashi K, Yamanaka S (2006) Induction of pluripotent stem cells from mouse embryonic and adult fibroblast cultures by defined factors. Cell 126(4):663–676
3. Zhang SC, Wernig M, Duncan ID, Brüstle O, Thomson JA (2001) In vitro differentiation of transplantable neural precursors from human embryonic stem cells. Nat Biotechnol 19 (12):1129–1133
4. Hattori N (2014) Cerebral organoids model human brain development and microcephaly. Nature 501(7467):373–379
5. van dan Ameele J, Tiberi L, Vanderhaeghen P, Espuny-Camcho I (2014) Thinking out of the dish: what to learn about cortical development using pluripotent stem cells. Trends Neurosci 37 (6):334–342
6. Shi Y, Kirwan P, Livesey FJ (2012) Directed differentiation of human pluripotent stem cells to cerebral cortex neurons and neural networks. Nat Protoc 7(10):1836–1846
7. Begum AN, Guoynes C, Cho J, Hao J, Lutfy K, Hong Y (2015) Rapid generation of sub-type, region-specific neurons and neural networks from human pluripotent stem cell-derived neurospheres. Stem Cell Res 15(3):731–741
8. Begum AN, Aguilar JS, Elias L, Hong Y (2016) Silver nanoparticles exhibit coating and dose-dependent neurotoxicity in glutamatergic neurons derived from human embryonic stem cells. Neurotoxicology 57:45–53

Chapter 5

Methods for Evaluation of Ovarian Granulosa Cells with Exposure to Nanoparticles

Jin Liu and Wenchang Zhang

Abstract

Increasing evidence demonstrates that a substantial number of chemicals including nanoparticles have potential toxic effects on human and wildlife reproductive health. Ovarian granulosa cells (GCs), the functional unit of the ovary, play a pivotal role in the regulation of ovarian reproductive health in females. They are considered to be the main target by the chemicals at all stages of their development. It has been reported that nanoparticles induced toxicity of GCs by interfering with cell cycle. Some basic methods for evaluation of GCs with exposure to nanoparticles are described in this chapter including isolation of GCs, determination of apoptosis by immunofluorescence, and measurement of progesterone level by ELISA.

Key words Ovarian granulosa cells, In vitro culture, Immunofluorescence, ELISA, Nanoparticles

1 Introduction

The ovary is a central to female reproductive function, and ovarian follicles are the functional and morphological units which are composed of oocytes and multiple surrounding somatic cells (theca and granulosa cells) [1, 2]. The granulosa cells produce hormones necessary for the regulation of the reproductive system, and support the maintenance, growth, and development of oocyte [3]. In vitro culture of rat ovarian granulosa cells has been widely used in endocrine research [4], especially in evaluation and prediction of potential reproductive toxicants [5, 6].

Along with the increasing application of nanoparticles (NPs) in various products, environmental exposure to NPs has raised considerable health concerns [7, 8]. The toxic effects of NPs have different mechanisms. It has been reported that calcium phosphate NPs may accumulate in human ovarian granulosa cells, resulting in increasing cell apoptosis, although exposure to calcium phosphate NPs at concentrations of 10–100 μM did not significantly change either the progesterone or estradiol levels in culture medium [9]. Studies also showed that NPs could interfere with the pathways

Qunwei Zhang (ed.), *Nanotoxicity: Methods and Protocols*, Methods in Molecular Biology, vol. 1894,
https://doi.org/10.1007/978-1-4939-8916-4_5,

of proliferation and apoptosis of porcine ovarian granulosa cells through hormonal and intracellular peptides such as cyclin B1 and caspase-3 [10]. Exposure of human granulosa cells KGN and granulosa cells from patients undergoing in vitro fertilization to different concentrations of carbon black nanoparticles (CB NPs) (1–100 μg/mL) caused inhibition of aromatase expression and estradiol secretion through ERK1/2 pathway [11]. Thus, it is interesting to use GCs to evaluate and predict the reproductive toxicity of NPs.

In this chapter, several methods are described to evaluate the functional and cellular states of GCs after exposure to NPs, including immunofluorescence to determine the apoptosis of GCs, as well as ELISA to determine the progesterone level of GCs due to NPs exposure.

2 Materials

Perform all media preparation, tissue dissection, and culture work in a lamina flow hood to ensure sterility. Diligently follow all waste disposal regulations when disposing of waste materials. All animal use in this protocol was reviewed and approved by the Fujian Medical University Institutional Animal Care and Use Committee.

2.1 Isolation of Rat Ovarian GCs and Assessment of Cell Maturity

1. 75% ethanol sprayer.
2. Sterile forceps and two sets of scissors.
3. Laminar flow cell culture hood.
4. Sterile 35 mm and 60 mm cell culture dishes.
5. Dissection microscope with heated stage (37 °C).
6. Cell culture incubator (37 °C/5% CO_2).
7. Complete rat ovarian GCs dissection or culture medium (*see* Subheading 2.2).
8. 0.22 μM filtration system.
9. Sterile 1 mL syringe and insulin needle.
10. Sterile 1000 μL and 200 μL pipette tips.
11. 15 mL sterile conical centrifuge tubes.
12. Micro centrifuge (Eppendorf 5415D).

2.2 Media, Buffers and Solutions

1. Dissection medium: Add 0.5 mL of 1% penicillin–streptomycin in 50 mL DMEM/F12 medium (*see* **Note 1**). Filter to sterilize through a 0.22 μm filtration system (*see* **Note 2**).
2. Culture medium: Add 5 mL of 10% FBS and 0.5 mL of 1% penicillin-streptomycin in 45 mL DMEM/F12 medium and filter to sterilize through a 0.22 μm filtration system (*see* **Note 3**).

2.3 Identification of GCs with Immunohistochemistry

1. 4% paraformaldehyde: add 4 g paraformaldehyde to 100 mL 1× PBS, and place in the thermostat water bath for overnight at 65 °C (*see* **Note 4**).
2. Thermostat water bath.
3. Polink-2 plus® polymer HRP detection for rabbit primary antibody kit: including Reagent 1 polymer helper and Reagent 2 poly HRP anti-rabbit IgG.
4. Anti-FSHR rabbit polyclonal antibody.
5. Deionized water.
6. 3% hydrogen peroxide (H_2O_2): Mix 30 mL of 10% H_2O_2 solution with 70 mL deionized water.
7. Coverslips.
8. Incubation box.
9. 1× PBS, pH 7.2–7.4: Add one bag of phosphate buffered saline powder (0.01 mol/L, pH 7.2–7.4) in 2 L distilled water. Autoclave and store at room temperature.
10. 4 °C refrigerator.
11. Light microscope.
12. Hematoxylin, different concentrations of ethanol and xylene for staining.
13. Neutral resin.

2.4 Determination of Apoptosis of Ovarian GCs by Immunofluorescence Staining

1. Hoechst Staining Kit: Including fixative, Hoechst 33258, and antifade medium (Beyotime).
2. Sterile 1.5 mL Eppendorf tubes.
3. Sterile 60 mm cell culture dish.
4. 1× PBS, pH 7.2–7.4: *see* Subheading 2.3, **item 9**.
5. Hemocytometer with coverslip.
6. Light microscope.
7. Fluorescent microscope.
8. Pipettes and sterile pipette tips.

2.5 Determination of the Progesterone Level in Ovarian GCs Culture Media Using ELISA

1. Progesterone ELISA Kit (Elabscience).
2. Pipette and sterile pipette tips.
3. 1× PBS, pH 7.2–7.4: *see* Subheading 2.3, **item 9**.
4. Sterile 1.5 mL Eppendorf tubes.
5. High speed freezing centrifuge.
6. 37 °C incubator.
7. Deionized or distilled water.
8. Absorbent paper.
9. Promega Multimode Microplate reader with 450 nm wavelength filter.

3 Methods

Treat cells or animal tissues with NPs according to experimental design (unless indicated otherwise). Prepare tissues and/or cells through standard exposure procedures as required [12, 13].

3.1 Collection of Ovary

1. Place 1 mL of dissection medium into each sterile 35 mm culture dish. Prewarm it in an incubator.
2. For in vitro nanoparticle exposure, each female SD rat is injected with 20 IU Pregnant Mare Serum Gonadotropin (PMSG) (*see* **Note 5**). After 48 h, rat is sacrificed. For in vivo nanoparticle exposure, female SD rat is directly sacrificed without PMSG (*see* **Note 6**).
3. Grasp the rat back skin using a pair of fine dissection forceps and make a large incision in the skin and body wall. Pull open the incision so that the entire back is exposed.
4. Push the muscle off the way using watchmaker forceps. The ovary is located just beside the kidney at the top of the uterus and appears as a cloud-like structure under the eyes.
5. Grasp the ovary gently with watchmaker forceps, and use scissors to sever its attachment to the uterus. Transfer the pair of ovaries into culture dishes containing prewarmed dissection medium.

3.2 Isolation of Ovarian GCs

1. Dissect ovaries under a dissection microscope on a heated stage (37 °C) (*see* **Note** 7). Use insulin needles to trim away the bursal sac and any excess tissues including the Fallopian tube, until only the ovary remains.
2. Transfer each ovary into a 60 mm cell culture dish. Puncture follicles under dissection microscope (*see* **Note 8**), then transfer the cells to a 15 mL conical tube using a 1000 μL pipette tip. And pellet the cells by centrifugation at 1000 × *g* for 5 min at 4 °C.
3. Discard the supernatant. Resuspend the cells with 2 mL culture medium.

3.3 Culture of Ovarian GCs

1. Transfer the cells by a 1000 μL pipette tip into a 60 mm culture dish with 2 mL culture medium. Incubate in an incubator at 37 °C with 5% CO_2.
2. After 24 h, change the medium and remove unattached cells.
3. On day 2 of culture, add nanoparticles to treat the cells.
4. Change the medium every day. Maintain cultures for up to 72 h.
5. Capture images of GCs in culture (Fig. 1).

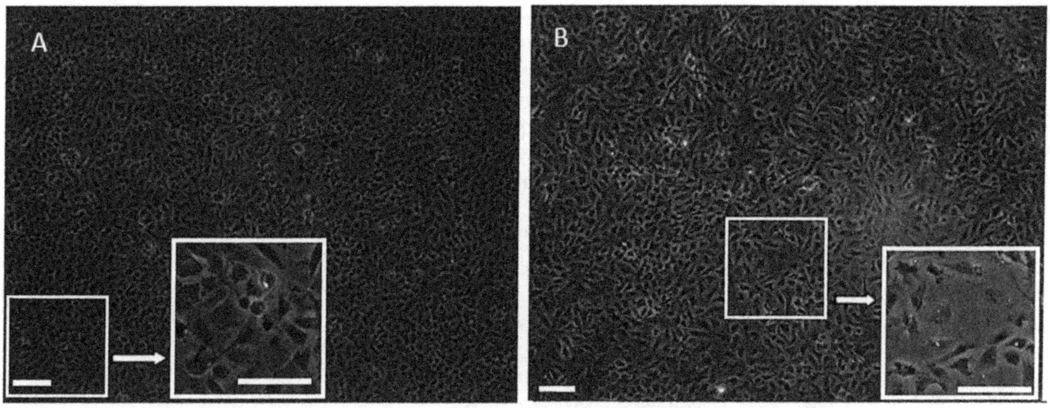

Fig. 1 Images of rat ovarian granulosa cells (GCs). (**a**) GCs in the control group which were cultured in vitro for 72 h. (**b**) GCs 48 h after nanoparticle exposure, showing decreased cell numbers in the culture. Bars represent 100 μm in (**a**) and (**b**) and 200 μm in insets of (**a**) and (**b**)

3.4 Identification GCs with Follicle-Stimulating Hormone Receptor (FSHR) Immuno-histochemistry

1. Culture GCs on coverslips. When it is confluent, fix cells with 4% paraformaldehyde solution (*see* **Note 9**).
2. Wash GCs with 1× PBS twice, 5 min each time.
3. Incubate cells with 3% H_2O_2 in deionized water for 10 min to block the endogenous peroxidase.
4. Wash with 1× PBS twice, 5 min each time.
5. Add anti-FSHR rabbit polyclonal antibody (1:100) and incubate overnight at 4 °C (*see* **Note 10**).
6. Wash GCs with 1× PBS twice, 5 min each time.
7. Add Reagent 1 and incubate the cells at room temperature for 20 min.
8. Wash with 1× PBS twice, 5 min each time.
9. Add Reagent 2 and incubate the cells at room temperature for 20 min.
10. Wash the cells with 1× PBS twice, 5 min each time.
11. Apply DAB solvent (*see* **Note 11**).
12. Wash the cells thoroughly with running water (*see* **Note 12**) and stain with hematoxylin for 1 min.
13. Wash the cells with 1× PBS for 5 min.
14. Dehydrate the cells with a series of ethanol solutions (70%, 80%, 90%, 95%, 100% and 100%, 3 min each) and xylene twice, 5 min each. Mount in neutral resin.
15. Capture the images.

3.5 Determination of the Apoptosis of GCs Using Immunofluorescence Staining

3.5.1 Determination of Cell Concentration

1. Transfer the cells by a 1000 μL pipette tip into a 1.5 mL tube and add mL culture medium to make 1 mL cell suspension (*see* **Note 13**).
2. Place the coverslip over the hemocytometer counting chamber, and load 10 μL of cell suspension to the hemocytometer chamber. Allow the cell suspension to be drawn into the chamber by capillary action (*see* **Note 14**).
3. Place the chamber on the microscope stage.
4. There are nine 1 × 1 mm squares on the hemocytometer. Each square is divided into smaller squares. One 1 × 1 mm square represents a volume of 0.1 mm^3 or 10^{-4} mL. Using the 10× objective, count the number of cells in four corner 1 × 1 mm squares.
5. To calculate the concentration of the cells, first calculate the average of four 1 × 1 mm areas, then apply this formula: $c = n/v$ (*see* **Note 15**).
6. Add culture medium to adjust the cell concentration to 1×10^6 cells/mL.

3.5.2 Immunofluorescence Staining of Apoptosis of GCs

1. Discard the medium and add 0.5 mL fixative. Incubate for 10 min.
2. Discard the fixative and wash the cells with 1× PBS twice, 5 min each time.
3. Add 0.5 mL Hoechst 33258 and incubate at room temperature for 5 min.
4. Discard the Hoechst solution and wash with 1× PBS twice, 5 min each time.
5. Add antifade to the cells.
6. Capture the images after 15 min.
7. Analyze images with ImageJ software (Fig. 2).

3.6 Determine the Progesterone Level in the Culture Media of GCs Using ELISA

1. After culture, transfer all the culture medium into a 1.5 mL tube (*see* **Note 16**).
2. Centrifuge at 1000 × *g* for 20 min at 4 °C.
3. Transfer the supernatant to a new tube (*see* **Note 17**). The samples then can be used to determine the progesterone level by using a kit (*see* **Note 18**).
4. Take out precoated plates. Set a blank well in which 100 μL of medium is added. Add 50 μL per well of corresponding standard into standard wells. Add 50 μL per well of sample to the sample wells. Each standard or sample is duplicated.
5. Cover the plate with the sealer provided and incubate the plate at 37 °C for 1 h.
6. Discard the content in the well.

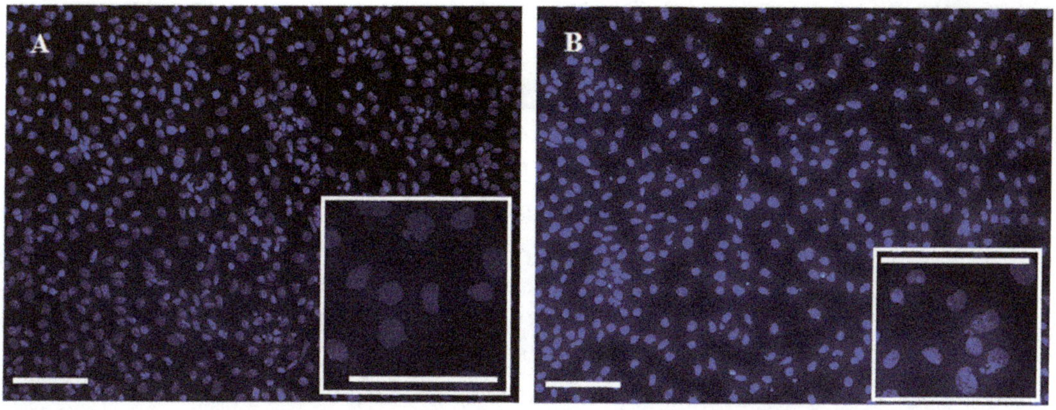

Fig. 2 Images from rat ovarian granulosa cells, showing cell apoptosis. (**a**) Rat ovarian granulosa cells in the control group exhibited a uniform light blue. (**b**) After exposure to nanoparticles, the cell nuclei showed strong blue fluorescence, indicating a high degree of shrinkage of the nuclei, or the nuclei were lobulated. Bars represent 200 μm in (**a**) and (**b**), and 400 μm in insets of (**a**) and (**b**)

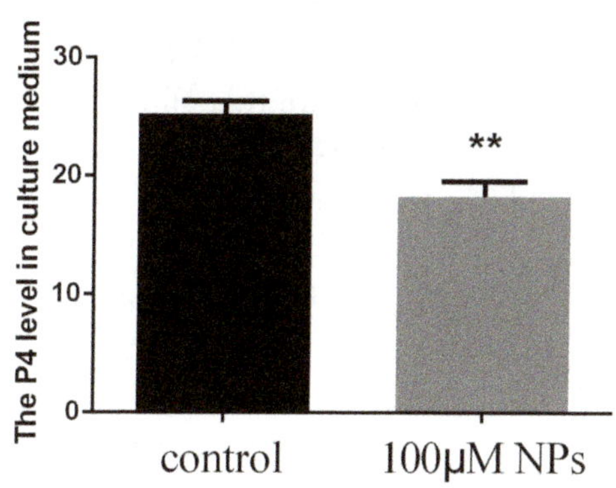

Fig. 3 Effects of nanoparticles on progesterone (P4) expression in rat ovarian granulosa cells in vitro. GCs were cultured as described in the text and P4 in culture medium of GCs was determined by ELASA. Data represent mean ± SD. $^{**}p < 0.01$ as compared with the control group

7. Add 100 μL of HRP-labeled progesterone antigen to each well, then add 50 μL anti-progesteron antibody to each well. Cover the plate with the sealer provided. Incubate at 37 °C for 1 h.
8. Discard the content in the well and add 350 μL Wash Buffer to each well to wash.
9. Repeat **step 8** three times.
10. Add 50 μL of substrate solution A and 50 μL of substrate solution B to each well. Mix and incubate at 37 °C for 15 min.
11. Add 50 μL of stop solution to each well.
12. Determine the absorbance at 450 nm by using a microplate reader.
13. Record and analyze the results (Fig. 3).

4 Notes

1. The specific total volume of transfer solution and culture medium are determined by samples, and the proportion of each reagent keeps same.
2. Add 2 mL of transfer solution to each 35 mm culture dish as a transfer dish.
3. If 35 mm culture dish is used to culture the cells, 2 mL culture medium will be added. If 60 mm culture dish is used 4 mL culture medium should be used.
4. The 4% paraformaldehyde may keep up to 2 weeks.
5. Ensure that the PMSG is fresh.
6. For in vivo experiment, make sure that the amount of nanoparticles is the only independent variable in the treated groups, so do not add another variable (for example PMSG) to rats.
7. All cell culture steps (e.g., isolation of GCs) should be done on the heated stage.
8. Ensure that all follicles are punctured by observing under the dissection microscope.
9. The time for fixation could be 10–20 min based on the number of cells, but do not exceed 30 min.
10. Cells can be incubated with primary antibody at room temperature for 2 h.
11. The reaction time should be controlled by observing under light microscope. When color change is observed, wash it in running water as soon as possible.
12. The washing time should be controlled by observing under light microscope. Make sure that the color is not too light or too dark. Usually, wash 3 times with 3–5 min each time.
13. Make sure that all the cells in the tube are suspended.
14. Care should be taken not to overfill or underfill the chamber.
15. $C =$ cell concentration in cells/mL; $n =$ average number of cells/mm^2 area; $v =$ volume (10^{-4} mL).
16. Ensure that the number of cells in each dish is same and the culture time is also the same.
17. In this step, only supernatant is saved for later analysis. Care should be taken not to disturb the cell debris.
18. Before experiment, pretest needs to be done to make sure that the concentrations of progesterone level in experimental samples will be within the optimum range (1–30 ng/mL). In this study, we did a pretest and found that the concentration of progesterone level in some samples was beyond the optimum range. Therefore, we diluted samples four times with 1× PBS.

Acknowledgments

This work was supported by NSFC grant (no. 81673212, 81373027, 30972514) and Fujian Provincial Key Laboratory of Environmental Factors and Cancer.

References

1. Lopes F, Smith R, Anderson RA, Spears N (2014) Docetaxel induces moderate ovarian toxicity in mice, primarily affecting granulosa cells of early growing follicles. Mol Hum Reprod 20:9489–9459
2. Holesh JE, Lord M (2017) Physiology, ovulation. StatPearls [Internet]. StatPearls Publishing, Treasure Island, FL. PMID: 28723025
3. Kranc W, Brązert M, Ożegowska K, Nawrocki MJ, Budna J, Celichowski P, Dyszkiewicz-Konwińska M, Jankowski M, Jeseta M, Pawelczyk L, Bruska M, Nowicki M, Zabel M, Kempisty B (2017) Expression profile of genes regulating steroid biosynthesis and metabolism in human ovarian granulosa cells—a primary culture approach. Int J Mol Sci 18: E2673
4. Gottschall PE1, Katsuura G, Arimura A (1989) Interleukin-1 suppresses follicle-stimulating hormone-induced estradiol secretion from cultured ovarian granulosa cells. J Reprod Immunol 15:281–290
5. Sun Y, Lin Y, Li H, Liu J, Sheng X, Zhang W (2012) 2,5-Hexanedione induces human ovarian granulosa cell apoptosis through BCL-2, BAX, and CASPASE-3 signaling pathways. Arch Toxicol 86:205–215
6. Miglietta S, Belli M, Bianchi S, Cecconi S, Di Nisio V, Familiari G, Macchiarelli G (2017) The pesticide Lindane induces dose-dependent damage to granulosa cells in an in vitro culture. Reprod Biol 17:349–356
7. Palmerini MG, Zhurabekova G, Balmagambetova A, Nottola SA, Nel A, Xia T, Mädler L, Li N (2006) Toxic potential of materials at the nanolevel. Science 311:622–627
8. Nohynek GJ, Dufour EK (2012) Nano-sized cosmetic formulations or solid nanoparticles in sunscreens: a risk to human health? Arch Toxicol 86:1063–1075
9. Liu X, Qin D, Cui Y, Chen L, Li H, Chen Z, Gao L, Li Y, Liu J (2010) The effect of calcium phosphate nanoparticles on hormone production and apoptosis in human granulosa cells. Reprod Biol Endocrinol 8:32
10. Kolesarova A, Capcarova M, Sirotkin AV, Medvedova M, Kovacik J (2011) In vitro assessment of silver effect on porcine ovarian granulosa cells. J Trace Elem Med Biol 25:166–170
11. Simon V, Avet C, Grange-Messent V, Wargnier R, Denoyelle C, Pierre A, Dairou J, Dupret JM, Cohen-Tannoudji J (2017) Carbon black nanoparticles inhibit aromatase expression and estradiol secretion in human granulosa cells through the ERK1/2 pathway. Endocrinology 158:3200–3211
12. Wang W, Chen J, Luo L, Li Y, Liu J, Zhang W (2018) Effect of cadmium on KITL pre-mRNA alternative splicing in murine ovarian granulosa cells and its associated regulation by miRNAs. J Appl Toxicol 38:227–239
13. Li H, Zhang C, Ni F, Guo S, Wang W, Liu J, Lu X, Huang H, Zhang W (2015) Gestational N-hexane inhalation alters the expression of genes related to ovarian hormone production and DNA methylation states in adult female F1 rat offspring. Toxicol Lett 239:141–151

Chapter 6

In Vitro Approaches for Assessing the Genotoxicity of Nanomaterials

Maria Dusinska, Espen Mariussen, Elise Rundén-Pran, Alexandra Misci Hudecova, Elisabeth Elje, Alena Kazimirova, Naouale El Yamani, Nils Dommershausen, Julian Tharmann, Dagmar Fieblinger, Frank Herzberg, Andreas Luch, and Andrea Haase

Abstract

Genotoxicity is associated with serious health effects and includes different types of DNA lesions, gene mutations, structural chromosome aberrations involving breakage and/or rearrangements of chromosomes (referred to as clastogenicity) and numerical chromosome aberrations (referred to as aneuploidy). Assessing the potential genotoxic properties of chemicals, including nanomaterials (NMs), is a key element in regulatory safety assessment. State-of-the-art genotoxicity testing includes a battery of assays covering gene mutations, structural and numerical chromosome aberrations. Typically various in vitro assays are performed in the first tier. It is not very likely that NMs may induce as yet unknown types of genotoxic damage beyond what is already known for chemicals. Thus, principles of genotoxicity testing as established for chemicals should be applicable to NMs as well. However, established test guidelines (i.e., OECD TG) may require adaptations for NM testing, as currently under discussion at the OECD. This chapter gives an overview of genotoxicity testing of NMs in vitro based on experiences from various research projects. We recommend a combination of a mammalian gene mutation assay (at either Tk or HPRT locus), the in vitro comet assay, and the cytokinesis-block micronucleus assay, which are discussed in detail here. In addition we also include the Cell Transformation Assay (CTA) as a promising novel test for predicting NM-induced cell transformation in vitro.

Key words Genotoxicity, Nanomaterials, Mammalian gene mutation assay, Comet assay, Micronucleus assay, Cell transformation assay, Cell lines, Human 3D tissue models

1 Introduction

Genotoxicity is a general term that refers to the alteration of the genetic information of a cell induced by a chemical. It includes different endpoints, that is, alteration of the structure, information content, or segregation of DNA, including those, which cause DNA damage by interfering with normal replication processes, or which in a nonphysiological manner (temporarily) alter its

Qunwei Zhang (ed.), *Nanotoxicity: Methods and Protocols*, Methods in Molecular Biology, vol. 1894,
https://doi.org/10.1007/978-1-4939-8916-4_6, © Springer Science+Business Media, LLC, part of Springer Nature 2019

replication. This covers different types of DNA lesions such as chromosome breakage and/or rearrangements (referred to as clastogenicity), numerical chromosome aberrations (referred to as aneuploidy) as well as gene mutations. Genotoxicity in germ cells may lead to heritable damage to the offspring while genotoxicity in somatic cells can induce carcinogenesis. In addition, various chronic diseases are associated with accumulation of DNA damage. Accordingly, genotoxicity is associated with serious health effects. It can become manifest already at very low exposure levels. Therefore, assessing the potential genotoxic properties of chemicals, including nanomaterials (NMs), is a key element in regulatory safety assessment [1]. It is required in the overarching chemicals regulations REACH and CLP, as well as in sector-specific regulations such as those for cosmetics, food, biocides, pesticides, or drugs. State-of-the-art genotoxicity testing typically includes a battery of assays covering gene mutations, structural and numerical chromosome aberrations. First tier testing usually is performed using various in vitro assays. If a chemical is without any effect in vitro it might be classified as nongenotoxic in chemicals legislations (e.g., REACH, CLP, Cosmetics Directive), while others (i.e., legislations for pharmaceuticals or veterinary drugs) always require an in vivo follow-up. A positive outcome in vitro may call for confirmation by appropriate in vivo testing. One of the biggest current challenges for in vitro genotoxicity testing is the high rate of irrelevant positive results, which cause a high number of in vivo follow-ups and can (in some cases) also lead to the rejection of substances wrongly incriminated as genotoxic as in the Cosmetics Directive in vivo assays are prohibited [2]. The high rate of irrelevant positives was addressed in an ECVAM workshop in April 2006 [3], which also included a discussion on strategies to improve in vitro genotoxicity testing. Overall, in vitro genotoxicity assays are of high importance in regulatory safety assessment for chemicals and for NMs.

NMs often display novel and enhanced properties compared to conventional chemicals, which make them interesting for many different applications but at the same time also cause concerns about their safety. Nanotechnology is regarded as a key enabling technology in Europe but also elsewhere. Thus, reliable methods to assess the safety of NMs are urgently needed. Clearly genotoxicity of NMs is one of the most important regulatory relevant endpoints to address. It is not very likely that NMs may induce as yet unknown types of genotoxic damage beyond what is already known for chemicals (i.e., gene mutations, structural or numerical chromosome aberrations). Thus, it is widely accepted that the principles of genotoxicity testing as established for chemicals are applicable to NMs as well [4, 5]. Regulatory relevant genotoxicity testing should always be performed according to the OECD test guidelines (OECD TGs). However, the focus of OECD TGs is on conventional chemicals [6], and their suitability for NM testing is now under discussion at the OECD. Genotoxicity testing of NMs has been discussed at an OECD WPMN workshop in 2013 [7]. The major conclusions were that most assays are in general suitable for NM testing (with the exception of the Ames test as discussed below) but NMs deserve special attention in some of the experimental details. In particular, comprehensive physico–chemical characterization and test item preparation (i.e., NM dispersion) are crucial for the test outcome. Furthermore, the test protocols have to be adapted to meet the special requirements of NM testing. To that end, the EU initiated a joint action project NanoGenoTox aiming to develop harmonized protocols for NM genotoxicity testing. Results from both activities (i.e., OECD and EU NanoGenoTox) were considered in the ECHA Guidance on information requirements and chemical safety assessment [8].

NMs that are taken up by mammalian cells can get into direct contact with the genetic material leading to direct physical or chemical damage or they can act indirectly (e.g., via inducing oxidative stress) [9–12]. As for chemicals, before undertaking any toxicological test it is crucial to comprehensively describe the physico-chemical properties of the test item and its behavior in the test environment, which requires taking into account additional parameters in the case of NMs. Moreover, some physico–chemical properties of a NM will change as soon as the material comes into contact with a biological environment. For instance, proteins will adsorb on its surface, which may cause alterations in size, surface charge and surface reactivity. A NM can also dissolve in biological fluids or may agglomerate. Properties that are dependent on the respective environment are referred to as "extrinsic" properties in contrast to invariable "intrinsic" properties of the material. For toxicological studies it is recommended to follow a stepwise approach for NM characterization [13] with phase one covering the powder state including an assessment of the chemical composition, size, size distribution, surface area, and morphology. Phase two covers characterization of the dispersion, typically in water, including tests on agglomeration or aggregation, as well as formation of reactive species. Phase three then includes a characterization of the material in the relevant biological fluid, also taking into account changes over time. Thus, when characterizing a NM in a biological fluid for a toxicological assay it is recommended to consider different time points, that is, before, during, and after the toxicological assay. Relevant properties for genotoxicity are in particular the particle size, the shape and the presence of contaminating known mutagens (i.e., "impurities"). One of the most important mechanisms for genotoxicity of NMs is the enhanced production of reactive oxygen species (ROS) [9, 11]. In fact, oxidative stress has often been described as a key mechanism underlying the ability of NMs to cause DNA damage [11]. Genotoxicity can also depend on surface properties, the presence of transition metals, intracellular iron mobilization, or lipid peroxidation processes. In addition, assessing the cellular uptake should be an integral part of genotoxicity testing for NMs. In order to obtain meaningful results, cytotoxicity must always be assessed alongside the genotoxicity assays. Cytotoxic effects of chemicals can be determined by different methods, based on (1) membrane integrity (trypan blue exclusion, neutral red uptake, lactate dehydrogenase (LDH) assay), (2) metabolic competence (resazurin or MTT assay), or (3) relative cell growth (reflecting cell death together with inhibition of cell proliferation). Within this chapter we therefore include a short description of three assays to determine cytotoxicity, AlamarBlue, colony forming efficiency (CFE) and ATP assay.

The **AlamarBlue® (AB) assay** is based on a nontoxic dye, resazurin, that yields colorimetric change and a fluorescent signal in response to metabolic activity [14]. It is used for analysis of cell viability and cell proliferation. Resazurin (oxidized form) is taken up by the cells and converted to resorufin (reduced form) due to the reducing environment of the cytosol of the cells. Resorufin produces bright red fluorescence, but can also be measured spectrophotometrically. The AB assay is a convenient and fast method to assess cell viability and it is often used in combination with other methods such as the comet assay. However, care must be taken as NMs can interfere with the spectrophotometric readout [15]. Therefore it is very important to check for possible interferences beforehand.

The **Colony Forming Efficiency (CFE) assay** is a label-free method for assessment of basal cytotoxicity by measuring the ability of surviving cells to form colonies. Cell survival is expressed as the number of colonies formed from surviving cells being exposed to a chemical relative to the number of colonies observed for unexposed control cells. Thus, the CFE assay can detect cytotoxic effects (reduction of the number of colonies formed) and cytostatic effects (reduction in colony size). Adherent mammalian cells are exposed at low density. Being noncolorimetric and nonfluorescent, CFE avoids possible interferences of NMs with toxicity assessments. The CFE assay protocol has been optimized and standardized for NMs testing by the JRC Nanobiosciences Unit and validated in an interlaboratory comparison study [16]. This assay has already been used with different in vitro systems to assess the cytotoxicity of a wide range of NMs such as gold NMs [17], silver NMs [18, 19], titanium oxide NMs [19–21], zinc oxide NMs [19, 20], silica NMs [22], multiwalled carbon nanotubes [23], and cerium oxide NMs [19].

The **ATP cell viability assay** is an Adenosine Triphosphate (ATP) monitoring system based on a readout using firefly (*Photinus pyralis*) luciferase. Luciferases are enzymes that under consumption of ATP catalyze the reaction of luciferin with oxygen to form high-energy, unstable dioxetanes or dioxetanones (oxidation) resulting into bioluminescence. This assay can be used as an early marker for effects of chemicals or NMs on cell viability. The major advantage of this assay is the high sensitivity. Here we include it as a suitable assay to evaluate cytotoxicity in human 3D cell models. It has been applied already to assess cytotoxicity of various different NMs (including SiO_2, TiO_2, nanosilver) in human 3D bronchial models in parallel to the assessment of the genotoxicity [24]. It also has been evaluated for applicability in various different cell lines to assess cytotoxicity of NMs [25].

Genotoxicity testing must cover all the important endpoints including gene mutations as well as structural or numerical DNA aberrations. The assessment of aneuploidy is particularly relevant in case of fiber-like NMs as they may interfere with the mitotic spindle formation [26]. Mutagenicity of chemicals in tier 1 is usually tested in bacteria using the "Ames test" according to the OECD TG 471 [27, 28]. The Ames test is based on induction of reverse-mutations in a defective histidine synthetase gene. However, this assay is not suitable for investigating NMs as bacteria do not efficiently take up NMs [28]. However, there are several mammalian mutation assays that can be used instead and that are better suited for NMs. They are based on mutations in specific genes—most commonly *HPRT* (hypoxanthine phosphoribosyltransferase) or *Tk* (thymidine kinase) [29–32]. For chemicals, procedures for mammalian gene mutation assays are described in OECD TG 476 [33] and OECD TG 490 [34]. Here we describe the mouse lymphoma assay (based on the *Tk* gene) for NMs that detects both point mutations as well as large deletions [35, 36].

The **mouse lymphoma assay (MLA)**, which is included in the OECD TG 490, uses the *Tk* gene. It is the most widely used of the various in vitro mammalian cell gene-mutation assays [35, 36]. This assay detects a wide spectrum of genetic damage, including gene and chromosomal mutations, as well as epigenetic silencing of the functional *Tk* allele due to promoter hypermethylation [37]. Here we describe a fluctuation assay using 96-well plates and trifluorothymidine (TFT) as the selective agent, which is based on Clements et al. [38]. Two distinct types of mutant colonies can be recognized, large and small ones. Large colonies grow at a normal rate and represent events within the gene (base-pair substitutions or small deletions) whilst small colonies represent large deletions and changes involving chromosome 11b (suggesting clastogenic activity).

The **comet assay** (single cell gel electrophoresis) is a simple method widely used to detect DNA breaks in vitro as well as in vivo. It is the most common test for assessing genotoxicity of NMs [11, 19, 24, 39, 40]. It detects DNA strand breaks and alkali-labile sites. When using modified versions based on incubating nucleoids (i.e., DNA attached to the nuclear matrix obtained after cell lysis and stripping of histones) with lesion-specific endonucleases, such as endonuclease III or formamidopyrimidine DNA glycosylase (Fpg) that recognize oxidized pyrimidines and purines respectively, this test can also detect damaged DNA bases [19, 30, 31, 41]. Recently, OECD released a TG for in vivo comet assay [42]. However, there is none for in vitro comet assay. Cosmetics Europe started an initiative to validate the comet assay in human 3D models for chemicals [43, 44]. Here we describe the comet assay for NMs in cell lines including modified versions (i.e., Fpg comet). For the comet assay the cells are embedded in agarose on a microscope slide and lysed in detergent solution with high concentration of salt (NaCl). The DNA of the cells remains as series of loops attached to the nuclear matrix. These loops are supercoiled as (although the histones have been removed) the nucleosome winding of the DNA remains. When subjected to an electrophoretic field, DNA tends to move towards the anode due to its negative charge. If a single break is present in the loop, the supercoiling is relaxed and the loop is free to extend under the electrophoretic field and moves toward the anode. Accordingly, after staining of the DNA, images resembling comets can be observed in microscopic evaluation. The tail consists of loops of DNA that have moved out from the head, which represents the former nucleus. The amount of DNA in the tail reflects the number of relaxed loops, reflecting the number of breaks in the DNA. Within a certain range there is a near-linear relationship between the proportion of DNA in the tail and the number of breaks. The standard comet assay measures single- and double-strand breaks. Modified versions using lesion-specific enzymes can, in addition, detect specific DNA lesions, such as oxidized purines (with formamidopyrimidine DNA glycosylase, Fpg, or the mammalian counterpart, 8-oxoguanine DNA glycosylase, OGG1) or oxidized pyrimidines (with endonuclease III, Endo III). The incubation with the enzyme takes place after lysis and removes the damaged base, leaving an apurinic/apyrimidinic (AP) site that is converted into a break by the AP lyase/endonuclease, which is normally associated with the repair enzyme, or by the alkaline conditions of the assay [45]. The % of DNA in the tail is proportional to the break frequency. Normally the mean or median % tail DNA from 50 or 100 comets is taken as the measure of DNA damage. If required this can be converted to a break frequency using a calibration curve based on X- or γ-irradiation, which has a known breakage rate per Gray. For genotoxicity testing of NMs different exposure times are recommended, that is, 3 and 24 h. The possibility of interference of NMs in the comet assay—causing additional damage to DNA during the performance of the assay, or inhibiting enzyme activity—has been discussed [46–48] but these concerns seem to be hypothetical. Some authors have described the presence of NMs in the comets, which implies that they were also present during the performance of the assay and thus, could have interacted with the naked DNA which might have resulted in artificial additional damage [49]. However, Magdolenova et al. [46] found with five NMs that their presence in the gel does not affect the comet tail. Caution is needed with photocatalytic NMs, as they can induce additional breaks when the slides are exposed to normal light during their processing [47]. To avoid any possible artifactual results, an additional control (such as NMs to be included in gel with control cells) should be considered.

The comet assay should always be performed alongside a cytotoxicity assay such as the AB and/or CFE assay. A high-throughput version of the comet assay involving 12 minigels per slide is also established [19, 50]. In this chapter we also include a protocol for the comet assay using human 3D skin and lung tissue models. The use of human 3D models is increasingly gaining importance for in vitro toxicity testing. Compared to cell lines, 3D models better reflect tissue architecture, barrier functions and the metabolic capacity of the target organ(s). Thus, using human 3D models can be one promising way of improving current in vitro genotoxicity tests. For genotoxicity testing of NMs in human 3D tissues we recommend longer exposure times than for cells (i.e., 48–72 h). The test should also be performed alongside a cytotoxicity test, where in our experience the ATP assay is best suited. The protocol for comet assay in human 3D tissue models has been established and verified for human 3D skin and bronchial lung models [24, 51].

Clastogenicity and aneugenicity can be evaluated with the **chromosomal aberration (CHA) test** that identifies agents causing structural chromosome or chromatid breaks, dicentrics, and other abnormal chromosomes. The in vitro **micronucleus assay (MN)** is a genotoxicity test for the detection of micronuclei (MN) in the cytoplasm of interphase cells. MN are formed from chromosome or chromatid fragments or from whole chromosomes that lag behind in cell division. Excluded from the nuclei of daughter cells, these structures form single or multiple micronuclei in the cytoplasm, which are detected by visual (or automated) examination after DNA staining. Therefore, the MN assay reveals the ability of the test materials to induce structural chromosome damage (clastogenic effect) or numerical chromosome alterations (aneugenic effect). Cytochalasin B is an agent that has been used to block cytokinesis because it inhibits actin assembly, and thus prevents separation of daughter cells after mitosis, leading to the formation of binucleated cells. By adding cytochalasin B, MN scoring can be limited to cells that have gone through mitosis during or after treatment. This is particularly relevant for relatively unsynchronized cells (e.g., from primary cultures). The appropriate concentration of cytochalasin B is usually between 3 and 6 μg/ml [52, 53]. In addition, it is possible to differentiate MN formed by clastogenic and aneugenic action in binucleated cells [54]. The MN test is less time-consuming compared to the CHA test. Thus, it is used more often, also for NM testing. For chemicals the MN test is usually performed according to the OECD TG 487 [53]. The OECD TG 487 describes the cytokinesis-block micronucleus (CBMN) assay in different cell models including cultured primary human or other mammalian peripheral blood lymphocytes and a number of rodent and human cell lines. It is important to consider the p53 status, genetic (karyotype) stability, DNA repair capacity, and origin (rodent versus human) of the cells chosen for testing. Recent considerations about the in vitro MN assay should also be applied when testing NMs, in particular when sub-toxic concentrations (not the 55 ± 5% toxicity as top dose) are tested to better reflect the real exposure situation and if an aneugenic mode of action is suspected. This means practically to enhance as much as possible the sensitivity of the assay and to maximize its capacity to detect aneugens [53, 55]. Here we also include the MN assay in human 3D tissue models. The most critical point when using human 3D tissue models for the MN test is to assure that a significant fraction of the cells is undergoing cell division. Human 3D models consist of differentiated primary human cells and typically only a low number of cells are still dividing. To that end it can be useful to test different cell culture media beforehand and to perform the cytokinesis-block micronucleus (CBMN) [53]. According to our experience, genotoxicity testing of NMs in human 3D tissues also requires longer exposure times than for cell lines (i.e., 48–72 h) and it can be useful to treat the tissues in a repeated dose system, that is, at 0, 24 and 48 h [56]. Furthermore, it is very important to assess whether the NMs have penetrated into a cell layer capable of cell division, in particular when using 3D skin models. The protocol for MN assay in human 3D tissue models has been established and verified for human 3D skin models and bronchial lung models [24, 51].

It needs to be acknowledged that any DNA lesion caused by chemicals and NMs can still be repaired by cellular DNA repair systems, which typically is not considered in standard in vitro tests. As stated above, the high number of irrelevant positive results is one of the biggest current challenges in in vitro genotoxicity testing. One possible strategy to overcome this could be the use of more complex systems. The **hen's egg test for micronucleus induction assay (HET-MN)** is an example of such a system as it includes toxicologically important features such as absorption, distribution, metabolic activation, and excretion ("ADME") of the test compound [57]. The HET-MN is a promising follow-up assay to complement existing in vitro test batteries for genotoxicity and is currently undergoing a formal validation [58]. However, so far it has not been applied or evaluated for applicability for NMs.

Finally, in this chapter we also include the **cell transformation assay (CTA)** as a promising novel test for predicting NM-induced cell transformation in vitro, which might be a promising approach toward predicting carcinogenicity in vitro [59]. The CTA with Bhas42 cells measures morphological transformation of cells as foci derived from a single cell [60, 61]. This assay can detect both genotoxic and non-genotoxic carcinogens. It aims to identify both tumor-initiating and tumor-promoting activity of a substance. As an initiation assay to test tumor-initiating activity, cells at low density are treated with a test chemical for three days. As a promotion assay to test for tumor promoting activity, near confluent cells are treated with a test chemical for 10 days. After 21 days the cells are fixed and stained. The CTA assay with Bhas42 cells has been validated and an OECD guidance document was developed in 2016. Several NMs have been already tested in CTA [32, 61]. The Bhas42 cell line is derived from the BALB/c 3T3 mouse whole embryo cell line and transfected with v-Ha-ras gene. Bhas42 cells proliferate exponentially and on reaching confluence they form a contact-inhibited monolayer. After exposure to carcinogenic stimuli, which induce cell transformation, cells are morphologically altered and form colonies referred to as foci on the confluent monolayer. The foci are characterized by criss-crossed, piled-up, and spindle shaped cells. The transformation frequency is quantified by microscopic scoring of the number of transformed foci in each well. Cytotoxicity of the chemical or NM is evaluated colorimetrically—this is performed concurrently with the CTA assay [60, 61]. It is recommended to do a cytotoxicity test ahead of the CTA to set doses.

It should be noted that the knowledge summarized in this chapter is based on experiences of the authors in the context of various European and national research projects such as NanoGenoTox (Project ID: 20092101), NanoTEST (Project ID: 201335), NANoREG (Project ID: 310584), NanoReg2 (Project ID: 646221), HISENTS (Project ID: 685817), ERA-NET EuroNanoMed II GEMNS and INNOCENT, BMBF nanoGEM (Grant Number 03X0105) or the Norwegian project NorNANoREG (239199/O70). An overview of a suitable NM testing strategy involving cytotoxicity and genotoxicity tests is schematically depicted in Fig. 1. Methods for characterization and for quantifying uptake are not part of this chapter, though this information would be highly useful when evaluating whether there is genotoxic potential induced by NMs.

2 Materials

2.1 Chemicals, Buffers, Kits

Chemicals should be purchased in p.a. quality. Most of the chemicals were obtained from Sigma-Aldrich, but they can also be purchased from other suppliers. The following chemicals are required:

Acetic acid glacial, agarose (MEEO or NEEO quality, Roth, Cat. No. 2267.2), low melting point (LMP) agarose (SeaPlaque

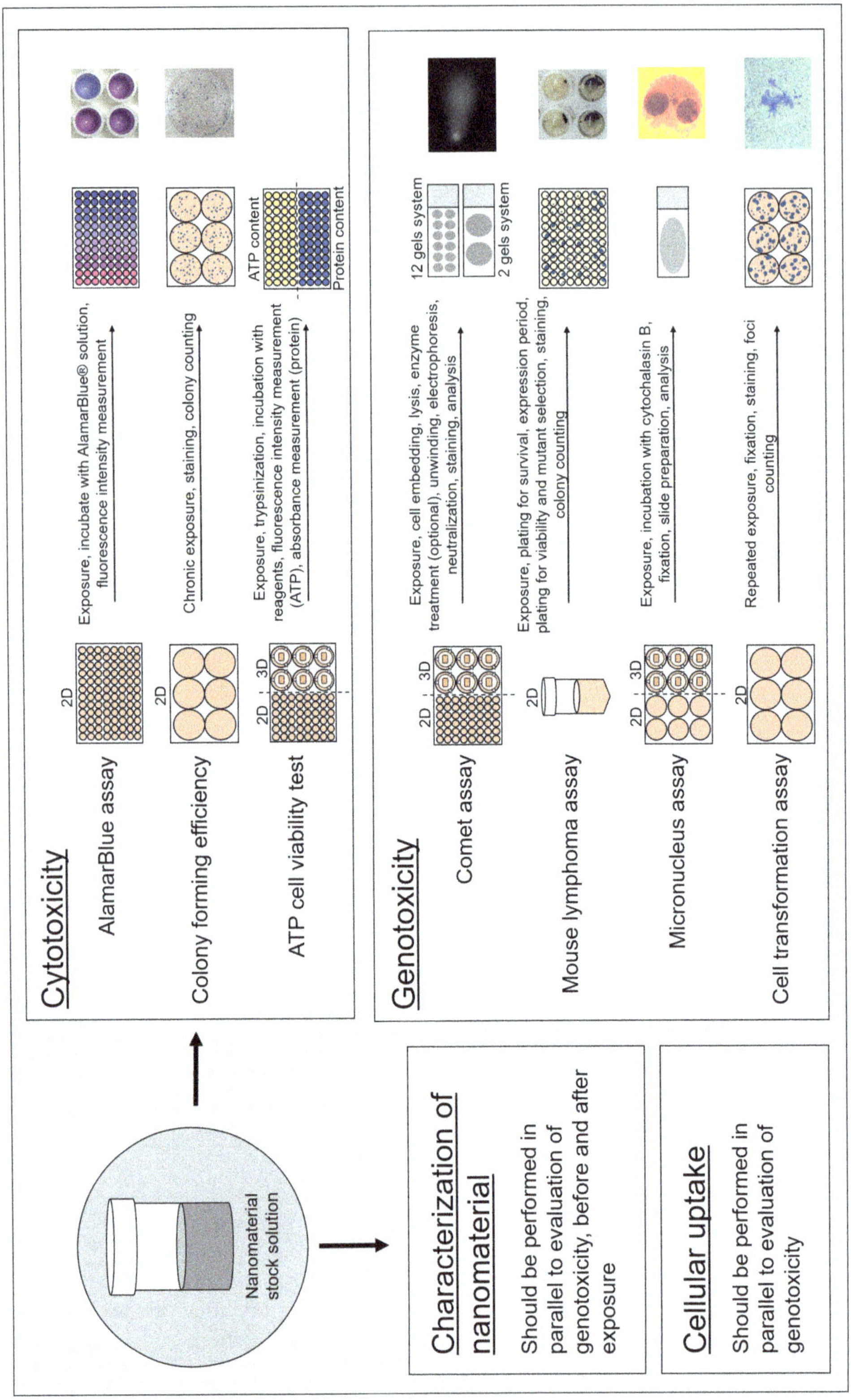

Fig. 1 Testing strategy for genotoxicity of nanomaterials

GTG agarose, Cambrex, Cat. No. 50111), bovine serum albumin (BSA) (Sigma-Aldrich, Cat. No. A5418), Cytochalasin B, DMSO (AppliChem), EDTA (Na2EDTA Dihydrat, Titriplex III, Sigma-Aldrich, Cat. No. E4884), Ethanol (absolute, 100%), Fetal Bovine Serum (FBS, Sigma-Aldrich, Cat. No. F6178), formaldehyde, Giemsa stain, glycerol (Sigma-Aldrich, Cat. No. G5516), HCl (37%, Sigma-Aldrich, Cat. No. 435570), HEPES (Sigma-Aldrich, Cat. No. H3375), dH_2O (distilled/deionized water, e.g., by using Millipore Water Purification Systems), horse serum, Hydrogen peroxide (H_2O_2) (30%, Sigma-Aldrich, Cat. No. H1009), KCl (Sigma-Aldrich, Cat. No. P4504), KOH (Sigma-Aldrich, Cat. No. P5958), 3-methylcholantrene (MCA), Methylene blue (1%), methanol, Mitomycin C, MMS (methyl methane-sulfonate), Phosphate buffered saline w/o Ca^{2+}/Mg^{2+} (Dulbecco PBS, purchase as a powder, Gibco, via Thermo Fisher, Cat. No. 21600069), Ro 19-8022 (Hoffmann La Roche), sodium chloride (NaCl), sodium hydroxide (NaOH) (Sigma-Aldrich, Cat. No. S5881), SYBR®-Gold (10,000× in DMSO, ThermoFisher, Cat. No. S11494), 12-O-tetradecanoylphorbol-13-acetate (TPA), Tris (Sigma-Aldrich, Cat. No.T1503), Triton X-100, Trypan blue cell stain (0.4%, Invitrogen).

In addition the following reagents/kits are required: AlamarBlue® reagent (Invitrogen), ATP-Kit (e.g., ATPlite™ kit, PerkinElmer), Bradford reagent (Bio-Rad).

2.1.1 Buffers and Solutions

Electrophoresis solution (comet assay): 300 mM NaOH/ 1 mM EDTA.

The electrophoresis solution is prepared using the following stock solutions: (a) 10 N NaOH (400 g/l dH_2O) and (b) 200 mM Disodium EDTA (Titriplex III) (14.89 g/200 ml dH_2O, adjust pH to 10 by adding approx. 20 NaOH pellets). These stocks can be stored at room temperature.

In order to obtain 1× electrophoresis solution mix 600 ml NaOH stock and 100 ml Na2EDTA stock, fill up to 20 l, mix well, check pH (should be >13). The 1× electrophoresis solution can be stored at 4 °C for approx. 1 month.

Enzyme reaction buffer for Endo III and Fpg (Buffer F, comet assay): Buffer F is prepared as a10× stock, which consists of 0.04 M HEPES, 0.10 M KCl, 0.0005 M EDTA, and 0.2 mg/ml BSA in sterile dH_2O. The pH is adjusted to 8.0 with 8 M KOH. Aliquot (50 ml) and store at −20 °C until use.

Fpg enzyme (comet assay): Titration should be performed to find the final working concentration. Follow supplier's instructions for dilution. If this is not provided follow these general guidelines: Thaw the received amount of enzyme on ice, make few aliquots as soon as possible (e.g., 50 μl/tube) and freeze at −80 °C. It is recommended to make a second stock solution immediately upon receipt from the original stock into buffer F with 10% glycerol (e.g., dilute the enzyme 1:100) and use it all after thawing. The final working dilution of Fpg used to incubate with nucleoids on gels depends on titration experiments. Do not refreeze the working solution!

H_2O_2 positive control (comet assay): Commercial H_2O_2 stock solution (9.82 M, 30% w/w) is kept in fridge. Out of this prepare 100 mM H_2O_2 working stock in PBS. Final concentration for cell exposure is 50–100 μM.

Low Melting Point Agarose (LMPA) (comet assay): 0.8% dissolved in water, small aliquots (ca. 10 ml) can be stored at 4 °C until used. For embedding the cells, prior to the experiment melt the LMP carefully in microwave, keep at 38 °C.

Lysis solution (comet assay): Lysis buffer consists of 2.50 M NaCl, 0.10 M Na2EDTA, and 0.01 M Tris–HCl. To prepare this buffer mix 146.1 g NaCl, 37.2 g Na2EDTA, and 1.2 g Tris, fill up to final volume of 1 l with dH_2O, consider when adding dH_2O that pH has to be adjusted to 10 (either by using NaOH pellets or by adding 8 M NaOH). It can take up to several hours to dissolve all reagents and to adjust pH. Keep at 4 °C. On the day of experiment, add 1 ml Triton X-100 per 100 ml lysis buffer before use and mix properly with magnetic blender.

Methyl methanesulfonate (MMS), (comet assay): Prepare a stock solution (11.8 M) in DMSO, dilute in DMSO (1 M), dilute further in PBS (1 mM). Working solutions (0.1–0.3 mM) are prepared by further dilution the appropriate culture medium.

MTT (Thiazolyl blue tetrazolium bromide solution): Prepare freshly before use (2.5 mg/ml in PBS).

Phosphate-buffered saline without Ca^{2+} and Mg^{2+}: Prepare 10× PBS by dissolving 95.5 g Dulbecco's PBS (w/o Ca^{2+} and Mg^{2+}) in 1 l dH2O, autoclave. For final use dilute 1:10 with dH_2O.

Ro 19-8022 (photosensitizer) positive control solution (comet assay): Dissolve stock (obtained from Hoffmann La Roche) in 70% ethanol at 1 mM, store in small aliquots at −20 °C. Avoid excessive light during preparation and wrap tubes in aluminum foil. Working solution is 1–2 μM Ro, diluted in PBS.

Trifluorothymidine (TFT), (comet assay): 400 μg/ml in Fischer's medium, sterile-filtered (0.22 μm filter), stored at −20 °C.

SYBR®Gold stock solution (comet assay): Thaw the purchased stock, aliquot, store at −20 °C. Then prepare 2000× SYBR®Gold working solution in TE buffer, store at 4 °C, cover to avoid light (Do not freeze the working solution!).

TRIS–EDTA (TE) buffer stock (comet assay): TE buffer consists of 10 mM Tris–HCl and 1 mM Na_2EDTA in dH2O, pH is adjusted to 7.5–7.8 using HCl. It can be prepared using stocks of Tris–HCl (500 mM) and Na_2EDTA (200 mM). The stocks can be stored at room temperature for months. TE buffer should be stored at 4 °C (for a few weeks).

2.2 Cell Models

The MLA was developed and characterized using the Tk+/− −3.7.2C subline of L5178Y cells. Thus, this specific subline has to be used for the MLA. The Comet assay and MN assay can be performed using a variety of different cell models. For MN assay suitable cell models are listed in OECD TG 487 [53]. Bhas42 cells for the CTA can be obtained from Japanese Collection of research Bioresources Cell Bank (No.: JCRB0601). Human 3D tissue models for comet and MN assay can be obtained from MatTek Corporation, USA (e.g., EpiAirway™, EpiDerm™, or EpiDermFT™), but also from other suppliers.

2.3 Cell Culture

Cell culture is done according to standard protocols as described by the supplier of the respective cell models. Standard consumables for cell culture (plasticware, cell culture medium, fetal calf serum, trypsin, etc.) can be purchased from different suppliers as well.

Heat-inactivated horse serum (hi-HS): Heated in water bath, 56 °C for 30 min, with turning of bottle every 5 min to ensure evenly heating. Stored in aliquots at −20 °C.

F5 cell culture medium (mouse lymphoma assay): Fischer's medium, supplemented with 2 mM glutamine, 1% sodium pyruvate, 5% hi-HS, and 100 U/ml penicillin and 100 μg/ml streptomycin.

F10 cell culture medium (mouse lymphoma assay): Fischer's medium, supplemented with 2 mM glutamine, 1% sodium pyruvate, 10% hi-HS, and 100 U/ml penicillin and 100 μg/ml streptomycin.

F20 cell culture medium (mouse lymphoma assay): Fischer's medium, supplemented with 2 mM glutamine, 1% sodium pyruvate, 20% hi-HS, and 100 U/ml penicillin and 100 μg/ml streptomycin.

2.4 Other Consumables

Black/white flat-bottom 96-well plate (ATP assay).

Centrifuge Tubes.

Coplin jars (comet assay).

Ice (comet assay).

Frozen ice packs (comet assay).

Microscope slides and coverslips (comet assay and MN).

2.5 Equipment

Standard equipment for cell culture (i.e., incubator, sterile hood, water bath, centrifuge) is needed.

Spectrophotometer or spectrofluorometer (AB assay and MN).

Cell counter (CFE assay).

Countess® Cell Counting Chamber Slides or Bürker chamber.

Cytospin (e.g., Shandon Cytospin 3) (MN assay).

Digital microscope or inverted phase contrast microscope (comet assay).

Fluorescence microscope (e.g., Zeiss Axioplan 2) (comet assay).

Heating block (optimal would be two heating blocks, comet assay).

Horizontal Electrophoresis Tank(s) (comet assay).

Luminometer (ATP assay).

Microwave oven.

Optical microscope (mouse lymphoma assay).

Power Unit.

2.6 Software

For analysis of comets different software is available, e.g., Komet 5,5 (Imaging program, Andor Bioimaging), Komet VI (Perceptive), Metafer, Comet Assay IV™ (Perceptive Instruments Ltd.)

3 Methods

3.1 AlamarBlue (AB) Assay

1. Cells are exposed to NMs for the desired period of time, typically in 96-well format. Untreated cells serve as negative controls. In addition, a positive chemical control may be included—the choice of the positive control depends on the cell model. After incubation the cell culture medium is removed, cells are washed with PBS, then the same volume of alamarBlue (AB) solution is added. AB solution is obtained by diluting AB reagent in cell culture medium, typically 1:10, but the final concentration can be optimized. The necessary incubation time depends on the test system, such as cell type or cell density. Typically 1–4 h are recommended. In our experience 3 h works well with most cell systems. However, cells can be incubated with AB even for days [62]. In addition, blank wells containing AB solution only and no cells are needed for background correction.
2. After incubation the fluorescence is read on a plate reader (excitation 530 nm, emission 590 nm). Alternatively, the absorbance of reagent can be read on a spectrophotometer at 540 and 630 nm. The fluorescence is typically read in black plates to avoid interference from adjacent wells. Transparent wells may also work well, interference and background fluorescence must be tested before use. Importantly, as there might be a risk of interferences of the NMs with the test system this has to be checked either beforehand or in parallel to the assay. Interference should be tested on both resazurin (oxidized form) and resorufin (reduced form) by adding increasing concentrations of NMs.
3. Results are analyzed by plotting fluorescence intensity versus compound concentration. The blank is subtracted from all samples (i.e., treated and untreated control cells). Cell viability is

calculated by the following formula: Cell viability (%) = (fluorescence from treated wells after blank subtraction/(fluorescence from untreated control wells after blank subtraction) × 100.

4. The experiment should be independently repeated, preferably to have three biological replicates.

3.2 Colony Forming Efficiency (CFE)

1. Seed cells, normally 50–200 cells per well in 6-well format in 1 ml cell culture medium, for 1–16 h (depending on the doubling time of respective the cell line) before exposure to allow for treatment of individual cells. Cells should be taken in the exponential growth phase (50–75% confluence) in a low passage number (<p15). NMs are prepared with 2× of the desired final test concentration in cell culture medium, then 1 ml of the 2× concentration is added directly to cells.
2. The test should include a negative control (i.e., untreated cells), a solvent control (i.e., the NM dispersion medium), a positive chemical control, and at least three concentrations of the test substance. For relatively non-cytotoxic compounds the maximum concentration should not be above 5 mg/ml, 5 ml/l, or 10 mM (whichever is the lowest). Steps of ~three-fold (e.g., 1, 3, 10, 30, 100) are often just right. Normally one 6-well plate per treatment is applied, resulting in six replica wells.
3. The cells are exposed to the test substance continuously (5–12 days), or alternatively for 72 h in total. In case of 72 h treatment, the test compound is removed and replaced with complete fresh medium and then the cells are cultured for additional 3–7 days, until colonies are visible. However, be aware that it will not be possible to wash out the NMs in case of 72 h exposure, as they will stick to the cells and the walls of the well.
4. Stain the colonies with 1% methylene blue when they are visible by eye (Fig. 2). Methylene blue can be added directly into the culture media in the wells. Alternatively, the colonies can be fixed in 4% (v/v) formaldehyde in PBS and then can be stained in 0.4% (v/v) of Giemsa in MilliQ water.
5. After drying, colonies composed of at least 50 cells are counted manually. It is advantageous to apply counting pen to avoid duplicate counting of colonies.
6. To calculate CFE, the number of colonies is expressed as % of the number of inoculated cells. The relative CFE (RCFE) is the ratio of colonies for treated cells to control (i.e., untreated) cells.
7. The experiment should be repeated twice in independent experiments.

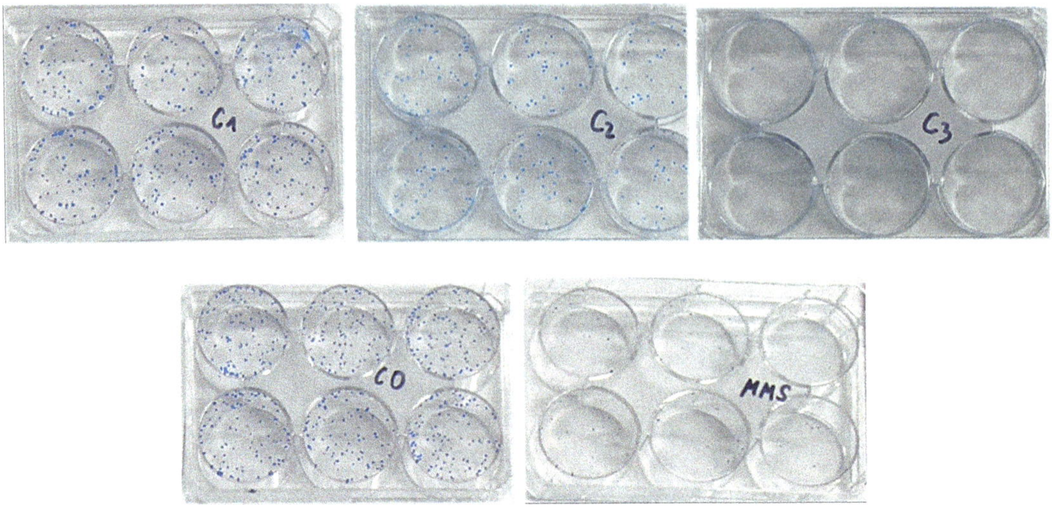

Fig. 2 CFE: Examples of 6-well plates with cell colonies stained with methylene blue. C_0 = negative control (left down) compared with cells exposed to a cytotoxic nanomaterial at increasing concentrations (C_1, C_2, C_3). MMS is positive control. Each independent sample has six replicates

8. Criteria for characterizing the tested compound as cytotoxic are:
   (a) Colony formation is reduced by at least 20% compared to negative control.
   (b) A concentration-dependent effect is observed.
   (c) The effect is reproducible.

   A test substance for which the results do not meet the above criteria is considered non-cytotoxic under the experimental conditions.

3.3 ATP Assay

1. The 3D models are cultivated as described by the supplier, typically grown in inserts in 6-well plates (diameter about 10 mm). For treatment, small volumes (i.e., up to 30 μl) of dispersed NMs are applied on top of the models and incubated for the desired period of time. Vehicle (i.e., NM dispersant) treated tissues are included as negative controls. A suitable chemical positive control should also be included (dependent on the tissue and/or the assay).
2. Cell harvest of 3D models: Please refer to the respective sections describing the protocols for comet assay and micronucleus assay in 3D tissue models for details how to digest the models and how to prepare single cell suspensions. Only a fraction of each tissue is used for the ATP assay, the remaining part is used for the assessment of genotoxicity (e.g., for comet assay or MN assay). Typically approx. 2/3 of the total cell suspension of each tissue is used for the ATP assay. These cells are lysed for ATP assay.

3. ATP measurement is performed as described by the manufacturer. Please note that as ATP is the universal energy carrier in nature, ATP is abundantly present everywhere. ATP is fairly heat-stable so mere autoclaving is not always sufficient for complete reduction. Therefore, it is important not to contaminate equipment to be used for that assay. In particular when pipetting the standards avoid direct contact of reagents and hands or fingertips. Open standard vials carefully and do not touch the mouth of the bottle. Be careful when removing the rubber stoppers from the vials. Use ATP-free pipette tips. Handle microplates carefully and use lids to avoid dust or other contamination. From each 3D model two technical repeats are measured in black/white flat-bottom 96-well plate. Perform all steps in the dark. The measurement is done at 22 °C.
4. Afterwards measure the protein content of each sample by using a standard protein assay such as Bradford assay.
5. For ATP content calculation: first determine the mean value for the blank. Subtract the mean blank from all other measurements (standards and samples). Calculate means for the standards and plot a calibration curve, use a linear regression. Determine ATP content in each sample from the standard curve, then calculate mean values from the repeats. Care must be taken as NMs can interfere with the readout of the assays. This has to be tested beforehand or in parallel to the assay.
6. For protein content calculation: first subtract the mean value of the blank from all other measures (standards and samples). Use the mean values of the standards to plot a calibration curve, use a linear regression. Determine protein content in each sample from the standard curve, then calculate mean values from the repeats.
7. Finally calculate the ratio of ATP content in relation to the protein content.

3.4 Mouse Lymphoma Assay (MLA)

1. L5178Y Tk +/− 3.7.2 mouse lymphoma cells should always be kept at cell densities below 1×10^6 cells/ml. Cells are ready for start of experiment at passage 3 and can be used for up to ten passages. The cells should have a low level of spontaneous mutation. If mutant frequency in solvent controls is too high, cells can cleansed from preexisting Tk mutants by treatment with methotrexate as described elsewhere [63]. After cleansing, cells should be frozen in aliquots to be used for mutation experiment.
2. A minimum of 6×10^6—1×10^7 live cells must be used for culturing each sample during the experiment. Aliquot cells in 50 ml centrifugation tubes, use 0.6–1×10^7 cells/tube.

Centrifuge at 300 × *g* for 5 min. Re-suspend the cell pellet in total 15 ml F10.

3. Prepare 2× concentrated dilutions of the test compound for the treatments, also include controls, i.e., solvent, negative and positive (MMS 0.1 mM) controls. At least 4 concentrations of the test compound should be tested in either single or replica samples. The highest test compound concentration should correspond to a cytotoxicity between 20% and 10% relative total growth rate (RTG). If the cytotoxicity of the test substance is unknown, a range-finding experiment should be performed first. If the substance is noncytotoxic and no precipitation is seen, the highest concentration should correspond to 10 mM, 2 mg/ml, or 2 μl/ml (whichever is the lowest).
4. Mix cells (in 15 ml medium) with 15 ml of either the test compound or controls. Seal the tubes with a cap and Parafilm. Incubate horizontally on a shaker (80 ± 10 orbits/min), for 24 h at 37 °C. The positive control cells are incubated with MMS (100 μM) for 3 h only, at the end of the 24 h.
5. Plating for survival and expression period: At the end of treatment, centrifuge the cells at 300 × *g* for 5 min, and resuspend the cells in 10 ml F10. Count the number of live cells twice in Countess, and transfer 0.6–1.0 × 10^7 live cells to a 25 cm^2 culture flask. Add F20 to a final cell density of 2 × 10^5 cells/ml. Be aware of potential interferences of NMs with countess, as some NM agglomerates can look as dead cells. However, no interferences of NMs with the test system are expected when care is taken with cell counting after NM exposure. A 24 h treatment is recommended only for incubation without metabolizing system (i.e., S9 fraction) to ensure cellular uptake of NMs. Adding S9 fraction is recommended only in combination with short treatment—it may alter NMs by protein corona formation and thus can change NM behavior and consequently, the observed effect.
6. Plating for survival: Dilute further by serial dilution to 1 × 10^4, then 1 × 10^3 ml^{-1}, and finally 8 cells/ml. Seed two 96-well plates per sample, with 200 μl/well from the suspension of 8 cells/ml using multipipette dispenser. There will be on average 1.6 cells/well. Incubate the plates at 37 °C, 5% CO_2 for 10–13 days before colony counting.
7. The remaining cell suspension of 2 × 10^5 cells/ml, at (0.6–1.0 × 10^7 live cells) is cultured at 37 °C, 5% CO_2 for and expression period of 48–72 h. Suspension growth during treatment and expression period should meet the test acceptance criteria (see below). After 24 and 48 h resuspend and count the cells, and adjust the cell density to 2 × 10^5 cells/ml.

8. At the end of expression period, resuspend cells and count. Dilute cells to 1×10^4 cells/ml in F20, 90 ml in total for procedure (a) and (b):
   (a) Plating for viability: Take 1 ml of cell suspension of 1×10^4 cells/ml and prepare a suspension of 1×10^3 cells/ml in F20, then 8 cells/ml. Seed two 96-well plates per sample, with 200 μl/well from the suspension of 8 cells/ml using multipipette dispenser. There will be on average 1.6 cells/well. Incubate the plates at 37 °C, 5% CO_2 for 10–13 days, before the colonies are counted.
   (b) Plating for mutants/TFT resistance: To the remaining 89 ml of the cell suspension (1×10^4 cells/ml), add 890 μl TFT solution (400 μg/ml) to give a final TFT concentration of 4 μg/ml (though 3 μg/ml of TFT is sufficient to kill normal cells). Seed four 96-well plates per sample with 200 μl/well using multipipette dispenser, resulting in 2000 cells/well. In case experiment is running without replica samples, prepare four 96-well plates for TFT resistance per sample (384 wells at 2×10^3 cells/well). In case experiment is running with replica samples, only two 96-well plates are necessary. Incubate the plates at 37 °C, 5% CO_2 for 12–14 days, before colony counting.
9. Counting of colonies: In plates for survival/cytotoxicity and plates for viability, count the number of wells with viable clones (Fig. 3). In plates for TFT resistance, the colonies are visualized by staining with freshly prepared MTT-solution (2.5 mg/ml), 25 μl/well, and incubation at 37 °C 5% CO_2 for 4 h or until all colonies are clearly stained. Mutant colonies are counted according to size. Count the number of wells with small colonies ($<1/4$ of well, compact morphology), with large colonies ($\geq 1/4$ of well, diffuse morphology in whole well or only in the periphery), and with both small and large colonies. It is important to separately count the *wells* with small, large, and both small and large colonies.
10. **Calculations of** plating efficiency (PE): Plates for survival and viability are used to calculate the $PE_{cytotoxicity}$ and $PE_{viability}$, respectively. The distribution of colony formation in wells is described by Poisson distribution; thus, the PE is calculated using the term 0 of Poisson distribution $\{P(0)\}$.

$$P(0) = -\ln \frac{\text{number of negative wells}}{\text{total number of wells}}.$$

$$\mathrm{PE} = \frac{P(0)}{\text{number of cells/well}} \text{ or PE (\%)} = \frac{\mathrm{P}(0) \times 100\%}{\text{number of cells/well}}.$$

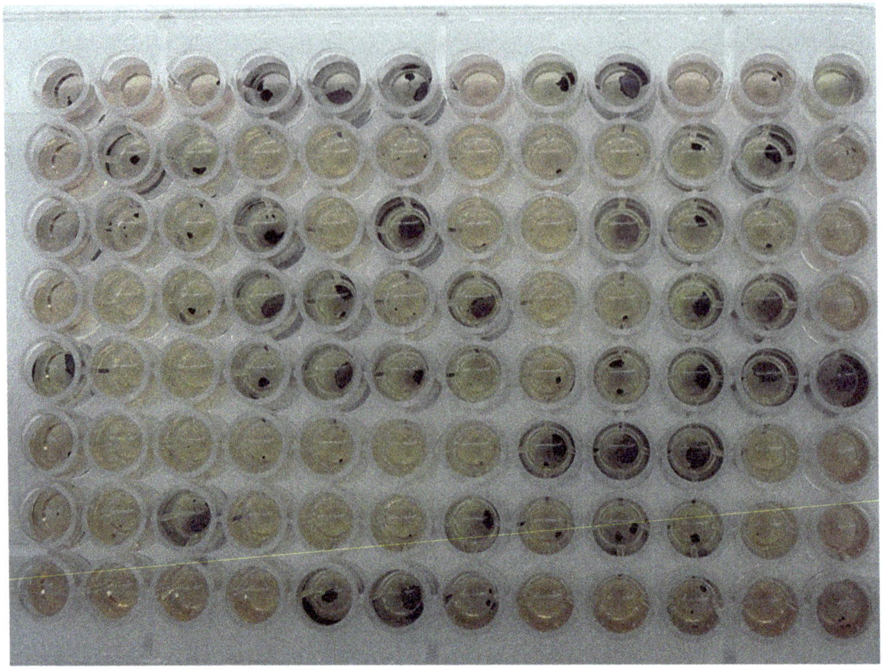

Fig. 3 MLA: Image of a 96-well plate with small and large mutant colonies of L5178Y cells in Tk locus after treatment with MMS (100 μM)

11. Calculation of mutant frequency (MF): The colonies in plates with TFT are used to calculate the MF of the test sample, per million viable cells. Calculate MF_{small}, MF_{large}, and MF_{total} separately.

$$\mathrm{MF}\left(10^{-6}\mathrm{cells}\right) = \frac{P(0)_{\mathrm{TFT\ resistance}}}{(\mathrm{number\ of\ cells/well})_{\mathrm{TFT\ resistance}} \times \mathrm{PE}_{\mathrm{viability}}}.$$

12. Calculation of relative suspension growth (RSG): RSG is calculated using the number of live cells per sample (live cells, LC) at beginning and end of treatment, and the cell counts during expression period. Use the number of live cells per sample, and not the cell density, unless the volumes of the samples are constant during cell counting in the whole experiment. In the formula B and A is noted as before and after adjusting the cell densities, respectively:

$$\mathrm{RSG}\ (\%) = \text{Relative suspension growth}$$
$$= \frac{\left[\frac{\mathrm{LC}_{2\mathrm{B}}}{\mathrm{LC}_1} \times \frac{\mathrm{LC}_{3\mathrm{B}}}{\mathrm{LC}_{2\mathrm{A}}} \times \frac{\mathrm{LC}_{4\mathrm{B}}}{\mathrm{LC}_{3\mathrm{A}}} \times \frac{\mathrm{LC}_{5\mathrm{B}}}{\mathrm{LC}_{4\mathrm{A}}}\right]_{\mathrm{treatment}}}{\left[\frac{\mathrm{LC}_{2\mathrm{B}}}{\mathrm{LC}_1} \times \frac{\mathrm{LC}_{3\mathrm{B}}}{\mathrm{LC}_{2\mathrm{A}}} \times \frac{\mathrm{LC}_{4\mathrm{B}}}{\mathrm{LC}_{3\mathrm{A}}} \times \frac{\mathrm{LC}_{5\mathrm{B}}}{\mathrm{LC}_{4\mathrm{A}}}\right]_{\mathrm{control}}} \times 100\%.$$

13. Cytotoxicity is defined as the relative total growth (RTG) which includes the RSG during the 2 day expression period

and the relative cloning efficiency (PE) obtained at the time of mutant selection.

$$\mathrm{RTG}\,(\%) = \mathrm{RSG}\,(\%) \times \text{Relative PE}$$

$$= \frac{\left[\frac{LC_{2B}}{LC_1} \times \frac{LC_{3B}}{LC_{2A}} \times \frac{LC_{4B}}{LC_{3A}} \times \frac{LC_{5B}}{LC_{4A}} \times PE_{\text{cytotoxicity}}\right]_{\text{treatment}}}{\left[\frac{LC_{2B}}{LC_1} \times \frac{LC_{3B}}{LC_{2A}} \times \frac{LC_{4B}}{LC_{3A}} \times \frac{LC_{5B}}{LC_{4A}} \times PE_{\text{cytotoxicity}}\right]_{\text{control}}} \times 100\%.$$

14. Test acceptance criteria: The assay is considered as valid if the following criteria are fulfilled: (a) Adequate number of cells and concentrations should be analyzable; (b) The MF for solvent control is above 50 and below 170 mutants per 10^6 viable cells but not more than three times the historical mean value of the respective laboratory. The PE and relative PE for solvent controls is between 65–120% and suspension growth is 32- to 180-fold. The positive control(s) should meet at least one of the following two criteria: (a) The positive control should demonstrate an absolute increase in total MF, that is, an increase above the spontaneous background MF of at least 300×10^{-6}. At least 40% of the increase should be reflected in the small colony MF; (b) The positive control has an increase in the small colony MF of at least 150×10^{-6} above that seen in the concurrent untreated/solvent control.

    The International Workshop on Genotoxicity Test mouse lymphoma work group [35, 36] states that biological relevance should be a major factor in data evaluation. Therefore, an approach for defining positive and negative responses is based on the distribution of the negative control MF (global evaluation factor, GEF) which is considered to be 126×10^{-6} for the microwell version [34]. The test sample is considered to be clearly positive in the assay (i.e., the test chemical is able to induce mutation in this test system) if all the following criteria are fulfilled:

    (a) The assay is valid.

    (b) The increase in MF above the concurrent background in any of the experimental conditions examined exceeds the GEF ($MF_{\text{test substance}} > MF_{\text{control}} + GEF$), and the increase is concentration related.

    The test sample is considered clearly negative (i.e., unable to induce mutations in this test system) if following criteria are fulfilled:

    (a) The assay is valid.

    (b) In all experimental conditions examined, there is no concentration related response, or the increase in MF does not exceed the GEF ($MF_{\text{test substance}} < MF_{\text{control}} + GEF$).

3.5 Comet Assay

1. Before starting the experiment, prepare precoated slides. The slides are dipped vertically into normal melting point agarose (0.5% NMP, 55 °C), then placed on a flat service to dry. Dried precoated slides can be stored together in slide boxes indefinitely.
2. Expose the cells to NMs for the desired period of time. Different cell models can be used for performing the in vitro comet assay. Before the end of exposure, melt the low melting point agarose (LMPA) carefully in the microwave oven and leave it on a heating block at about 37–40 °C. Make sure that the LMPA is at the right temperature before adding it to the cells—temperature should not be too high. At the end of exposure, remove the test compound and wash cells with PBS. Take an appropriate number of cells (adherent cells need to be trypsinized) into a 96-well plate. About 5–10 × 10^4 cells should be appropriate (i.e., approx. 200–300 cells/5 μl LMPA gel). The ratio for embedding the cells in agarose should be 1:3–4× agarose. Add agarose into the wells with cells, and mix properly. Add 5–10 μl drops of gels on the slide placed on top of cooled metal blocks. Use a multichannel pipette to make 12 gels per slide. Work quickly as the agarose sets fast.
3. Lysis: Place the slides in lysis solution in a (vertical) staining jar. Leave at 4 °C for at least 1 h. The slides can also stay in lysis solution overnight (24 h) or longer.
4. Treatment with H_2O_2 as a positive control for strand breaks: Put the slides with the embedded cells into a jar with 100 μM H_2O_2 in PBS for 5 min. Wash 2 × 2 min in PBS and place them in lysis buffer.
5. Enzyme treatment (optional, only for modified version of the comet assay): Get Fpg from freezer and keep on ice. Wash slides 2 × 10 min in Buffer F. Meanwhile, dilute enzyme in Buffer F according to procedure described above. Keep on ice until use. Add about 200 μl of enzyme solution (or buffer alone, as control) on top of each slide, and cover with thin plastic foil. Put slides into moist box (prevents desiccation) and incubate at 37 °C for 30 min with Fpg. Place slides into fridge for 5–10 min for the gels to stabilize.
6. Alkaline treatment: Place the slides on platform in the tank, forming complete rows (gaps should be filled with blank slides). It is also recommended to place one slide at the end of the tank (Fig. 4) to avoid moving of slides when you fill the tank with electrophoresis solution. Put the tank into the cooling incubator. Gently add appropriate volume of cold electrophoresis solution into the tank until slides are immersed, just enough to be covered. Make sure that tank is leveled. Leave for 20 min to equilibrate.

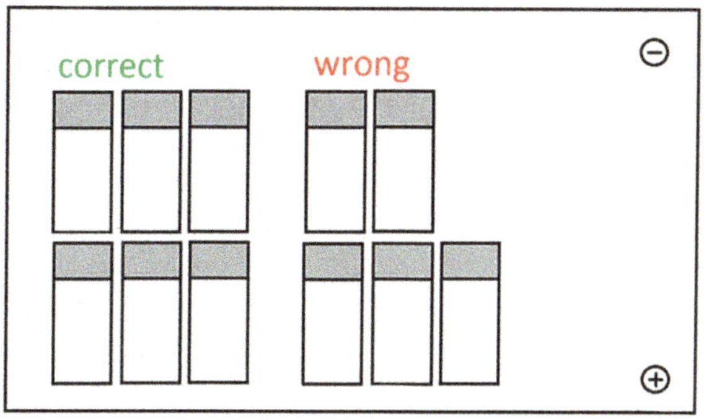

Fig. 4 Comet assay: Correct placement of the slides in the electrophoresis chamber

7. Electrophoresis: Put lid with cables onto the tank in right position. The tank should be kept in the cooling incubator or cold room. Start the power supply and run the electrophoresis at 1.2 V/cm (25 V) for 20 min. If 25 V is not reached, remove some solution using a pipette. The current should be around 300 mA; however, this is not crucial.
8. Neutralization: After electrophoresis, gently move the slides into a jar and wash 5 min with cold PBS. Then wash the slides in a jar with cold ddH_2O for 5 min. Dry the slides horizontally laying at room temperature (normally overnight). The slides can be stored in a slide box until stained and scored.
9. Staining for scoring: Stain only dried slides. Use 2000× SYBR®Gold (in TE buffer) to stain DNA. However, DAPI, Ethidium bromide or other DNA dyes can be used as well. Spread approx. 50 μl of 2000× SYBR®Gold evenly in small droplets to cover the whole 12 gels and cover with large cover slip (22 × 60 mm). Leave in dark for 5–10 min before visualization and scoring in the fluorescence microscope.
10. Scoring: Slides are analyzed using a fluorescent microscope and appropriate image analysis software (e.g., Comet assay IV (Perceptive instruments) or Metasystem (Metafer)). Score 50 comets per gel (two gels per concentration). These software systems operate with a charge-coupled device camera mounted on the microscope, and can automatically analyze individual comet images. The programs are designed to differentiate comet head from tail, and to measure a variety of parameters including tail length; % of total fluorescence in head and tail; and "tail moment." The most informative parameter that always should be used is % DNA in tail.
11. Statistical analyses of the data**:** For statistical analysis the widely preferred measurement is the tail intensity or per cent of DNA in tail (% tail DNA), since those can be "standardized" over studies while other measures of DNA (i.e., tail length and tail

moment), although consistent within a study, may not be comparable across studies [64, 65]. At least three concentrations of NMs plus the corresponding positive and negative controls should be used for statistical analysis. It is advised to use two replicates or cultures per concentrations and to score 50 cells per slide with two slides per culture. Every in vitro experiment is repeated at least twice, preferably to have three biological replicates. Measurements made on 50 cells per slide have appeared as a recommendation following extensive realistic simulations of both in vitro and in vivo studies that compared measurements on different number of cells per slide [65]. The data can be analyzed by ANOVA, using the mean or median value of 50 cells (mean or median % tail DNA per slide). In addition, linear regression analysis is also recommended to find out a linear concentration-response effect. As recommended by Bright et al. [65], the focus should be on the confidence intervals for the treatment effects and not on the p-values because the former conveys the sizes of effects consistent with the study data.

3.6 Comet Assay in Human 3D Models

1. As commercial human 3D models are rather costly one may consider to first use a cell line for screening and then to test selected NMs only in 3D models.
2. For NM exposure, a small volume of the NM dispersion (i.e., 30 μl) is pipetted on top of the cell model (diameter around 10 mm), which typically is grown in an insert in a 6-well format. Note that typically longer exposure times are needed for 3D models compared to cell lines (i.e., 48–72 h). We recommend 60 h. Typically at least two tissues should be treated under identical conditions to have two technical repeats. In addition a negative control (i.e., vehicle treated tissue) is needed. As a positive control MMS can be applied at 5 mM but should be incubated only for 1 h, at the end of the treatment time. At the end of the treatment, the models are washed three times in PBS.
3. Cell harvest of 3D models (i.e., EpiAirway™, EpiDermTM): Cells embedding on slides: Microcentrifuge tubes are prepared with 100 μl cold PBS on ice (one tube per sample). Low Melting Point Agarose (LMPA) is carefully heated in a microwave oven and then put into a heating block at 37 °C for later use (carefully check the temperature before adding LMPA to the cells). To lyse the tissues, 100 μl of trypsin /EDTA are added to each 3D model and incubated for 15 min in an incubator (37 °C, 5% CO_2, 95% relative humidity). A cell suspension is obtained by pipetting up and down several times and the suspension is transferred to the prepared tubes. The remaining inserts where the 3D models were contained are

washed with another 100 μl cold PBS, which is combined with the cell suspension. The total obtained cell suspension is split—one-third to be used for the comet assay and 2/3 to be used for the ATP assay as cytotoxicity has to be assessed in parallel in the same samples. The ATP assay samples are immediately frozen in liquid nitrogen and can be stored at −80 °C. The cell suspension for the comet assay is centrifuged at 400 × *g* and 4 °C for 5 min. The supernatant is removed and discarded. The cell pellet is resuspended in 300 μl LMP agarose (37 °C) and evenly distributed (70 μl each) on three coated slides. A coverslip is placed on the slide and afterwards left on a flat cooling pack until agarose has set.

4. Cell harvest of full thickness skin models (i.e., EpiDerm FT™): Every full thickness skin tissue is placed in a well of a 6-well plate containing 5 ml of dPBS (w/o Ca^{2+} and Mg^{2+}) for 5–15 min at room temperature. Then, dPBS is discarded, each tissue is picked up from the insert and mechanically (i.e., using a pincette) the dermis is separated from the epidermis. Each part (i.e., epidermis and dermis) of each tissue is incubated in a 6-well plate in 2 ml 0.1% EDTA/PBS for 5 min at room temperature, then EDTA/PBS is removed and the tissues are incubated in 2 ml 0.25% trypsin (prewarmed at 37 °C) for 15 min at 37 °C. Then, 1 ml of cold MEM with 10% FBS (or any other medium containing FBS, pure FBS is also possible) is added to each well. In order to ensure that all cell aggregates are separated, the cell suspension is pipetted up and down several times and agitated in between (4–6 times). Cell suspensions are then filtrated through a 40 μm cell strainer, which is put on a 50 ml Falcon tube. The cell strainer is washed with 1.5 ml cold MEM with 10% FBS. Filtrates are centrifuged at 200 × *g* for 5 min, the supernatant is discarded and the remaining cell pellets are resuspended in 2.5 ml of DMEM with 10% FBS each. Store on ice. The total obtained cell suspension is split to obtain 100 μl that will be used for the comet assay and 200 μl that will be used for the ATP assay as cytotoxicity has to be assessed in parallel in the same samples. The ATP assay samples are immediately frozen in liquid nitrogen and can be stored at −80 °C. The cell suspension for the comet assay is centrifuged at 400 × *g* and 4 °C for 5 min. The supernatant is removed and discarded. The cell pellet is resuspended in 300 μl LMP agarose (37 °C) and evenly distributed (70 μl each) on three coated slides. A coverslip is placed on the slide and afterward left on a flat cooling pack until agarose has set.
5. Lysis: Place the slides in lysis solution in a (vertical) staining jar. Leave at 4 °C for at least overnight (24 h) or longer (if needed, this may depend on the cell type).

6. Alkaline treatment and Electrophoresis: Place the slides on platform in the chamber, forming complete rows (gaps should be filled with blank slides) Distribute the slides statistically on the tray (for example: not always put the controls at the bottom left). This way, methodological errors can be minimized. The frosted end of the slide has to be aligned facing the cathode. The chamber must be perfectly horizontal. (Use a spirit level.) Carefully fill the chamber with electrophoresis solution. The chamber should be either in a cold room (4 °C) or placed in an ice bath. Equilibrate for 20 min for alkaline denaturation. Put lid with cables onto the chamber in the correct position (correct placement of anode and cathode). Start the power supply and run the electrophoresis at 1.2 V/cm (25 V) for 20 min. If 25 V is not reached, adjust of volume of electrophoresis solution using a syringe. The current should be around 300 mA.
7. Neutralization: After Electrophoresis, gently move the slides into a glass jar and equilibrate 5 min with neutralization buffer (0.4 M Tris) at room temperature. Repeat this step once, resulting in an equilibration time of 10 min. Do not exceed this time, otherwise the cells in the gel will begin to swell. After the second wash, slides are immersed in a cuvette filled with 100% ethanol for 5 min or longer (the ethanol is reusable up to five times). They are then placed at an angle and dried at room temperature. The slides can be stored for months until staining.
8. Staining and Scoring is identical to the procedures described above.
9. Statistical analyses of the data are identical to the procedures described above.

   It is advised to use two technical replicates per concentrations and to score 50 cells per slide (having two slides per sample). Every in vitro experiment should be repeated in at least two independent biological repeats using a new batch of 3D models.

3.7 Micronucleus Assay (MN Assay)

1. At least three concentrations of a test compound that meet the acceptability criteria should be evaluated in MN assay. Thus, several concentrations of the test compound or NMs should be included. If the maximum chosen test concentration is based on cytotoxicity, the highest concentration should aim to achieve 55 ± 5% cytotoxicity using the recommended cytotoxicity parameters (i.e., reduction in cytokinesis-block proliferation index (CBPI) to 45 ± 5% of the concurrent negative control). Negative controls (solvent alone in the treatment medium and processed in the same way as the treatment cultures) should be included for every harvest time. Positive controls (e.g., Mitomycin C, or MMS) are needed to demonstrate

the ability of the laboratory to identify clastogens and aneugens under the conditions of the test protocol used [53]. It is recommended to perform the cytokinesis-block MN (CBMN) using cytochalasin B, which inhibits actin assembly and prevents separation of daughter cells after mitosis, leading to the formation of binucleated cells [53]. Scoring then can be limited to cells that have gone through mitosis during or after treatment, which is in particular relevant for little synchronized cells (e.g., from primary cultures). Cytochalasin B also inhibits endocytosis, which is an important cellular uptake mechanism favored by some NMs. Therefore, the cells need to be exposed to NMs several hours before adding cytochalasin B [28, 46, 55, 66]. However, also serum levels in the cell culture medium can modulate the uptake of NMs and the cellular response, in a cell type- and NM-dependent manner. This can affect the level of intracellular damage induced [66, 67]. Thus, it might be advisable to assess the genotoxicity of NMs in parallel both complete and reduced serum content in their medium [55, 68].

2. During or after exposure to the test compound, the cells are grown for a period sufficient to allow chromosome damage or other effects on cell cycle/cell division to lead to the formation of micronuclei in interphase cells. Cells should be exposed to the NMs for minimum period of 3–6 h and continuously. However, longer exposure times are more informative as they allow for uptake of NMs, which has been shown to be time-dependent. Furthermore, it is recommended to expose cells during mitosis, in particular for those NMs that cannot cross the nuclear membrane and might need to be in contact with the chromatin to exert their effect [28, 55, 66].
3. Cells should be sampled at a time equivalent to about 1.5–2.0 normal cell cycle lengths after the beginning of treatment [52, 53]. Two replica samples should be done for each dose. Each culture should be harvested and processed separately. Cell preparation may involve hypotonic treatment, but this step is not necessary if adequate cell spreading is otherwise achieved. Different techniques can be used in slide preparation provided that high-quality cell preparations for scoring are obtained. Cells with intact cell membrane and intact cytoplasm should be retained to allow the detection of micronuclei and reliable identification of binucleate cells [53].
4. The slides can be stained using various DNA staining methods, such as Giemsa or fluorescent DNA-specific dyes.
5. Micronucleus frequencies should be analyzed in at least 2000 binucleate cells per concentration and control, equally divided among the replicates. Care should be taken not to score binucleate cells with irregular shapes or where the two nuclei differ

greatly in size. In addition, binucleate cells should not be confused with poorly spread multinucleate cells [53].

6. Scoring MN in mononucleated cells in cytokinesis-blocked cultures may add an additional parameter in the CBMN assay when aneugenic effects are suspected [53, 69]. Aneugenic compounds may induce mitotic slippage resulting in an increase of mononucleated cells with MN and almost no increase of MN in binucleated cells [53, 55]. Five hundred viable cells are scored to determine the frequency of cells with 1, 2, or more nuclei and calculate the cytokinesis-block proliferation index (CBPI) using the formula: CBPI $= ((M1) + 2. (M2) + 3. (M3))/N$; where M1–M3 represent the number of cells with one ($M1$), two ($M2$), and multi nuclei, and N is the total number of viable cells scored [52, 53, 70].
7. Criteria for selecting binucleated cells which can be scored for micronucleus frequency: The cytokinesis-blocked cells that may be scored for MN frequency should have the following characteristics:
   (a) The cells should be binucleated.
   (b) The two nuclei in a binucleated cell should have intact nuclear membranes and be situated within the same cytoplasmic boundary.
   (c) The two nuclei in a binucleated cell should be approximately equal in size, staining pattern and staining intensity.
   (d) The two nuclei within a BN cell may be attached by a fine nucleoplasmic bridge, which is no wider than one-fourth of the nuclear diameter.
   (e) The two main nuclei in a BN cell may touch but ideally should not overlap each other. A cell with two overlapping nuclei can be scored only if the nuclear boundaries of each nucleus are distinguishable.
   (f) The cytoplasmic boundary or membrane of a binucleated cell should be intact and clearly distinguishable from the cytoplasmic boundary of adjacent cells [70].
8. Criteria for scoring micronuclei: MN are morphologically identical to but smaller than nuclei. They also have the following characteristics:
   (a) The diameter of MN in human lymphocytes usually varies between 1/16th and one-third of the mean diameter of the main nuclei, which corresponds to 1/256th and one-ninth of the area of one of the main nuclei in a BN cell, respectively.

(b) MN are nonrefractile and they can therefore be readily distinguished from artifact such as staining particles.

(c) MN are not linked or connected to the main nuclei.

(d) MN may touch but not overlap the main nuclei and the micronuclear boundary should be distinguishable from the nuclear boundary.

(e) MN usually have the same staining intensity as the main nuclei, but occasionally staining may be more intense [70].

3.8 Micronucleus Assay in Human 3D Models

1. As commercial human 3D models are rather costly one may consider to first use a cell line for screening and then to test selected NMs only in 3D models.
2. At least three test concentrations that meet the acceptability criteria should be evaluated. If the maximum concentration is based on cytotoxicity, the highest concentration should aim to achieve 55 ± 5% cytotoxicity. Negative controls (i.e., tissues treated with the vehicle only that was used to disperse the NMs and that were processed in the same way as the treated tissues) should be included. Positive controls (e.g., Mitomycin C or MMS) are needed. The most critical point when using human 3D tissue models is to assure that a significant fraction of the cells is undergoing cell division, which might be difficult to achieve. Human 3D models consist of differentiated primary human cells and typically only a low number of cells are still dividing. Thus, it can be useful to test different cell culture media beforehand and to perform the cytokinesis-block micronucleus (CBMN) using cytochalasin B [53]. Cytochalasin B prevents separation of daughter cells after mitosis, leading to the formation of binucleated cells. Scoring then can be limited to cells that have gone through mitosis during or after treatment, which is in particular relevant for primary cells. However, cytochalasin B also inhibits endocytosis, which is an important cellular uptake mechanism favored by some NMs. Therefore, the cells need to be exposed to NMs several hours before adding cytochalasin B. According to our experience longer exposure times with NMs are needed in order to perform meaningful MN assays (i.e., 48–72 h). It also is advisable to carry out the treatments in the repeated dose system, i.e., at 0, 24 and 48 h. For treatment the NM dispersions are applied in small volumes (i.e., 30–60 μl) directly on top of the tissues. According to the manufacturer's instructions the medium has to be exchanged at specific time points (depending on the type of tissue used). However, when refeeding the tissues the fresh medium should always contain 3 μg/ml Cytochalasin B. After a total time period of 72 h the preparation of the tissues starts.
3. Cell isolation: After the treatment several washing steps are required. The tissues should be handled with a maximum

number of six models at a time. If more tissues have been treated, they should be treated with trypsin in several groups. It is important not to increase the number of tissues to be handled at the same time in order to maintain consistency of the resulting single cell suspensions.

4. Cell harvest of 3D models (EpiAirway™, EpiDerm™): Every 3D tissue is placed in a well of a 12-well plate containing 5 ml of dPBS (Ca^{2+}, Mg^{2+} free) for 5–15 min at room temperature. Then, dPBS is discarded and tissues are transferred into another 12-well plate and incubated in 5 ml of 0.1% EDTA for another 15 min. Then transfer the tissues into another 12-well plate with 1 ml warm (37 °C) trypsin-EDTA solution in each well, in addition put 0.5 ml of warm trypsin-EDTA solution inside each transwell insert (i.e., on top of each tissue). Place plate with the tissues in an incubator for 15 min (37 °C). A new 12-well plate containing 1 ml warm (37 °C) trypsin-EDTA solution is needed for the next step. Hold the insert over the new plate using tweezers. The model is then carefully separated from the membrane of the insert with a second pair of tweezers and placed into a well of the new 12-well plate. The membrane is rinsed with the trypsin-EDTA solution several times and can be discarded afterward. The last remaining adherent cells are separated from the stratum corneum by rinsing with trypsin-EDTA solution. In order to ensure that all cell aggregates are separated, the cell suspension is pipetted up and down several times. To inactivate the trypsin 1.0 ml of warm DMEM with 10% FBS added directly into the well.

5. Cell harvest of full skin models (EpiDerm FT™): Every full thickness skin tissue is placed in a well of a 6-well plate containing 5 ml of dPBS (Ca^{2+}, Mg^{2+} free) for 5—15 min at room temperature. Then, dPBS is discarded, each tissue is picked up from the insert and mechanically (i.e., using a pincette) the dermis is separated from the epidermis. Each part (i.e., epidermis and dermis) of each tissue is incubated in a 6-well plate in 2 ml 0.1% EDTA/PBS for 5 min at room temperature, then EDTA/PBS is removed and the tissues are incubated in 2 ml 0.25% trypsin (prewarmed at 37 °C) for 15 min at 37 °C. Thereafter, 1 ml of cold MEM with 10% FBS (or any other medium containing FBS, pure FBS also possible) is added to each well. In order to ensure that all cell aggregates are separated, the cell suspension is pipetted up and down several times and agitated in between (4–6 times). Cell suspensions are then filtrated through a 40 μm cell strainer, which is put on a 50 ml Falcon tube. The cell strainer is washed with 1.5 ml cold MEM with 10% FBS. Filtrates are centrifuged at 200 × *g* for 5 min, the supernatant is discarded and the remaining cell pellets are resuspended in 2.5 ml of DMEM with 10% FBS each. Store on ice.

6. Fixation and staining.

   Subsequently, an aliquot is taken and used for cell counting and vitality determination using a cell counter device (e.g., Multisizer III, Beckmann Coulter). To transfer the cells to the slides for evaluation, a cytospin device is used. Prepare the chambers for the slides und put them in the cytospin centrifuge. Add 50–200 μl of the cell suspension (containing ~30,000 cells) and spin for 5 min at 500 rpm. Air-dry the slides. However, different other techniques (e. g. hypotonic treatment and cell fixation before pipetting on slides) can be used instead to prepare the slides provided that high-quality cell preparations are obtained. The slides are then fixed in fresh methanol for 5 min, rinsed with tab water and stained for 15 min in 8% Giemsa solution. Rinse again with tab water and then air-dry the slides at an angle on a tray. The slides can be stored before analysis at room temperature in the dark even for years.

7. Evaluation, scoring, and analysis are done identical to the procedures described above.

3.9 Bhas42 Cell Transformation Assay

1. Experimental Design: The CTA consists of both an initiation (CTA-initiation) test and a promotion test (CTA-promotion). In the initiation assay the cells are treated with substances in the beginning of the growth phase with low cell density, whereas in the promotion assay the treatment is started at sub-confluence growth. The concentrations of the test substance may differ between the CTA-initiation and CTA-promotion experiments due to the difference in the cell amount used in the two assays. Both tests have two steps. In the first step a cell growth assay (CGA) is performed to select the correct doses for the CTA. The CGA is a cell viability experiment and a broad dose range is used. The second step is the cell transformation assay and a concurrent CGA is performed to verify the effects of the selected doses. In any case, CTA has to be performed with cells at low passage and the cells have to be passaged at confluence $\leq$70%. This is to prevent spontaneous transformation. Frozen working cell stocks are rapidly thawed and suspended in 10% FBS in DMEM/F12 (DF10F). The cultivation medium can be prepared with 5% or 10% FBS and streptomycin/penicillin is added (final concentration 100 U/ml penicillin, 100 μg/ml streptomycin). When the cells reach approximately 70% confluence, they are trypsinized and plated in 5% FBS in DMEM/F12 (DF5F). Freshly prepared, 2–3 passage cells derived from the cryopreserved cell working stocks are used for each transformation assay. However, cells at higher passages (within a maximum number of ten passages) can be used for dose finding. The procedure described below is adapted to 6-wells plates, but may also be performed on 96-well plates.

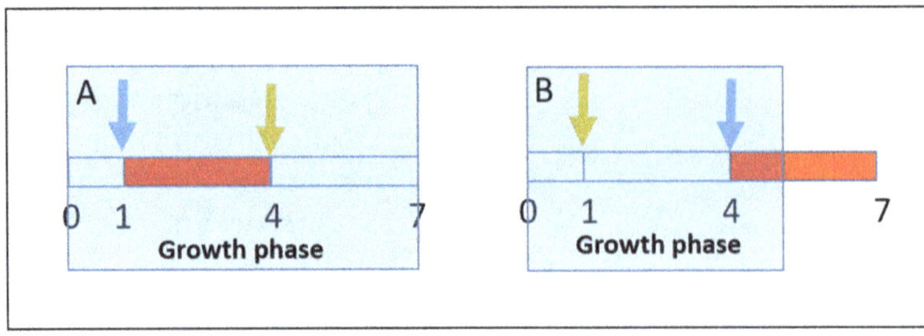

Fig. 5 CTA: Time lines for the CGA-initiation (**a**) and CGA-promotion (**b**). Cells are seeded with two different densities at day 0. Blue arrow and red box indicate chemical treatment; the yellow arrow indicates change into fresh medium. At day 7 the cells are prepared for cell viability experiment

2. Dose Finding-Cell Growth Assay (CGA):
   (a) Cells at a density of ≤70% confluence in DF5F are trypsinized and 4000 and 14,000 cells respectively are plated onto each well of a 6-well plate with 2 ml DF5F (Day 0).
   (b) After 20–24 h (Day 1), the culture medium of plates with 4000 cells (CGA-Initiation) is replaced with fresh medium containing different concentrations of the test substance. According to the OECD 2016 guidance document, final solvent concentrations of water, DMSO, acetone, and ethanol should not exceed 5%, 0.5%, 0.5%, and 0.1% respectively. However, we recommend a final DMSO concentration of 0.1% (if possible). Three wells are prepared for each concentration. The medium is changed with fresh medium on Day 4 (Fig. 5a).
   (c) On Day 4 the culture medium of plates with 14,000 cells (CGA-promotion) is replaced with fresh medium containing different concentrations of the test substance (Fig. 5b). On Day 7 the cultures are prepared for cell viability assay with AlamarBlue® or equivalent.
   (d) The assay is performed similar in 96-wells with some differences. In 96-wells plate, 200 cells are plated in each well with 0.05 ml DF5F for the CGA-initiation assay, and 400 cells are plated in each well with 0.1 ml DF5F for the CGA-promotion assay. At day 1, the cells prepared for the CGA-initiation are exposed by addition of 0.05 ml of medium containing the substances (final volume 0.1 ml). At day 4, the cells prepared for the CGA-promotion are exposed by addition of 0.1 ml of medium containing the substances (final volume 0.1 ml). Eight wells are prepared for each concentrations of test substance. Cell viability is measured by AlamarBlue® or equivalent with a final volume in each well of 0.1 ml.

3. Cell Transformation Assay: Based on the results from the CGA, five to nine concentrations are prepared for the CTA. These concentrations should cover a range from little toxicity to high toxicity. At least one concentration should be below nontoxic levels (80–120% cell growth), two concentrations between nontoxic levels and 50% inhibitory concentrations and two concentrations between 50% and 90% inhibition of cell growth. A factor of 3 between subsequent concentrations may be suggested, but will depend on the concentration—response curve. For both the CTA-initiation and CTA-promotion assay, one plate with six wells is prepared for each concentrations, and three wells are prepared for each concentration for the concurrent CGA.

3.9.1 CTA-Initiation Assay

1. At Day 0, 4000 cells are plated onto each well of 6-well plate at a volume of 2 ml for both CTA and the concurrent CGA.
2. Approximately 24 h later (20–24 h) after seeding (Day 1) the cells are exposed to the substance for three consecutive days (Day1–4). 3-methylcholantrene (MCA, 1 μg/ml in DMSO) can be used as a positive control for the CTA-initiation.
3. The medium is changed with fresh medium (DF5F) on Day 4, 7, 10 (or 11), and 14 (Fig. 6).
4. On day 7 the cultures for the CGA are prepared for cell viability assay as described above.
5. On day 21 the cells for the CTA are fixed with ethanol or methanol (1–2 ml) in at least 10 min and stained with 5% Giemsa solution (1–2 ml) for approximately 30 min. The cells may not be washed before Giemsa treatment. After Giemsa treatment, the cells are washed with ultrapure water. The timeline for the CTA-Initiation is shown in Fig. 6.
6. The assay is performed similar in 96-wells with some differences. In 96-well plate, 200 cells are plated in each well with

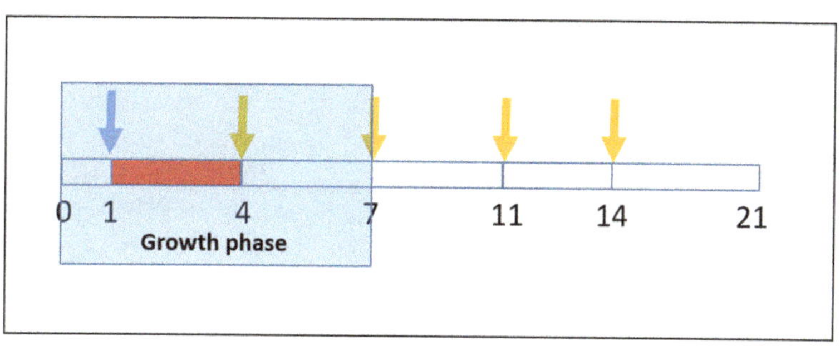

Fig. 6 CTA: Time line for the CTA-initiation test. Cells are seeded at day 0. Blue arrow and red box indicate chemical (or nanomaterial) treatment; yellow arrows indicate change into fresh medium. At day 21 the cells are fixed and stained

0.05 ml DF5F. At day 1, the cells are exposed by addition of 0.05 ml of medium containing the substances (final volume 0.1 ml). One plate is prepared for each concentration for the CTA, whereas eight wells are prepared for each concentration for the concurrent CGA.

3.9.2 CTA-Promotion Assay

1. At Day 0, 14,000 cells are plated onto each well of 6-well plates at a volume of 2 ml for both CTA and the concurrent CGA.
2. On Day 4 the cells are exposed to the substance. 12-O-tetradecanoylphorbol-13-acetate (TPA, 50 ng/ml in DMSO) can be used as a positive control for the CTA-promotion.
3. On day 7 the cultures for the cell growth assay are prepared for cell viability assay as described above.
4. The medium is changed with fresh medium (DF5F) containing the substance on Day 7 and 10 (or 11).
5. On day 14 the treatment medium is replaced with fresh medium (DF5F).
6. On day 21 the cells for the transformation assay are fixed with ethanol or methanol (1–2 ml) for at least 10 min and stained with 5% Giemsa solution (1–2 ml) for approximately 30 min. The cells may not be washed before Giemsa treatment. After Giemsa treatment, the cells are washed with ultrapure water. The timeline for the CTA-Promotion is shown in Fig. 7.
7. The assay is performed similarly in 96-wells with some differences. In 96-well plate, 400 cells are plated in each well with 0.1 ml DF5F. At day 4, the cells are exposed by addition of 0.1 ml of medium containing the substances (final volume 0.1 ml). One plate is prepared for each concentration for the CTA, whereas eight wells are prepared for each concentration for the concurrent CGA.

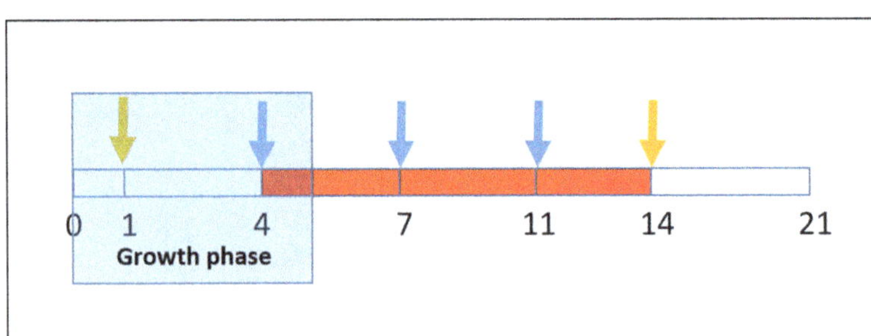

Fig. 7 CTA: Time line for the CTA-promotion test. Cells are seeded at day 0. Blue arrows and red boxes indicate chemical treatment, yellow arrows indicate change into fresh medium. At day 21 the cells are fixed and stained

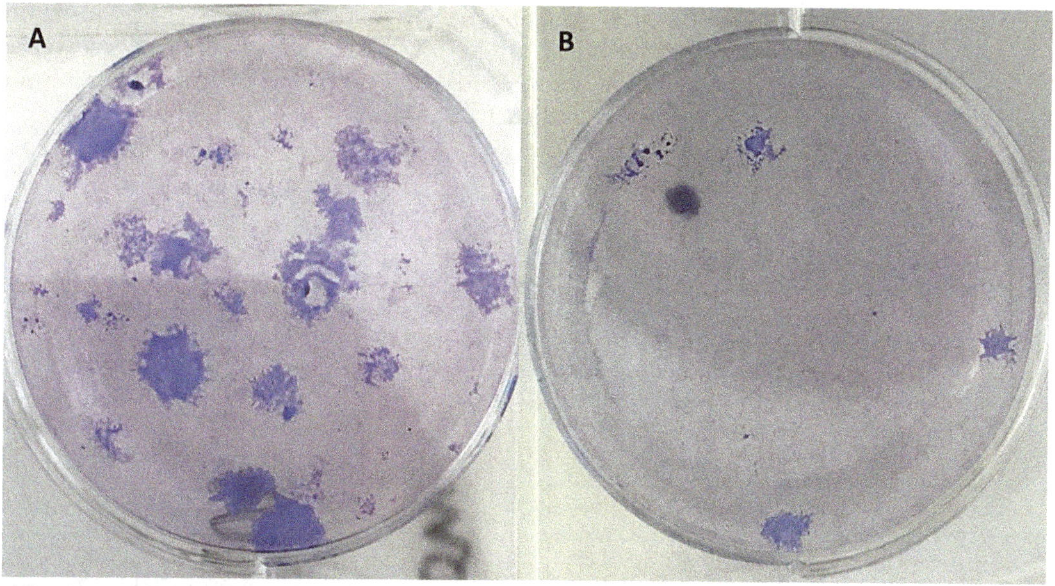

Fig. 8 CTA: Stained well of (**a**) TPA-treated cells and (**b**) control cells from a CTA-promotion experiment

3.9.3 Determination of the Transformation Frequency

1. Transformation frequency is expressed as the number of transformed foci per well. Transformed foci are counted visually under a microscope and can be viewed as shown in Fig. 8. Transformed foci have different morphological characteristics: (a) more than 100 cells, (b) spindle-shaped cells, (c) deep basophilic staining, (d) criss-cross, (e) piling up, and (f) invasive growth into the monolayer of surrounding contact-inhibited cells. Not all transformed foci have these characteristics and some subjective judgment must be considered. For the solvent control, the number of transformed foci must be ≤ 10 per well in the initiation test and ≤ 12 per well in the promotion test. The reason why the acceptability criteria for spontaneous transformation is different in the initiation and promotion assays is that a higher density of plated cells (as is used in the promotion test) increases the spontaneous transformation frequency. (For 96-wells: In 96-wells each well with one focus or more, is counted as one. For the solvent control, the number of transformed foci must be ≤ 15 per plate in the initiation test and ≤ 20 per well in the promotion test.) The positive control must have a statistically significant increase in the transformation incidence compared to the corresponding negative control. The transformation frequency is statistically determined from the relative increase in the number of morphologically transformed foci observed in the treated group compared to the number of foci appearing in the solvent controls. After scoring foci, averages are calculated and results are

assessed by an appropriate statistical analysis. For in-depth information about interpretation of the result and acceptance criteria for the method, we recommend the work by [61] and the OECD guidance document published in 2016.

References

1. Committee ES (2011) Scientific opinion on genotoxicity testing strategies applicable to food and feed safety assessment. EFSA J 9 (9):2379. https://doi.org/10.2903/j.efsa.2011.2379
2. Adler S, Basketter D, Creton S, Pelkonen O, van Benthem J, Zuang V, Andersen KE, Angers-Loustau A, Aptula A, Bal-Price A, Benfenati E, Bernauer U, Bessems J, Bois FY, Boobis A, Brandon E, Bremer S, Broschard T, Casati S, Coecke S, Corvi R, Cronin M, Daston G, Dekant W, Felter S, Grignard E, Gundert-Remy U, Heinonen T, Kimber I, Kleinjans J, Komulainen H, Kreiling R, Kreysa J, Leite SB, Loizou G, Maxwell G, Mazzatorta P, Munn S, Pfuhler S, Phrakonkham P, Piersma A, Poth A, Prieto P, Repetto G, Rogiers V, Schoeters G, Schwarz M, Serafimova R, Tahti H, Testai E, van Delft J, van Loveren H, Vinken M, Worth A, Zaldivar JM (2011) Alternative (non-animal) methods for cosmetics testing: current status and future prospects—2010. Arch Toxicol 85(5):367–485. https://doi.org/10.1007/s00204-011-0693-2
3. Kirkland D, Pfuhler S, Tweats D, Aardema M, Corvi R, Darroudi F, Elhajouji A, Glatt H, Hastwell P, Hayashi M, Kasper P, Kirchner S, Lynch A, Marzin D, Maurici D, Meunier JR, Muller L, Nohynek G, Parry J, Parry E, Thybaud V, Tice R, van Benthem J, Vanparys P, White P (2007) How to reduce false positive results when undertaking in vitro genotoxicity testing and thus avoid unnecessary follow-up animal tests: report of an ECVAM workshop. Mutat Res 628(1):31–55. https://doi.org/10.1016/j.mrgentox.2006.11.008
4. Oesch F, Landsiedel R (2012) Genotoxicity investigations on nanomaterials. Arch Toxicol 86(7):985–994. https://doi.org/10.1007/s00204-012-0838-y
5. Pfuhler S, Elespuru R, Aardema MJ, Doak SH, Maria Donner E, Honma M, Kirsch-Volders M, Landsiedel R, Manjanatha M, Singer T, Kim JH (2013) Genotoxicity of nanomaterials: refining strategies and tests for hazard identification. Environ Mol Mutagen 54(4):229–239. https://doi.org/10.1002/em.21770
6. Warheit DB, Donner EM (2010) Rationale of genotoxicity testing of nanomaterials: regulatory requirements and appropriateness of available OECD test guidelines. Nanotoxicology 4:409–413. https://doi.org/10.3109/17435390.2010.485704
7. OECD (2014) Genotoxicity of manufactured nanomaterials: report of the OECD expert meeting (ENV/JM/MONO(2014)34). http://www.oecd.org/officialdocuments/publicdisplaydocumentpdf/?cote=env/jm/mono(2014)34&doclanguage=en
8. ECHA (2017) Appendix R7-1 for nanomaterials applicable to Chapter R7a—Endpoint specific guidance, v. 2.0, May 2017. https://echa.europa.eu/documents/10162/13632/appendix_r7a_nanomaterials_en.pdf
9. Donaldson K, Poland CA, Schins RP (2010) Possible genotoxic mechanisms of nanoparticles: criteria for improved test strategies. Nanotoxicology 4:414–420. https://doi.org/10.3109/17435390.2010.482751
10. Sood A, Salih S, Roh D, Lacharme-Lora L, Parry M, Hardiman B, Keehan R, Grummer R, Winterhager E, Gokhale PJ, Andrews PW, Abbott C, Forbes K, Westwood M, Aplin JD, Ingham E, Papageorgiou I, Berry M, Liu J, Dick AD, Garland RJ, Williams N, Singh R, Simon AK, Lewis M, Ham J, Roger L, Baird DM, Crompton LA, Caldwell MA, Swalwell H, Birch-Machin M, Lopez-Castejon G, Randall A, Lin H, Suleiman MS, Evans WH, Newson R, Case CP (2011) Signalling of DNA damage and cytokines across cell barriers exposed to nanoparticles depends on barrier thickness. Nat Nanotechnol 6(12):824–833. https://doi.org/10.1038/nnano.2011.188
11. Magdolenova Z, Collins A, Kumar A, Dhawan A, Stone V, Dusinska M (2014) Mechanisms of genotoxicity. A review of in vitro and in vivo studies with engineered nanoparticles. Nanotoxicology 8(3):233–278. https://doi.org/10.3109/17435390.2013.773464
12. Doak SH, Dusinska M (2017) NanoGenotoxicology: present and the future. Mutagenesis 32(1):1–4. https://doi.org/10.1093/mutage/gew066
13. Sayes CM, Reed KL, Subramoney S, Abrams L, Warheit DB (2009) Can in vitro assays substitute for in vivo studies in assessing the pulmonary hazards of fine and nanoscale materials. J

Nanopart Res 11(2):421–431. https://doi.org/10.1007/s11051-008-9471-3

14. Ahmed SA, Gogal RM Jr, Walsh JE (1994) A new rapid and simple non-radioactive assay to monitor and determine the proliferation of lymphocytes: an alternative to [3H]thymidine incorporation assay. J Immunol Methods 170 (2):211–224
15. Kroll A, Pillukat MH, Hahn D, Schnekenburger J (2012) Interference of engineered nanoparticles with in vitro toxicity assays. Arch Toxicol 86(7):1123–1136. https://doi.org/10.1007/s00204-012-0837-z
16. Ponti J, Kinser-Ovaskainen A, Norlen H, Altmeyer S, Andreoli C, Bogni A, Chevillard S, De Angelis I, Chung S-T, Eom I, al. e (2014) Interlaboratory comparison study of the Colony Forming Efficiency assay for assessing cytotoxicity of nanomaterials. JRC Sci Policy Rep (JRC92910). doi: https://doi.org/10.2788/406937
17. Coradeghini R, Gioria S, Garcia CP, Nativo P, Franchini F, Gilliland D, Ponti J, Rossi F (2013) Size-dependent toxicity and cell interaction mechanisms of gold nanoparticles on mouse fibroblasts. Toxicol Lett 217 (3):205–216. https://doi.org/10.1016/j.toxlet.2012.11.022
18. Locatelli E, Broggi F, Ponti J, Marmorato P, Franchini F, Lena S, Franchini MC (2012) Lipophilic silver nanoparticles and their polymeric entrapment into targeted-PEG-based micelles for the treatment of glioblastoma. Adv Healthc Mater 1(3):342–347. https://doi.org/10.1002/adhm.201100047
19. El Yamani N, Collins AR, Runden-Pran E, Fjellsbo LM, Shaposhnikov S, Zienolddiny S, Dusinska M (2017) In vitro genotoxicity testing of four reference metal nanomaterials, titanium dioxide, zinc oxide, cerium oxide and silver: towards reliable hazard assessment. Mutagenesis 32(1):117–126. https://doi.org/10.1093/mutage/gew060
20. De Angelis I, Barone F, Zijno A, Bizzarri L, Russo MT, Pozzi R, Franchini F, Giudetti G, Uboldi C, Ponti J, Rossi F, De Berardis B (2013) Comparative study of ZnO and TiO (2) nanoparticles: physicochemical characterisation and toxicological effects on human colon carcinoma cells. Nanotoxicology 7 (8):1361–1372. https://doi.org/10.3109/17435390.2012.741724
21. Fenoglio I, Ponti J, Alloa E, Ghiazza M, Corazzari I, Capomaccio R, Rembges D, Oliaro-Bosso S, Rossi F (2013) Singlet oxygen plays a key role in the toxicity and DNA damage caused by nanometric TiO2 in human keratinocytes. Nanoscale 5(14):6567–6576. https://doi.org/10.1039/c3nr01191g
22. Uboldi C, Giudetti G, Broggi F, Gilliland D, Ponti J, Rossi F (2012) Amorphous silica nanoparticles do not induce cytotoxicity, cell transformation or genotoxicity in Balb/3T3 mouse fibroblasts. Mutat Res 745(1–2):11–20. https://doi.org/10.1016/j.mrgentox.2011.10.010
23. Ponti J, Colognato R, Rauscher H, Gioria S, Broggi F, Franchini F, Pascual C, Giudetti G, Rossi F (2010) Colony Forming Efficiency and microscopy analysis of multi-wall carbon nanotubes cell interaction. Toxicol Lett 197 (1):29–37. https://doi.org/10.1016/j.toxlet.2010.04.018
24. Haase A, Dommershausen N, Schulz M, Landsiedel R, Reichardt P, Krause BC, Tentschert J, Luch A (2017) Genotoxicity testing of different surface-functionalized SiO2, ZrO2 and silver nanomaterials in 3D human bronchial models. Arch Toxicol 91 (12):3991–4007. https://doi.org/10.1007/s00204-017-2015-9
25. Riebeling C, Piret J-P, Trouiller B, Nelissen I, Saout C, Toussaint O, Haase A (2018) A guide to nanosafety testing: Considerations on cytotoxicity testing in different cell models. NanoImpact 10:1–10. https://doi.org/10.1016/j.impact.2017.11.004
26. Siegrist KJ, Reynolds SH, Kashon ML, Lowry DT, Dong C, Hubbs AF, Young SH, Salisbury JL, Porter DW, Benkovic SA, McCawley M, Keane MJ, Mastovich JT, Bunker KL, Cena LG, Sparrow MC, Sturgeon JL, Dinu CZ, Sargent LM (2014) Genotoxicity of multi-walled carbon nanotubes at occupationally relevant doses. Part Fibre Toxicol 11:6. https://doi.org/10.1186/1743-8977-11-6
27. OECD (1997) Test no. 471: bacterial reverse mutation test. OECD, Paris
28. Doak SH, Manshian B, Jenkins GJ, Singh N (2012) In vitro genotoxicity testing strategy for nanomaterials and the adaptation of current OECD guidelines. Mutat Res 745 (1–2):104–111. https://doi.org/10.1016/j.mrgentox.2011.09.013
29. Wang JJ, Sanderson BJ, Wang H (2007) Cyto- and genotoxicity of ultrafine TiO2 particles in cultured human lymphoblastoid cells. Mutat Res 628(2):99–106. https://doi.org/10.1016/j.mrgentox.2006.12.003
30. Huk A, Izak-Nau E, Reidy B, Boyles M, Duschl A, Lynch I, Dusinska M (2014) Is the toxic potential of nanosilver dependent on its size? Part Fibre Toxicol 11:65. https://doi.org/10.1186/s12989-014-0065-1

31. Huk A, Izak-Nau E, El Yamani N, Uggerud H, Vadset M, Zasonska B, Duschl A, Dusinska M (2015) Impact of nanosilver on various DNA lesions and HPRT gene mutations—effects of charge and surface coating. Part Fibre Toxicol 12:25. https://doi.org/10.1186/s12989-015-0100-x
32. Gabelova A, El Yamani N, Alonso TI, Buliakova B, Srancikova A, Babelova A, Pran ER, Fjellsbo LM, Elje E, Yazdani M, Silva MJ, Dusinska M (2017) Fibrous shape underlies the mutagenic and carcinogenic potential of nanosilver while surface chemistry affects the biosafety of iron oxide nanoparticles. Mutagenesis 32(1):193–202. https://doi.org/10.1093/mutage/gew045
33. OECD. Test no. 476: in vitro mammalian cell gene mutation test. OECD, Paris
34. OECD. Test no. 490: in vitro mammalian cell gene mutation tests using the thymidine kinase gene. OECD, Paris
35. Moore MM, Honma M, Clements J, Awogi T, Bolcsfoldi G, Cole J, Gollapudi B, Harrington-Brock K, Mitchell A, Muster W, Myhr B, O'Donovan M, Ouldelhkim MC, San R, Shimada H, Stankowski LF Jr (2000) Mouse lymphoma thymidine kinase locus gene mutation assay: international workshop on genotoxicity test procedures workgroup report. Environ Mol Mutagen 35(3):185–190
36. Moore MM, Honma M, Clements J, Bolcsfoldi G, Burlinson B, Cifone M, Clarke J, Delongchamp R, Durward R, Fellows M, Gollapudi B, Hou S, Jenkinson P, Lloyd M, Majeska J, Myhr B, O'Donovan M, Omori T, Riach C, San R, Stankowski LF Jr, Thakur AK, Van Goethem F, Wakuri S, Yoshimura I (2006) Mouse lymphoma thymidine kinase gene mutation assay: follow-up meeting of the international workshop on genotoxicity testing—Aberdeen, Scotland, 2003—assay acceptance criteria, positive controls, and data evaluation. Environ Mol Mutagen 47(1):1–5. https://doi.org/10.1002/em.20159
37. Cheng TF, Patton GW, Muldoon-Jacobs K (2013) Can the L5178Y Tk+/− mouse lymphoma assay detect epigenetic silencing? Food and chemical toxicology: an international journal published for the. British Industrial Biological Research Association 59:187–190. https://doi.org/10.1016/j.fct.2013.06.007
38. Clements J (2000) The mouse lymphoma assay. Mutat Res 455(1–2):97–110
39. Cowie H, Magdolenova Z, Saunders M, Drlickova M, Correia Carreira S, Halamoda Kenzaoi B, Gombau L, Guadagnini R, Lorenzo Y, Walker L, Fjellsbo LM, Huk A, Rinna A, Tran L, Volkovova K, Boland S, Juillerat-Jeanneret L, Marano F, Collins AR, Dusinska M (2015) Suitability of human and mammalian cells of different origin for the assessment of genotoxicity of metal and polymeric engineered nanoparticles. Nanotoxicology 9(Suppl 1):57–65. https://doi.org/10.3109/17435390.2014.940407
40. Collins A, El Yamani N, Dusinska M (2017) Sensitive detection of DNA oxidation damage induced by nanomaterials. Free Radic Biol Med 107:69–76. https://doi.org/10.1016/j.freeradbiomed.2017.02.001
41. Dusinska M (1996) Detection of oxidised purines and UV induced photoproducts in DNA of single cells, by inclusion of lesion-specific enzymes in the comet assay. Alternat Lab Anim 24:405–411
42. OECD. Test no. 489: in vivo mammalian alkaline comet assay. OECD, Paris
43. Aardema MJ, Barnett BC, Khambatta Z, Reisinger K, Ouedraogo-Arras G, Faquet B, Ginestet AC, Mun GC, Dahl EL, Hewitt NJ, Corvi R, Curren RD (2010) International prevalidation studies of the EpiDerm 3D human reconstructed skin micronucleus (RSMN) assay: transferability and reproducibility. Mutat Res 701(2):123–131. https://doi.org/10.1016/j.mrgentox.2010.05.017
44. Reus AA, Reisinger K, Downs TR, Carr GJ, Zeller A, Corvi R, Krul CA, Pfuhler S (2013) Comet assay in reconstructed 3D human epidermal skin models—investigation of intra- and inter-laboratory reproducibility with coded chemicals. Mutagenesis 28 (6):709–720. https://doi.org/10.1093/mutage/get051
45. Collins AR, Dusinska M, Gedik CM, Stetina R (1996) Oxidative damage to DNA: do we have a reliable biomarker? Environ Health Perspect 104(Suppl 3):465–469
46. Magdolenova Z, Lorenzo Y, Collins A, Dusinska M (2012) Can standard genotoxicity tests be applied to nanoparticles? J Toxicol Environ Health A 75(13–15):800–806. https://doi.org/10.1080/15287394.2012.690326
47. Karlsson HL, Di Bucchianico S, Collins AR, Dusinska M (2015) Can the comet assay be used reliably to detect nanoparticle-induced genotoxicity? Environ Mol Mutagen 56 (2):82–96. https://doi.org/10.1002/em.21933
48. Azqueta A, Dusinska M (2015) The use of the comet assay for the evaluation of the genotoxicity of nanomaterials. Front Genet 6:239. https://doi.org/10.3389/fgene.2015.00239

49. Karlsson HL (2010) The comet assay in nanotoxicology research. Anal Bioanal Chem 398 (2):651–666. https://doi.org/10.1007/s00216-010-3977-0
50. Collins AR, Annangi B, Rubio L, Marcos R, Dorn M, Merker C, Estrela-Lopis I, Cimpan MR, Ibrahim M, Cimpan E, Ostermann M, Sauter A, Yamani NE, Shaposhnikov S, Chevillard S, Paget V, Grall R, Delic J, de-Cerio FG, Suarez-Merino B, Fessard V, Hogeveen KN, Fjellsbo LM, Pran ER, Brzicova T, Topinka J, Silva MJ, Leite PE, Ribeiro AR, Granjeiro JM, Grafstrom R, Prina-Mello A, Dusinska M (2017) High throughput toxicity screening and intracellular detection of nanomaterials. Wiley Interdiscip Rev Nanomed Nanobiotechnol 9(1). https://doi.org/10.1002/wnan.1413
51. Final Report NanoGenoTox (2013) https://www.anses.fr/en/content/nanogenotox-final-report
52. Fenech M (2000) The in vitro micronucleus technique. Mutat Res 455(1–2):81–95
53. OECD. Test no. 487: in vitro mammalian cell micronucleus test. OECD, Paris
54. Fenech M, Morley A (1985) Solutions to the kinetic problem in the micronucleus assay. Cytobios 43(172–173):233–246
55. Gonzalez L, Sanderson BJ, Kirsch-Volders M (2011) Adaptations of the in vitro MN assay for the genotoxicity assessment of nanomaterials. Mutagenesis 26(1):185–191. https://doi.org/10.1093/mutage/geq088
56. Dahl EL, Curren R, Barnett BC, Khambatta Z, Reisinger K, Ouedraogo G, Faquet B, Ginestet AC, Mun G, Hewitt NJ, Carr G, Pfuhler S, Aardema MJ (2011) The reconstructed skin micronucleus assay (RSMN) in EpiDerm: detailed protocol and harmonized scoring atlas. Mutat Res 720(1–2):42–52. https://doi.org/10.1016/j.mrgentox.2010.12.001
57. Wolf T, Niehaus-Rolf C, Banduhn N, Eschrich D, Scheel J, Luepke NP (2008) The hen's egg test for micronucleus induction (HET-MN): novel analyses with a series of well-characterized substances support the further evaluation of the test system. Mutat Res 650(2):150–164. https://doi.org/10.1016/j.mrgentox.2007.11.009
58. Hothorn LA, Reisinger K, Wolf T, Poth A, Fieblinger D, Liebsch M, Pirow R (2013) Statistical analysis of the hen's egg test for micronucleus induction (HET-MN assay). Mutat Res 757(1):68–78. https://doi.org/10.1016/j.mrgentox.2013.04.023
59. Dusinska M, Tulinska J, El Yamani N, Kuricova M, Liskova A, Rollerova E, Runden-Pran E, Smolkova B (2017) Immunotoxicity, genotoxicity and epigenetic toxicity of nanomaterials: New strategies for toxicity testing? Food and chemical toxicology : an international journal published for the British Industrial. Biol Res Assoc 109(Pt 1):797–811. https://doi.org/10.1016/j.fct.2017.08.030
60. Sasaki K, Mizusawa H, Ishidate M (1988) Isolation and characterization of ras-transfected BALB/3T3 clone showing morphological transformation by 12-O-tetradecanoyl-phorbol-13-acetate. Jpn J Cancer Res 79 (8):921–930
61. Sasaki K, Umeda M, Sakai A, Yamazaki S, Tanaka N (2015) Transformation assay in Bhas 42 cells: a model using initiated cells to study mechanisms of carcinogenesis and predict carcinogenic potential of chemicals. J Environ Sci Health C Environ Carcinogen Ecotoxicol Rev 33(1):1–35. https://doi.org/10.1080/10590501.2014.967058
62. Al-Nasiry S, Geusens N, Hanssens M, Luyten C, Pijnenborg R (2007) The use of Alamar Blue assay for quantitative analysis of viability, migration and invasion of choriocarcinoma cells. Hum Reprod 22(5):1304–1309. https://doi.org/10.1093/humrep/dem011
63. Lloyd M, Kidd D (2012) The mouse lymphoma assay. In: Parry JM, Parry EM (eds) Genetic toxicology: principles and methods. Humana, New York, NY, pp 35–54
64. Lovell DP, Omori T (2008) Statistical issues in the use of the comet assay. Mutagenesis 23 (3):171–182. https://doi.org/10.1093/mutage/gen015
65. Bright J, Aylott M, Bate S, Geys H, Jarvis P, Saul J, Vonk R (2011) Recommendations on the statistical analysis of the comet assay. Pharm Stat 10(6):485–493. https://doi.org/10.1002/pst.530
66. Doak SH, Griffiths SM, Manshian B, Singh N, Williams PM, Brown AP, Jenkins GJ (2009) Confounding experimental considerations in nanogenotoxicology. Mutagenesis 24 (4):285–293. https://doi.org/10.1093/mutage/gep010
67. Prasad RY, Wallace K, Daniel KM, Tennant AH, Zucker RM, Strickland J, Dreher K, Kligerman AD, Blackman CF, Demarini DM (2013) Effect of treatment media on the agglomeration of titanium dioxide nanoparticles: impact on genotoxicity, cellular interaction, and cell cycle. ACS Nano 7 (3):1929–1942. https://doi.org/10.1021/nn302280n
68. Li Y, Doak SH, Yan J, Chen DH, Zhou M, Mittelstaedt RA, Chen Y, Li C, Chen T (2017) Factors affecting the in vitro micronucleus

assay for evaluation of nanomaterials. Mutagenesis 32(1):151–159. https://doi.org/10.1093/mutage/gew040

69. Elhajouji A, Cunha M, Kirsch-Volders M (1998) Spindle poisons can induce polyploidy by mitotic slippage and micronucleate mononucleates in the cytokinesis-block assay. Mutagenesis 13(2):193–198

70. Fenech M, Chang WP, Kirsch-Volders M, Holland N, Bonassi S, Zeiger E (2003) HUMN project: detailed description of the scoring criteria for the cytokinesis-block micronucleus assay using isolated human lymphocyte cultures. Mutat Res 534(1–2):65–75

Chapter 7

Measurement of Nanoparticle-Induced Mitochondrial Membrane Potential Alterations

Salik Hussain

Abstract

Mitochondria hold a critical role in cell metabolism and homeostasis. Mitochondrial injury plays central part in deciding cell fate especially in programmed cell death pathways. Various nanomaterials lead to different cell death modalities by inducing mitochondrial injury. Mitochondrial injury is manifested as multiple biochemical events ranging from altered energy production, mitochondrial outer membrane permeability, release of pro-apoptotic BCl-2 family proteins, loss of mitochondrial inner membrane potential, mitochondrial swelling, and disruption of mitochondrial structure leading to eventual lysis of mitochondria. Mitochondrial membrane permeability (loss of mitochondrial membrane potential) is a critical event in deciding cell fate. This chapter presents an overview of nanomaterial-induced loss of mitochondrial membrane potential and discusses potential nano-specific artifacts in these assays. Finally, a detailed methodology to accurately quantify and validate the loss of mitochondrial membrane potential after nanomaterial exposures is presented.

Key words Mitochondria, Apoptosis, Nanomaterials, Membrane potential, Flow cytometry, Immunocytochemistry

1 Introduction

Cell death mechanisms are crucial not only in deciding the fate of cells but also in maintaining the ability of the body to respond appropriately to the environmental injury. Cell death modalities are critical element of multiple human pathologies like cancer, cardiovascular diseases, neurodegeneration, pulmonary and autoimmune disorders [1–4]. Surprisingly, these mechanisms are often overlooked in terms of their homeostatic potentials. Programmed or regulated cell death offers significant advantages in maintaining homeostasis in health as well as disease conditions. It acts as a measure to control the exuberant injury induced by the exogenous or endogenous stimuli by removing the dead and dying cells in a controlled fashion as and also perform important functions of alerting immune system by controlling the release of alarmins/

Qunwei Zhang (ed.), *Nanotoxicity: Methods and Protocols*, Methods in Molecular Biology, vol. 1894,
https://doi.org/10.1007/978-1-4939-8916-4_7,

danger associated molecular patterns from dying cells. Cell death manifests as both cellular as well as organelle level changes that in many instances are tightly controlled (in regulated cell death modalities), represent ongoing biochemical processes, and indicate particular phase of cell death pathway. Mitochondrial injury plays a central role in majority of the cell death routines (especially the programmed cell death pathways). Mitochondrial injury is manifested as multiple biochemical events ranging from altered energy production, mitochondrial outer membrane permeability, release of proapoptotic BCl-2 family proteins, loss of mitochondrial inner membrane potential, mitochondrial swelling, and disruption of mitochondrial structure leading to eventual lysis of mitochondria.

Engineered nanomaterials present significant advantages in multiple sectors of daily life and are gaining increasing biomedical applications. These potential applications increase the possibilities of human exposures and thus warrant a deeper understanding of how nanomaterials can influence organismal and cellular function. It is a now a well-known fact that engineered nanomaterials can induce cell injury through multiple pathways after accidental and/intentional exposures. These cell death modalities include both programmed/regulated cell death pathways as well as accidental cellular demise. Within the past decade and a half, a significant number of publications described the interactions of nanomaterials with biological systems; however, mechanistic understanding of nano–bio interactions is still rudimentary.

Multiple engineered nanomaterials target mitochondria and this property is of significant use in delivering drugs especially in cases of chemotherapy resistance cancers [5–9]. However, environmental and/or occupational exposures to multiple nanomaterials also provoke sustained mitochondrial injury leading to cell death [10–16]. Majority of these publications employed a variety of methods to study the impact of various nanoparticles with mitochondria. These methods range from plate reader based assays to flow cytometry and immunostaining. While majority of the methods that are developed for chemicals can be used for studying nanomaterial-induced effects, a special attention is warranted to avoid potential artifacts.

Mitochondrial membrane potential ($\Delta\Psi m$) or specifically inner mitochondrial membrane potential is a sensitive indicator of mitochondrial injury and mostly represents an early event in the mitochondrial/intrinsic cell death pathway. It is indispensable for maintaining the physiological ATP generation by the electron transport chain and a significant loss of $\Delta\Psi m$ causes energy depletion and cell death. Loss of $\Delta\Psi m$ may occur due to opening of the so-called "permeability transition pore complex" (PTPC). PTPC is a supramolecular complex assembled at the junction of outer and inner mitochondrial membranes [17, 18]. It is still unclear which the components of this PTPC are and how it is regulated [19].

Cellular energy production at the mitochondria level generates strong proton gradient, which is responsible for ΔΨm. When cell enters apoptosis this there is loss of energy production, which leads to a decrease in ΔΨm. Majority of the commercially available probes for ΔΨm are lipophilic cationic chemicals that are sometimes termed as redistribution dyes. These compounds accumulate in mitochondrial matrix according to their charge and solubility. Cell permeable dyes such as MitoTrackers® are an effective mean of measuring mitochondrial health by relying on mildly thiol reactive chloromethyl moiety. These dyes offer an additional advantage in terms of ability to withstand aldehyde fixation. This chapter presents a strategy for accurate quantification of number of cells demonstrating a loss of ΔΨm after nanomaterial exposure using Mitotracker® based dye (CMXRos®).

2 Materials

2.1 Cell Culture

1. Human Bronchial Epithelial Cells:
   (a) 16HBE14o- cell line: Immortalized primary human bronchial epithelial cells (16HBE140-) were a kind gift from Dr. C. Grunert (Vermont University Colchester) [20].
   (b) Primary Human Bronchial Epithelial cells (NHBE): These cells were purchased from Lonza (Basel, Switzerland) and were maintained in the recommended Bronchial Epithelial Growth Medium (BEGM) media.
2. Growth Media Preparation:
   (a) 16HBE cells growth medium—DMEM/F12 (Dulbecco Modified Eagle Medium Nutrient Mix F-12 (Gibco, Gaithersburg, MD) was supplemented with 10% fetal calf serum (Sigma St. Louis, MO), 100 μg/mL penicillin and 100 μg/mL streptomycin (Sigma St. Louis, MO) agents, and 1% glutamine (Sigma St. Louis, MO). Growth media was prepared fresh for each media change and reagents were stored at appropriate storage conditions.
   (b) NHBE growth medium—These cells were cultivated in bronchial epithelial basal medium (BEBM) supplemented with 10 μg/mL transferrin, 0.5 μg/mL epinephrine, 5 μg/mL insulin, 0.5 ng/mL hEGF, 6.5 ng/mL triiodothyronine, 0.5 μg/mL hydrocortisone, 50 μg/mL gentamycin, 50 μg/mL amphotericin B, 0.13 mg/mL bovine pituitary extract (all supplied by Lonza). Culture conditions were similar between 16HBe and NHBE cells. All the experiments were performed between passage 1 and 5 (*see* **Note 1**).

2.2 Nanomaterials

Nanoparticles of amorphous carbon black (FW2) were purchased from Evonik (formerly Degussa, Frankfurt, Germany). These particles were extensively characterized for impurities, size distribution, zeta potential, surface area, and morphology, and these data have been reported previously [12, 21, 22]. In brief, these particles are 23 ± 6 nm in diameter, had 350 m^2/g specific surface area, and exhibited 253 nm hydrodynamic diameter in exposure media. Stock solution of the nanomaterials was made at a concentration of 2 mg/mL cell culture media and stored at −20 °C till further use. Before use in experiments, sonicated three times for 20 s each at 60 kW with the help of an ultrasonic probe (Ultrasonic Processor, Bioblock Scientific) equipped with a cup horn accessory. Particles added to the cells within 3 min of sonication.

2.3 MitoTracker® Red (CMXRos)

CMXRos (Chloromethyl Xarosamine, $C_{32}H_{32}Cl_2N_2O$) purchased from molecular probes. Stock suspension made by dissolving in cell culture grade, anhydrous dimethylsulfoxide (DMSO) (Sigma St. Louis, MO) to a final concentration of 1 mM. Stock suspension was stored at −20 °C and thawed on ice before labeling.

2.4 Phosphate Buffer Saline (PBS)

Phosphate Buffer Saline (PBS) (Life Technologies, Carlsbad, CA).

2.5 Trypsin-EDTA

Trypsin (0.05%)-EDTA (ThermoFisher Scientific, Waltham, MA).

2.6 Hydrogen Peroxide (H_2O_2)

Hydrogen peroxide (H_2O_2) (Sigma, St. Louis, MO).

2.7 Carbonyl Cyanide 4-(Trifluoromethoxy) phenylhydrazone (FCCP)

Carbonyl cyanide 4-(trifluoromethoxy)phenylhydrazone (FCCP) (Sigma, St. Louis, MO).

2.8 12-Well Cell Culture Plates and Polystyrene Tubes with Cell Strainer Snap Cap

12-Well Cell Culture Plates and polystyrene tubes with cell strainer snap cap (Corning, Tewksbury, MA).

2.9 Forma™ Series II Water-Jacketed CO_2 Incubators

Forma™ Series II Water-Jacketed CO_2 Incubators (ThermoFisher Scientific, Waltham, MA).

2.10 Catalase and Peg-Catalase

Catalase and Peg-Catalase (Sigma, St. Louis, MO).

2.11 CyAn ADP LX

CyAn ADP LX (Dako Cytomation, Beckman Coulter, Villepinte, France).

3 Methods

3.1 Cell Culture and Nanoparticle Exposure

1. Grow16HBE14o- cells either in cell culture plates (12 well plates, 10,000 cells/cm^2). Growth conditions were 37 °C temperature, 5%CO_2 concentration and pH 7.4 for 48 h.
2. Sonicate nanoparticles stocks and disperse in cell culture medium to deliver different doses of particles (5–80 μg/cm^2).

3.2 Positive and Negative Control Exposures

1. DMSO as vehicle control, 500 nm H_2O_2 or 10 μM FCCP as positive controls for loss of mitochondrial membrane potential.
2. Pretreated cells with 1000 I.U. of either catalase or polyethylene glycol catalase (increased cell penetration abilities) for 30 min and then treat with nanoparticles in the presence of these inhibitors of oxidative stress.

3.3 Labeling with CMXRos and Flow Analysis

1. At the end of desired incubation times (4 h), collect culture supernatants and in polystyrene tubes with cell strainer snap cap.
2. Wash cell layer gently with warm PBS and harvest cells by trypsin (*see* **Note 2**).
3. Block the activity of trypsin by adding 10% FBS, pool supernatant and cells and keep tube on ice.
4. Centrifuge at 400 × *g* for 5 min at 4 °C.
5. Discard the supernatant and resuspend cells gently in a prewarmed cell culture medium containing 150 nm of CMXros.
6. Incubate cells for optimal duration for labeling (depending upon cells). For 16HBE 14o- cells 20 min is sufficient and for NHBE cells 25 min is recommended.
7. Proceed to flow analysis and record at least 10,000 cells at 488 nm excitation and 615 nm emission wavelength. Carefully draw flow gates to eliminate debris but still taking into account the scatter changes induced by particles. Figure 1 shows typical flowcharts. (*See* **Notes 3–8**).

4 Notes

1. Many cell lines have altered energy production and mitochondrial function and where possible the measurement of mitochondrial function should be performed/validated using primary representing more physiologically relevant model.

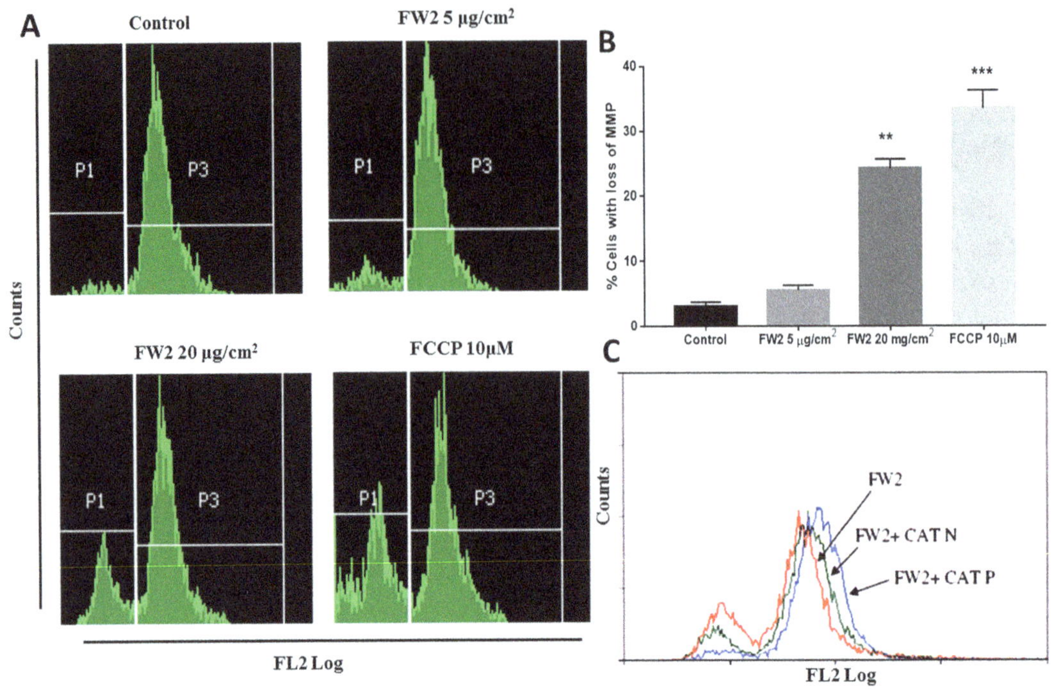

Fig. 1 Measurement of ΔΨm after carbon black nanoparticle exposure in human bronchial epithelial cells. Human bronchial epithelial cells treated with CB nanoparticles (5 or 20 μg/cm^2 for 4 h, labeled with CMXRos dye and analyzed by flow cytometry. (**a**) Flowcharts of labeled cells two distinct populations P1(cells with low ΔΨm) and P3(cells with normal ΔΨm). (**b**) Graphic representation of the results and statistical analyses performed using Graphpad Prism software. Control represents cells with DMSO and FCCP as positive control. (**c**) Demonstration of effective modulation of MMP by using pharmacological agents. Overlay charts of cells treated with either FW2 alone, with regular catalase (CAT N), or with peg-catalase (CAT-P)

2. Do not overtrypsinize cells as it may cause changes in membrane structure and potentials. It is important to observe cells every minute while they are in trypsin.
3. Nanomaterials can pose significant challenges with these chemicals by either interacting with the dye or interfering with the fluorescence measurements. The interaction with the dye can be unanticipated. Nanomaterials (owing to their large available surface area) can bind the dye and make it less available but can also lead to nonspecific accumulation in either mitochondria or lysosomes (by acting as Trojan horse).
4. While it is possible to optimize one technique (e.g., flow cytometry and/or immunochemistry), it may not address all the potential confounding factors. It is recommended that immunochemistry must accompany flow cytometry measurements to visually validate the findings. In recent years imaging flow cytometers are increasingly used and thus can speed the process of visual assessment. However, this will not replace the need to use two independent assay reagents for assessing MMP.

5. In our experience, some nanomaterials specifically interfere particular wavelengths (majority of the commercially available probes are available in different wavelengths). It is recommended that a test for interference be conducted prior to full scale study.
6. The conditions described in the protocol's for $\Delta\Psi m$ measurement for chemicals are not always optimal for nanoparticle exposures. It is recommended that a dose response of dye concentration and time course of incubation time is performed with each nanomaterial being tested.
7. Nanoparticles cause changes in scatter properties of the cells and thus gating strategy must be optimized to account for these changes.
8. It is recommended that a dose dependence of the biological response is established. In addition, know positive and negative modulators of the response should be used and the directionality of the response should be validated.

References

1. Fine A, Janssen-Heininger Y, Soultanakis RP, Swisher SG, Uhal BD (2000) Apoptosis in lung pathophysiology. Am J Physiol Lung Cell Mol Physiol 279(3):L423–L427. https://doi.org/10.1152/ajplung.2000.279.3.L423
2. Favaloro B, Allocati N, Graziano V, Di Ilio C, De Laurenzi V (2012) Role of apoptosis in disease. Aging (Albany NY) 4(5):330–349. https://doi.org/10.18632/aging.100459
3. Duprez L, Wirawan E, Vanden Berghe T, Vandenabeele P (2009) Major cell death pathways at a glance. Microbes Infect 11(13):1050–1062. https://doi.org/10.1016/j.micinf.2009.08.013
4. Galluzzi L, Maiuri MC, Vitale I, Zischka H, Castedo M, Zitvogel L, Kroemer G (2007) Cell death modalities: classification and pathophysiological implications. Cell Death Differ 14(7):1237–1243. https://doi.org/10.1038/sj.cdd.4402148
5. Preedia Babu E, Subastri A, Suyavaran A, Nithyananthan S, Suresh Kumar M, Premkumar K, Bharathidasan R, Thirunavukkarasu C (2017) Anticancer potential of ZnO nanoparticle-ferulic acid conjugate on Huh-7 and HepG2 cells and diethyl nitrosamine induced hepatocellular cancer on Wistar albino rat. Nanomedicine 14(2):415–428. https://doi.org/10.1016/j.nano.2017.11.003
6. Wang Y, Wei G, Zhang X, Huang X, Zhao J, Guo X, Zhou S (2018) Multistage targeting strategy using magnetic composite nanoparticles for synergism of photothermal therapy and chemotherapy. Small 14(12):e1702994. https://doi.org/10.1002/smll.201702994
7. Alavi AS, Meshkini A (2018) Fabrication of poly(ethylene glycol)-coated mesoporous nanocomposite ZnO@Fe2O3 for methotrexate delivery: an integrated nanoplatform for dual-mode cancer therapy. Eur J Pharm Sci 115:144–157. https://doi.org/10.1016/j.ejps.2018.01.027
8. Madala HR, Punganuru SR, Ali-Osman F, Zhang R, Srivenugopal KS (2018) Brain- and brain tumor-penetrating disulfiram nanoparticles: sequence of cytotoxic events and efficacy in human glioma cell lines and intracranial xenografts. Oncotarget 9(3):3459–3482. https://doi.org/10.18632/oncotarget.23320
9. Lu J, Liu X, Liao YP, Salazar F, Sun B, Jiang W, Chang CH, Jiang J, Wang X, Wu AM, Meng H, Nel AE (2017) Nano-enabled pancreas cancer immunotherapy using immunogenic cell death and reversing immunosuppression. Nat Commun 8(1):1811. https://doi.org/10.1038/s41467-017-01651-9
10. Hussain S, Al-Nsour F, Rice AB, Marshburn J, Yingling B, Ji Z, Zink JI, Walker NJ, Garantziotis S (2012) Cerium dioxide nanoparticles induce apoptosis and autophagy in human peripheral blood monocytes. ACS Nano 6

(7):5820–5829. https://doi.org/10.1021/nn302235u

11. Hussain S, Sangtian S, Anderson SM, Snyder RJ, Marshburn JD, Rice AB, Bonner JC, Garantziotis S (2014) Inflammasome activation in airway epithelial cells after multi-walled carbon nanotube exposure mediates a profibrotic response in lung fibroblasts. Part Fibre Toxicol 11:28. https://doi.org/10.1186/1743-8977-11-28
12. Hussain S, Thomassen LC, Ferecatu I, Borot MC, Andreau K, Martens JA, Fleury J, Baeza-Squiban A, Marano F, Boland S (2010) Carbon black and titanium dioxide nanoparticles elicit distinct apoptotic pathways in bronchial epithelial cells. Part Fibre Toxicol 7:10. https://doi.org/10.1186/1743-8977-7-10
13. Li L, Cui J, Liu Z, Zhou X, Li Z, Yu Y, Jia Y, Zuo D, Wu Y (2018) Silver nanoparticles induce SH-SY5Y cell apoptosis via endoplasmic reticulum- and mitochondrial pathways that lengthen endoplasmic reticulum-mitochondria contact sites and alter inositol-3-phosphate receptor function. Toxicol Lett 285:156–167. https://doi.org/10.1016/j.toxlet.2018.01.004
14. Liu J, Yang M, Jing L, Ren L, Wei J, Zhang J, Zhang F, Duan J, Zhou X, Sun Z (2018) Silica nanoparticle exposure inducing granulosa cell apoptosis and follicular atresia in female Balb/c mice. Environ Sci Pollut Res Int 25 (4):3423–3434. https://doi.org/10.1007/s11356-017-0724-5
15. Paesano L, Perotti A, Buschini A, Carubbi C, Marmiroli M, Maestri E, Iannotta S, Marmiroli N (2016) Markers for toxicity to HepG2 exposed to cadmium sulphide quantum dots; damage to mitochondria. Toxicology 374:18–28. https://doi.org/10.1016/j.tox.2016.11.012
16. Yang Y, Yu Y, Wang J, Li Y, Li Y, Wei J, Zheng T, Jin M, Sun Z (2017) Silica nanoparticles induced intrinsic apoptosis in neuroblastoma SH-SY5Y cells via CytC/Apaf-1 pathway. Environ Toxicol Pharmacol 52:161–169. https://doi.org/10.1016/j.etap.2017.01.010
17. Galluzzi L, Vitale I, Aaronson SA, Abrams JM, Adam D, Agostinis P, Alnemri ES, Altucci L, Amelio I, Andrews DW, Annicchiarico-Petruzzelli M, Antonov AV, Arama E, Baehrecke EH, Barlev NA, Bazan NG, Bernassola F, Bertrand MJM, Bianchi K, Blagosklonny MV, Blomgren K, Borner C, Boya P, Brenner C, Campanella M, Candi E, Carmona-Gutierrez D, Cecconi F, Chan FK, Chandel NS, Cheng EH, Chipuk JE, Cidlowski JA, Ciechanover A, Cohen GM, Conrad M, Cubillos-Ruiz JR, Czabotar PE, D'Angiolella V, Dawson TM, Dawson VL, De Laurenzi V, De Maria R, Debatin KM, DeBerardinis RJ, Deshmukh M, Di Daniele N, Di Virgilio F, Dixit VM, Dixon SJ, Duckett CS, Dynlacht BD, El-Deiry WS, Elrod JW, Fimia GM, Fulda S, Garcia-Saez AJ, Garg AD, Garrido C, Gavathiotis E, Golstein P, Gottlieb E, Green DR, Greene LA, Gronemeyer H, Gross A, Hajnoczky G, Hardwick JM, Harris IS, Hengartner MO, Hetz C, Ichijo H, Jaattela M, Joseph B, Jost PJ, Juin PP, Kaiser WJ, Karin M, Kaufmann T, Kepp O, Kimchi A, Kitsis RN, Klionsky DJ, Knight RA, Kumar S, Lee SW, Lemasters JJ, Levine B, Linkermann A, Lipton SA, Lockshin RA, Lopez-Otin C, Lowe SW, Luedde T, Lugli E, MacFarlane M, Madeo F, Malewicz M, Malorni W, Manic G, Marine JC, Martin SJ, Martinou JC, Medema JP, Mehlen P, Meier P, Melino S, Miao EA, Molkentin JD, Moll UM, Munoz-Pinedo C, Nagata S, Nunez G, Oberst A, Oren M, Overholtzer M, Pagano M, Panaretakis T, Pasparakis M, Penninger JM, Pereira DM, Pervaiz S, Peter ME, Piacentini M, Pinton P, Prehn JHM, Puthalakath H, Rabinovich GA, Rehm M, Rizzuto R, Rodrigues CMP, Rubinsztein DC, Rudel T, Ryan KM, Sayan E, Scorrano L, Shao F, Shi Y, Silke J, Simon HU, Sistigu A, Stockwell BR, Strasser A, Szabadkai G, Tait SWG, Tang D, Tavernarakis N, Thorburn A, Tsujimoto Y, Turk B, Vanden Berghe T, Vandenabeele P, Vander Heiden MG, Villunger A, Virgin HW, Vousden KH, Vucic D, Wagner EF, Walczak H, Wallach D, Wang Y, Wells JA, Wood W, Yuan J, Zakeri Z, Zhivotovsky B, Zitvogel L, Melino G, Kroemer G (2018) Molecular mechanisms of cell death: recommendations of the Nomenclature Committee on Cell Death 2018. Cell Death Differ 25 (3):486–541. https://doi.org/10.1038/s41418-017-0012-4
18. Bonora M, Wieckowski MR, Chinopoulos C, Kepp O, Kroemer G, Galluzzi L, Pinton P (2015) Molecular mechanisms of cell death: central implication of ATP synthase in mitochondrial permeability transition. Oncogene 34(12):1475–1486. https://doi.org/10.1038/onc.2014.96
19. Giorgio V, Guo L, Bassot C, Petronilli V, Bernardi P (2018) Calcium and regulation of the mitochondrial permeability transition. Cell Calcium 70:56–63. https://doi.org/10.1016/j.ceca.2017.05.004
20. Cozens AL, Yezzi MJ, Kunzelmann K, Ohrui T, Chin L, Eng K, Finkbeiner WE, Widdicombe JH, Gruenert DC (1994) CFTR expression and chloride secretion in polarized

immortal human bronchial epithelial cells. Am J Respir Cell Mol Biol 10(1):38–47. https://doi.org/10.1165/ajrcmb.10.1.7507342

21. Hussain S, Boland S, Baeza-Squiban A, Hamel R, Thomassen LC, Martens JA, Billon-Galland MA, Fleury-Feith J, Moisan F, Pairon JC, Marano F (2009) Oxidative stress and proinflammatory effects of carbon black and titanium dioxide nanoparticles: role of particle surface area and internalized amount. Toxicology 260(1–3):142–149. https://doi.org/10.1016/j.tox.2009.04.001
22. Val S, Hussain S, Boland S, Hamel R, Baeza-Squiban A, Marano F (2009) Carbon black and titanium dioxide nanoparticles induce pro-inflammatory responses in bronchial epithelial cells: need for multiparametric evaluation due to adsorption artifacts. Inhal Toxicol 21(Suppl 1):115–122. https://doi.org/10.1080/08958370902942533

Chapter 8

Application of Gelatin Zymography in Nanotoxicity Research

Yue Zhang, Rong Wan, Qunwei Zhang, and Yiqun Mo

Abstract

Gelatin zymography is a relatively simple, inexpensive, and powerful technique to detect proteolytic enzymes capable of degrading gelatin from various biological sources. It has been used particularly to detect the two members of the matrix metalloproteinase family, MMP-2 (gelatinase A) and MMP-9 (gelatinase B), due to their potent gelatin-degrading activity. MMP-2 and MMP-9 are also able to degrade a number of extracellular matrix molecules including type IV, V, and XI collagens, laminin, and aggrecan core protein, thus making them important in the nanotoxicity research. In this technique, proteins are separated by sodium dodecyl sulfate (SDS)–polyacrylamide gel electrophoresis (PAGE), and gelatinases, activated by SDS, digest gelatin embedded in the gel. After staining with Coomassie Brilliant Blue R-250, areas of degradation are visible as clear bands against a blue-stained background. Here, we describe the detailed procedure for gelatin zymography.

Key words Matrix metalloproteinases, MMP-2, MMP-9, Nanoparticles, Zymography, Gelatin

1 Introduction

The matrix metalloproteinases (MMPs), which are able to degrade extracellular matrix (ECM) proteins, are a family of zinc-dependent endopeptidases that consists of 25 members in mice and 24 in humans [1–3]. A typical MMP contains a catalytic metalloproteinase domain of about 170 amino acids, a propeptide of about 80 amino acids, a linker peptide of variable lengths (also called the "hinge region"), and a hemopexin (Hpx) domain of about 200 amino acids [4]. Loosely based on the order of discovery, MMPs are assigned numbers; while based on their domain organization and preferred substrate specificities, the MMPs can be classified as collagenases, gelatinases, stromelysins, matrilysins, membrane-type MMPs, and others [4]. Two gelatinases, gelatinase A (MMP-2, 72 kD) and gelatinase B (MMP-9, 92 kD), readily digest gelatin and a number of ECM molecules including type IV, V and XI collagens, laminin, and aggrecan core protein. A large number of studies have shown that MMPs play critical roles in

Qunwei Zhang (ed.), *Nanotoxicity: Methods and Protocols*, Methods in Molecular Biology, vol. 1894,
https://doi.org/10.1007/978-1-4939-8916-4_8,

both biological and pathological processes such as development, tissue repair, and immune response [1–3].

With the development of nanotechnology, a large number of nanoparticles are being produced. Nanoparticles can enter the human body via inhalation, the digestive tract, and the skin, resulting in local and systemic health effects [5]. Nanoparticles can cause dysregulation of MMPs. For example, our and other studies have shown that nanoparticles such as nickel or cobalt nanoparticles caused MMP-2 and MMP-9 mRNA upregulation and increased activity in human monocytes U937 [6, 7] or mouse embryonic fibroblasts [8]. In this chapter, we discuss how to determine MMP-2 and MMP-9 activity by gelatin zymography.

Zymography is a technique to assess the enzymatic activity of proteins in situ or by separating them with electrophoresis [9]. Gelatin zymography is a simple and popular technique in which proteins are separated by sodium dodecyl sulfate (SDS)–polyacrylamide gel electrophoresis (PAGE) with gelatin incorporated within the polyacrylamide gels. SDS is used to activate the gelatinases such as MMP-2 and MMP-9. While gelatin in the gel is degraded by the proteolytic enzymes such as gelatinases MMP-2 and MMP-9 in the sample, staining of the gel with Coomassie Brilliant Blue R-250 shows the areas of degradation as clear bands against a dark blue background. Below we will describe the detailed procedure for gelatin zymography that is commonly used in our laboratory.

2 Materials

All solutions are prepared by using analytical grade reagents and ultrapure water that is commercially available or purified deionized water produced by a water purification system, in which water is processed through purification cartridges to reach a resistivity of 18.2 MΩ·cm at 25 °C. A clean lab coat and disposable gloves should be worn, and the bench should be clean.

2.1 Sample Preparation

1. Complete media: Media containing 100 U/mL penicillin, 100 μg/mL streptomycin, and 10% fetal bovine serum (FBS).
2. FBS-free media: Media containing 100 U/mL penicillin and 100 μg/mL streptomycin.
3. Phosphate-buffered saline (1 × PBS): Weigh 8 g NaCl, 0.2 g KCl, 1.44 g Na_2HPO_4, and 0.24 g KH_2PO_4, and dissolve them in 800 mL water. Adjust pH to 7.4 with HCl. Add water to 1000 mL by using a graduated cylinder. Autoclave and store at room temperature.
4. Lysis buffer: RIPA Lysis Buffer System (Santa Cruz Biotechnology, Santa Cruz, CA). Store at −20 °C.
5. Bio-Rad protein assay: Store at 4 °C.

2.2 Preparation of SDS–Polyacrylamide Gel Incorporated with Gelatin

1. 10 mg/mL Gelatin: Weigh 100 mg gelatin and dissolve in 10 mL water by heating the solution at 60 °C in a water bath for at least 20 min. Mix well and ensure the gelatin is completely dissolved. Cool down the gelatin solution to room temperature before use. It is recommended to prepare it fresh (*see* **Note 1**).
2. 30% acrylamide–bis-acrylamide solution (29.2:0.8): Weigh 29.2 g acrylamide and 0.8 g bis-acrylamide (*see* **Note 2**) and dissolve them in 60 mL water. Mix well and adjust the volume to 100 mL with water. Filter through a 0.45 μm filter. Store in a dark bottle or a bottle wrapped with aluminum foil at 4 °C (*see* **Note 3**).
3. 1.5 M Tris–HCl, pH 8.8: Weigh 18.2 g Tris base and dissolve in 80 mL water. Mix well and adjust pH to 8.8 with HCl (*see* **Note 4**). Add water to 100 mL. Autoclave and store at 4 °C. It is stable for at least 6 months.
4. 1 M Tris–HCl, pH 6.8: Weigh 12.1 g Tris base and dissolve in 80 mL water. Mix well and adjust pH to 6.8 with HCl (*see* **Note 4**). Make up to 100 mL with water. Autoclave and store at 4 °C. It is stable for at least 6 months.
5. 10% Ammonium persulfate (AP): Weigh 500 mg ammonium persulfate and dissolve in 5 mL water. Mix well. Aliquot and store at 4 °C. It is stable for several weeks (*see* **Note 5**).
6. 10% SDS: Weigh 10 g SDS and dissolve in 80 mL water (*see* **Note 6**). Heat to 68 °C if necessary. Adjust the volume to 100 mL with water (*see* **Note 7**). Store at room temperature (*see* **Note 8**).
7. N, N, N′, N′-Tetramethylethylenediamine (TEMED): Store at room temperature (*see* **Note 9**).
8. Mini-PROTEAN® tetra cell casting stand with clamp kit (Bio-Rad), Mini-PROTEAN® short plates (Bio-Rad) and spacer plates with 1.5 mm integrated spacer (Bio-Rad), and Mini-PROTEAN® comb (10-well, 1.5 mm) (Bio-Rad).

2.3 Gel Running

1. 10× Running buffer: 0.25 M Tris–HCl, pH 8.3, 1.92 M glycine, 1% SDS. Weigh 30.3 g Tris base, 144.1 g glycine, and 10 g SDS. Dissolve them in 800 mL water. Add water to 1000 mL (*see* **Notes 6** and **10**). Store at room temperature.
2. Working running buffer (1×): 0.025 M Tris–HCl, pH 8.3, 0.192 M glycine, 0.1% SDS. Dilute 100 mL of 10× running buffer to 1000 mL with water (*see* **Note 10**). Store at room temperature.
3. 1.25% Bromophenol blue (BPB): Dissolve 0.125 g BPB in 10 mL water. Store at −20 °C.

4. 5× Loading buffer: 0.4 M Tris–HCl, pH 6.8, 5% SDS, 20% glycerol, 0.03% bromophenol blue. For a total volume of 50 mL, mix 20 mL of 1 M Tris–HCl, pH 6.8, 12.5 mL of 20% SDS, 10 mL of glycerol, 1.2 mL of 1.25% bromophenol blue, and 6.3 mL water. Aliquot and leave one aliquot at room temperature for current use and store the remaining aliquots at −20 °C (*see* **Note 11**).
5. Mini-PROTEAN® Tetra Vertical Electrophoresis Cell (For 1.5 mm thick gel, 4 gels, Bio-Rad).

2.4 Gel Washing and Incubation

1. Washing buffer: 50 mM Tris–HCl, pH 7.5, 2.5% Triton X-100. Weigh 6.06 g Tris base and dissolve in 900 mL water. Adjust pH to 7.5 with HCl. Add 25 mL Triton X-100 and mix well. Add water to 1000 mL. Store at room temperature.
2. 20 mM $ZnCl_2$: At first, prepare 5 mL of 400 mM $ZnCl_2$ by dissolving 0.273 g $ZnCl_2$ in 5 mL water. Aliquot and store at −20 °C. Then dilute to 20 mM by mixing 50 μL of 400 mM $ZnCl_2$ and 950 μL of water. Store at −20 °C.
3. Incubation buffer: 50 mM Tris–HCl, pH 7.5, 0.2 M NaCl, 7.55 mM $CaCl_2$, 1 μM $ZnCl_2$, 1% Triton X-100. Weigh 6.06 g Tris base, 11.7 g NaCl, and 1.11 g $CaCl_2$. Dissolve them in 900 mL water. Add 10 mL Triton X-100 and 50 μL of 20 mM $ZnCl_2$. Mix well and adjust pH to 7.5. Make a total volume to 1000 mL. Store at room temperature.

2.5 Gel Staining and Destaining

1. 0.1% Coomassie Brilliant Blue R-250: Dissolve 0.5 g Coomassie Brilliant Blue R-250 in 200 mL water (This will require warming to approximately 50 °C.). Cool and add 250 mL methanol and 50 mL acetic acid to a total volume of 500 mL. Filter the solution through a Whatman No. 1 filter paper to remove any particulate matter. Store in a dark bottle or a bottle wrapped with aluminum foil at room temperature (*see* **Note 12**).
2. 10% Acetic acid: Mix 50 mL acetic acid and 450 mL water to a total volume of 500 mL. Store at room temperature.

3 Methods

3.1 Sample Preparation

3.1.1 Preparation of Conditioned Media of Cultured Cells

The gelatinases, MMP-2 and MMP-9, are secreted enzymes [1–3, 10]. Thus, they can be detected in the media of cultured cells. Because of their presence in the serum, we suggest preparing serum-free conditioned media for gelatin zymography.

1. Culture same amount of cells per well in complete media in a six-well plate (2 mL/well) (*see* **Note 13**).

2. After overnight culture, remove complete media. Wash cells twice with FBS-free media. Treat cells with nanoparticles and continue to grow cells in 1 mL of FBS-free media (*see* **Notes 14** and **15**).
3. At the end of the experiment, collect conditioned media and centrifuge at 200 × *g* for 10 min to remove cells and debris. Collect supernatant for gelatin zymography analysis.

3.1.2 Preparation of Bronchoalveolar Lavage Fluid (BALF)

Nanoparticles can enter the body via inhalation (inhalative uptake), via the digestive tract (oral uptake), and via the skin (dermal uptake) [5]. Analysis of the cellular and biochemical parameters in the BALF is a useful tool to study the effects of nanoparticles on the lungs. The detailed procedure about how to obtain BALF from animals with or without nanoparticle treatment can be found in Chapter 18.

3.1.3 Preparation of Cell Lysates

Regulation of MMPs may occur at multiple levels, either by gene transcription and synthesis of inactive proenzymes, posttranslational activation of proenzymes, or via the interaction of secreted MMPs with their inhibitors called tissue inhibitor of metalloproteinases (TIMPs) [1–4, 10, 11]. In addition to being secreted, MMP-2 and MMP-9 are also cell-associated. Analysis of MMP-2 and MMP-9 activity in the cell lysates or tissue extracts (Subheading 3.1.4) can provide valuable information on the rate of synthesis, cell surface–matrix association, and activation status of surface-associated gelatinases.

Monolayer Cells

1. Wash the cells twice with ice-cold 1× PBS.
2. Add ice-cold lysis buffer with protease inhibitors (RIPA Lysis Buffer System) directly on the culture dish or plate according to the manufacturer's instruction.
3. Scrape the cells into the lysis buffer with a rubber policeman.
4. Collect the lysate.
5. Incubate the lysate on ice for at least 15 min.
6. Vortex-mix and centrifuge at 10,000 × *g* for 15 min at 4 °C in a microcentrifuge.
7. Collect the supernatant and measure protein concentration by using Bio-Rad protein assay.

Suspension Cells

1. Isolate cells by centrifugation at 200 × *g* for 10 min at 4 °C.
2. Wash the cells twice with ice-cold 1× PBS.
3. Add ice-cold lysis buffer with protease inhibitors into cells.
4. Incubate on ice for at least 15 min.

5. Vortex-mix and centrifuge at 10,000 × *g* for 15 min at 4 °C in a microcentrifuge.
6. Collect the supernatant and determine protein concentration by using Bio-Rad protein assay.

3.1.4 Preparation of Tissue Extracts (See Note 16)

1. Weigh the tissue (~25 mg) and cut the tissue into small pieces.
2. Place the tissue in a 12 × 75 mm tube which contains 20 volumes of ice-cold lysis buffer with protease inhibitors.
3. Homogenize the tissue by a homogenizer (*see* **Note 17**).
4. Transfer the tissue homogenate to a new 1.5 mL Eppendorf tube.
5. Centrifuge the homogenate at 10,000 × *g* for 15 min at 4 °C.
6. Collect the supernatant and determine the protein concentration by using Bio-Rad protein assay.

3.2 Gel Preparation

1. Mix the reagents in Table 1 for two 10% acrylamide separating gels containing gelatin. Add TEMED last to initiate polymerization. Swirl the solution rapidly without causing bubble formation or aeration.
2. Immediately, pipet 7.5 mL of separating gel solution into each cassette avoiding the formation of bubbles. Use spacer plates with 1.5 mm integrated spacer.
3. Carefully overlay the separating gel solution with 1 mL of 0.1% SDS. Try not to disturb the surface of the separating gel solution.

Table 1
Preparation of SDS polyacrylamide gel incorporated with gelatin

	Separating gel (10%)	Stacking gel
1.5 M Tris–HCI, pH 8.8	4 mL	
1.0 M Tris–HCI, pH 6.8		0.75 mL
30% Acrylamide/Bis-acrylamide	5.3 mL	1.0 mL
H_2O	5.6 mL	4.1 mL
Gelatin (10 mg/mL)	0.8 mL	
10% SDS	160 μL	60 μL
10% AP	160 μL	60 μL
TEMED	10 μL	6 μL
Total (for 2 gels)	~16 mL	~6 mL

4. Let the gel polymerize for at least 40 min at room temperature. Polymerization is complete when a discrete line of separation can be observed between the gel and the 0.1% SDS solution.
5. Prepare stacking gel solution according to Table 1 without adding TEMED.
6. Discard the overlay of 0.1% SDS solution from the separating gel.
7. Add TEMED to the stacking gel solution, swirl rapidly, and immediately pipet the solution on top of the polymerized separating gels until it reaches the top of the front plate.
8. Rapidly, insert the combs (10-well, 1.5 mm thick) into the liquid stacking gel, making sure that no bubbles remain trapped under the comb.
9. Let the stacking gel polymerize at room temperature for at least 40 min.

3.3 Gel Running

1. Gently pull the comb out of the stacking gel. Place the cassette into the gel apparatus. Fill the buffer chambers with 1× working running buffer.
2. Add 5× loading buffer into samples such as conditioned media, BALF, cell lysate, or tissue extract (*see* **Notes 18** and **19**).
3. Load the samples and run the gel at constant 25 mA until the bromophenol blue tracking dye runs into the separating gel.
4. Increase the electric current to 40 mA and run the gel until the bromophenol blue tracking dye runs out of the gel (*see* **Note 20**).

3.4 Gel Washing and Incubation

1. Carefully remove the gel from the cassette after cutting a notch at the bottom left corner of the gel for identification of the order of the samples.
2. Place the gel in a plastic tray containing 100 mL of washing buffer.
3. Incubate the gel for 60 min at room temperature with gentle agitation by using a Rocker. Change the washing buffer every 15 min (*see* **Note 21**).
4. Decant the solution and incubate the gel at room temperature for an additional 10 min in 100 mL of incubation buffer with gentle agitation.
5. Decant the incubation buffer and replace it with 150 mL of fresh incubation buffer. Incubate the gel in a closed tray placed in a 37 °C water bath with gentle agitation overnight (~16 h) (*see* **Note 22**).

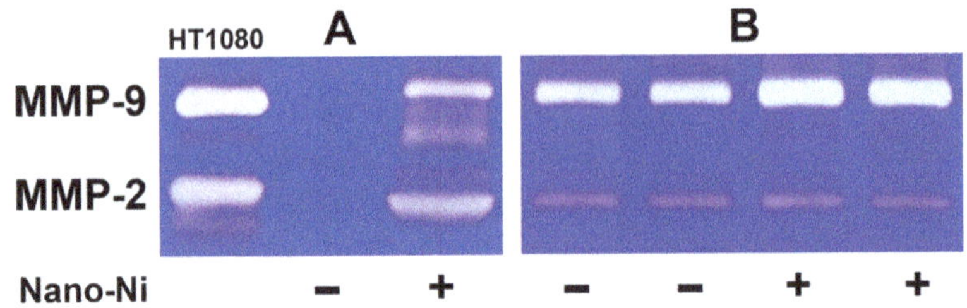

Fig. 1 MMP-2 and MMP-9 activity in mouse bronchoalveolar lavage fluid (BALF) (**a**) and lung tissue extracts (**b**). C57BL/6J mice were intratracheally instilled with 50 μg per mouse of nickel nanoparticles (Nano-Ni). Control mice were instilled with normal saline. Bronchoalveolar lavage fluid (BALF) or lung tissues were collected from mice at day 3 after Nano-Ni exposure. Gelatinolytic activity of MMP-2 and MMP-9 in the BALF (**a**) or lung tissue extracts (**b**) was determined by gelatin zymography as described in this chapter. Conditioned media collected from cultured HT1080 cells was used as a molecular weight marker for MMP-2 and MMP-9 (**a**, lane 1)

3.5 Gel Staining and Destaining

1. Decant the incubation buffer and wash the gel twice with water, 5 min each time.
2. Stain the gel in staining solution for at least 1 h at room temperature or until the gel is uniformly dark blue (*see* **Note 23**). Decant the staining solution.
3. Rinse with water until excess staining solution is removed.
4. Destain the gel with destaining solution until areas of gelatinolytic activity appear as clear sharp bands over the blue background (*see* **Note 24**).
5. Capture the image (Fig. 1). Analyze the bands by Quantity One (Bio-Rad) or other software if necessary.

4 Notes

1. The gelatin solution can also be aliquoted (1 mL/tube) and stored at −20 °C for later use. Only take out the required amount for each use.
2. Wear a face mask and operate gently when weighing acrylamide and bis-acrylamide. Unpolymerized acrylamide is a neurotoxin and can be absorbed via skin, thus care should be taken to avoid skin contact.
3. The 30% acrylamide–bis-acrylamide solution can be stored at 4 °C for up to 1 month. It is better to make the acrylamide–bis-acrylamide solution fresh about every month since acrylamide hydrolyzes to acrylic acid.
4. Use concentrated HCl (12 N) at first to narrow the gap from the starting pH to the required pH. When it is near the

required pH, it would be better to use a series of HCl (e.g., 6 N and 1 N) with lower ionic strengths to avoid a sudden drop in pH below the required pH.

5. 10% ammonium persulfate can also be prepared, aliquoted, and stored at −20 °C for later use. It is stable for at least 6 months at −20 °C. Remove only the required amount for each use.
6. Wear a face mask to avoid inhalation of SDS dust during preparation of the solution. Try to avoid frothing.
7. Do not autoclave 10% SDS solution.
8. Do not store the solution at 4 °C. SDS will precipitate at temperature below 15 °C. If there is any precipitate, redissolve by warming the solution (68 °C for 10 min).
9. Transfer a small amount of TEMED from the original bottle to an Eppendorf tube for current use, and store it dark at 4 °C to reduce its pungent smell.
10. The pH of the running buffer should be 8.3 and no pH adjustment is required.
11. SDS precipitates at temperature below 15 °C. Therefore, the loading buffer needs to be warmed up prior to use.
12. 0.1% Coomassie Brilliant Blue R-250 solution can be reused, but using old dye solution will take longer time for staining. Staining is complete when the gel is a uniform blue color. We suggest using new dye solution every time.
13. The amount of cells seeded at the beginning of the experiment must be optimized for the cell line. In order to obtain conditioned media containing higher concentrated enzymes, it is ideal to seed cells as dense as possible, but keep cells at less than 100% confluence at the end of the experiment.
14. We suggest using FBS-free media. However, some cells cannot survive in FBS-free media; thus, it is better to test before the experiment. If culture of cells in FBS-free media affects cell viability, media containing 1% FBS could be used.
15. In order to obtain more concentrated samples, a minimum amount of FBS-free media (~50–60% of the amount of growth media) will be used to culture the cells.
16. The tissues need to be processed or frozen in liquid N_2 immediately after removing from the animal to prevent proteins from degradation. If not used immediately, the samples need to be stored at −70 °C.
17. We usually put the tube containing tissues and lysis buffer on ice for 1–5 min after homogenizing for 10 s each time. Repeat homogenization for several times or until no tissue pieces are visible.

18. For each sample, test one aliquot at a low protein concentration and one at a high protein concentration to find the appropriate amount of protein for loading.
19. The maximum loading volume for a well (10-well, 1.5 mm) is 66 μL. We usually load 50 μL or less.
20. These running conditions will prevent overheating of the gel.
21. Soaking the gel in washing buffer removes SDS from the gel.
22. The incubation buffer contains cofactors necessary for the gelatinase reaction to occur.
23. The staining solution can be reused. However, it may require a longer staining time. We suggest using fresh staining solution each time.
24. Areas of enzyme activity appear as white bands against a dark blue background.

Acknowledgment

This work was partly supported by the NIESH/NIH (ES023693 and ES028911), KSEF-148-502-16-381, Kentucky Lung Cancer Research Program, and an Intramural Research Incentive Grants (50992) from UofL to Dr. Qunwei Zhang.

References

1. Greenlee KJ, Werb Z, Kheradmand F (2007) Matrix metalloproteinases in lung: multiple, multifarious, and multifaceted. Physiol Rev 87(1):69–98. https://doi.org/10.1152/physrev.00022.2006
2. Murphy G, Willenbrock F, Crabbe T, O'Shea M, Ward R, Atkinson S, O'Connell J, Docherty A (1994) Regulation of matrix metalloproteinase activity. Ann N Y Acad Sci 732:31–41. https://doi.org/10.1111/j.1749-6632.1994.tb24722.x
3. Parsons SL, Watson SA, Brown PD, Collins HM, Steele RJ (1997) Matrix metalloproteinase. Br J Surg 84(2):160–166
4. Nagase H, Visse R, Murphy G (2006) Structure and function of matrix metalloproteinases and TIMPs. Cardiovasc Res 69(3):562–573. https://doi.org/10.1016/j.cardiores.2005.12.002
5. Medina C, Santos-Martinez MJ, Radomski A, Corrigan OI, Radomski MW (2007) Nanoparticles: pharmacological and toxicological significance. Br J Pharmacol 150(5):552–558. https://doi.org/10.1038/sj.bjp.0707130
6. Wan R, Mo Y, Zhang X, Chien S, Tollerud DJ, Zhang Q (2008) Matrix metalloproteinase-2 and -9 are induced differently by metal nanoparticles in human monocytes: the role of oxidative stress and protein tyrosine kinase activation. Toxicol Appl Pharmacol 233(2):276–285. https://doi.org/10.1016/j.taap.2008.08.022
7. Wan R, Mo Y, Chien S, Li Y, Li Y, Tollerud DJ, Zhang Q (2011) The role of hypoxia inducible factor-1α in the increased MMP-2 and MMP-9 production by human monocytes exposed to nickel nanoparticles. Nanotoxicology 5(4):568–582. https://doi.org/10.3109/17435390.2010.537791
8. Annangi B, Bach J, Vales G, Rubio L, Marcos R (2015) Long-term exposures to low doses of cobalt nanoparticles induce cell transformation enhanced by oxidative damage. Nanotoxicology 9(2):138–147. https://doi.org/10.3109/17435390.2014.900582
9. Kaberdin VR, McDowall KJ (2003) Expanding the use of zymography by the chemical linkage of small, defined substrates to the gel matrix.

Genome Res 13(8):1961–1965. https://doi.org/10.1101/gr.1277303

10. Hadler-Olsen E, Fadnes B, Sylte I, Uhlin-Hansen L, Winberg JO (2011) Regulation of matrix metalloproteinase activity in health and disease. FEBS J 278(1):28–45. https://doi.org/10.1111/j.1742-4658.2010.07920.x

11. Oum'hamed Z, Garnotel R, Josset Y, Trenteseaux C, Lauren-Maquin D (2004) Matrix metalloproteinases MMP-2, -9 and tissue inhibitors TIMP-1, -2 expression and secretion by primary human osteoblast cells in response to titanium, zirconia, and alumina ceramics. J Biomed Mater Res A 68((1):114–122. https://doi.org/10.1002/jbm.a.20001

Chapter 9

Determination of Phosphorylated Histone H2AX in Nanoparticle-Induced Genotoxic Studies

Rong Wan, Yiqun Mo, Ruirui Tong, Meiqin Gao, and Qunwei Zhang

Abstract

DNA double-strand breaks (DSBs), one of the most severe lesions of DNA damage triggered by various genotoxic insults, can lead to chromosome change, genomic instability, and even tumorigenesis if not repaired efficiently. In response to DNA damage, histone H2AX molecules are rapidly phosphorylated at serine 139 near the site of DNA DSBs and form γ-H2AX foci. As an early important cellular event linked to DNA damage and repair, γ-H2AX is a highly sensitive biomarker for "monitoring" DNA damage and consequently is a useful tool in genetic toxicology screen. We and other researchers have used γ-H2AX as a marker to assess the potential genotoxic effects of some nanoparticles in vitro and in vivo. In this chapter, we describe several useful methods for γ-H2AX detection, which can be used to evaluate the potential genotoxic effects of nanoparticles.

Key words DNA, Double-strand breaks, Histone H2AX, Phosphorylation, Genotoxicity, Nanoparticles, Immunofluorescence, Immunoblotting, Immunohistochemistry, Flow cytometry

1 Introduction

Histones are key components of eukaryotic cell nuclei; genomic DNA winds around core families of histones, namely, the H2A, H2B, H3, and H4 histones, to form nucleosomes, a fundamental unit of chromatin. The histone variant H2AX is a minor component in the core H2A histone family, but plays an important role in DNA damage signaling and chromatin remodeling [1].

A variety of internal or external cellular stress signals, such as DNA replication and recombination in physiological processes, ionizing radiation, and genotoxic agents, may trigger various types of DNA damage in cells, including DNA adduct formation, base mismatch, DNA strand breaks, and interstrand or intrastrand DNA cross-links. Among these different forms of DNA damage, DNA double-strand breaks (DSBs) is the most severe one that could cause genomic instability, leading to tumorigenesis through loss or rearrangements in chromosomes [2].

Qunwei Zhang (ed.), *Nanotoxicity: Methods and Protocols*, Methods in Molecular Biology, vol. 1894, https://doi.org/10.1007/978-1-4939-8916-4_9,

DNA DSBs activate a cascade of DNA damage signals. Once DSB happens, hundreds to thousands of H2AX molecules are phosphorylated rapidly at serine 139 near the damage sites to form H2AX foci, named gamma-H2AX (γ-H2AX) [3]. This histone H2AX modification results in chromatin remodeling and may provide a platform for the recruitment of other enzymes responsible for DSB signaling and DNA repair in order to maintain the integrity of genome [4]. The phosphorylation of H2AX in response to DSBs is mediated by members of the phosphatidylinositol 3-kinase-like-kinase (PIKK) family, including Ataxia Telangiectasia Mutated (ATM), Ataxia Telangiectasia and Rad3 related (ATR), and DNA dependent protein kinase catalytic subunit (DNA-PKcs) [5, 6]. Absence of H2AX or inhibition of the phosphorylation of H2AX enhances radiosensitivity and impairs DNA repair, which results in genomic instability [7, 8]. Since phosphorylation of H2AX closely correlates with each DNA DSB, γ-H2AX is served as a highly sensitive monitor for DNA damage [9]. Many studies have demonstrated that γ-H2AX is a reliable biomarker for genotoxic assessment [10, 11]. Due to the fast growth of nanotechnology and wide use of related nanoproducts in various fields, the assessment of health risks of nanoparticles is of great critical. Some studies have shown the potential genotoxic effects of some nanomaterials [12, 13]. In addition, γ-H2AX detection has been used to assess the potential genotoxicity effects of a variety of nanoparticles [14–16]. For example, we have employed γ-H2AX as a DNA damage molecular marker to investigate genotoxic effects of nanoparticles such as cobalt nanoparticles in vitro and in vivo [17, 18]. Below, we describe several general and standard protocols for γ-H2AX detection.

2 Materials

2.1 Immunofluorescence Staining

1. 2-well Nunc™ Lab-Tek™ II chamber slides (Nalge Nunc).
2. Tissue-Tek staining rack and dish with lid (dark color) (SAKURA).
3. 1× Phosphate-buffered saline (1× PBS): Weigh 8 g NaCl, 0.2 g KCl, 1.44 g Na_2HPO_4, and 0.24 g KH_2PO_4, and dissolve in 800 mL distilled water. Adjust pH to 7.4 with HCl and add distilled water to 1000 mL.
4. PBS-T: 1× PBS containing 0.05% Tween 20, pH 7.4.
5. Acetone: Store at −20 °C.
6. Cytospin ™ 4 Cytocentrifuge (Thermo Scientific).
7. Superfrost Plus™ adhesion microscope slides and coverslip (Thermo Scientific).
8. Mini PAP pen (Thermo Scientific).

9. Antigen retrieval buffer: 10 mM sodium citrate, pH 6.0, 0.05% Tween 20. Weigh 2.94 g trisodium citrate (dihydrate) and dissolve in 1 L distilled water. Mix and adjust pH to 6.0 with 1 N HCl. Add 0.5 mL Tween 20 and mix well. Store at room temperature for 3 months or at 4 °C for longer storage.
10. Blocking solution: 1× PBS containing 5% normal goat serum and 0.3% Triton X-100. To prepare 10 mL, add 500 μL normal goat serum to 9.5 mL of 1× PBS. Mix well. While stirring, add 30 μL Triton X-100. Store at 4 °C.
11. Primary antibody: Mouse monoclonal anti-γ-H2AX (Millipore). Store at −20 °C.
12. Secondary antibody: Goat anti-mouse IgG (H + L), Rhodamine-conjugated (Invitrogen). Store at 4 °C.
13. ProLong Diamond Antifade Mountant with DAPI (Invitrogen).
14. Fluorescence microscope (Nikon, Tokyo, Japan).

2.2 Immunohistochemical Staining

1. Methanol-free formaldehyde: 10% (v/v) in aqueous solution (VWR).
2. Ethanol, xylene, Histoplast paraffin (Thermo Scientific).
3. Lab Vision™ mayer's Hematoxylin (Thermo Scientific).
4. Tissue-Tek staining rack and dish with lid (dark color) (SAKURA).
5. 30% H_2O_2 (Thermo Scientific).
6. Permount (Sigma).
7. Primary antibody: Mouse anti-γ-H2AX antibody (Millipore). Store at −20 °C.
8. VECTASTAIN® ABC Kit: Containing Blocking Serum, Biotinylated Secondary Antibody, Avidin DH-Reagent A and Biotinylated Horseradish Peroxidase H-Reagent B (Vector Laboratories). Store at 4 °C.
9. DAB peroxidase substrate (Vector Laboratories): Prepare working solution and use immediately.

2.3 Immunoblotting

1. NE-PER Nuclear and Cytoplasmic Extraction Reagent (Thermo Scientific): Store at 4 °C.
2. Protease Inhibitor Cocktail Kit (Thermo Scientific): Store at −20 °C.
3. 30% acrylamide–bis-acrylamide solution (29.2:0.8): 29.2 g acrylamide and 0.8 g bis-acrylamide in a total of 100 mL distilled water. Filter through a 0.45 μm filter. Store in a dark bottle or a bottle wrapped with aluminum foil at 4 °C (*see* **Note 1**).
4. 1.5 M Tris–HCl, pH 8.8: 18.2 g Tris base in a total of 100 mL distilled water, pH 8.8. Autoclave and store at 4 °C. It is stable for at least 6 months.

5. 1 M Tris–HCl, pH 6.8: 12.1 g Tris base in a total of 100 mL distilled water, pH 6.8. Autoclave and store at 4 °C. It is stable for at least 6 months.
6. 10% ammonium persulfate (AP): 500 mg ammonium persulfate in 5 mL distilled water. Mix well. Store at 4 °C. It is stable for several weeks (*see* **Note 2**).
7. 10% SDS: 10 g SDS in a total of 100 mL distilled water (*see* **Note 3**). Heat to 68 °C if necessary. Adjust the volume to 100 mL with water. Store at room temperature (*see* **Note 4**).
8. N, N, N′, N′-Tetramethylethylenediamine (TEMED): Store at room temperature.
9. 10× Running buffer: 0.25 M Tris–HCl, pH 8.3, 1.92 M glycine, 1% SDS. 30.3 g Tris base, 144.1 g glycine, and 10 g SDS in a total of 1 L distilled water. Store at room temperature.
10. Mini-PROTEAN® Tetra Vertical Electrophoresis Cell System (Bio-Rad).
11. Mini Trans-Blot Cell (Bio-Rad).
12. 1.25% Bromophenol blue (BPB): Dissolve 0.125 g BPB in 10 mL distilled water. Store at −20 °C.
13. Loading buffer: 0.4 M Tris–HCl, pH 6.8, 5% SDS, 20% glycerol, 0.03% bromophenol blue. For a total volume of 50 mL, mix 20 mL of 1 M Tris–HCl, pH 6.8, 12.5 mL of 20% SDS, 10 mL of glycerol, 1.2 mL of 1.25% bromophenol blue, and 6.3 mL distilled water. Store at −20 °C.
14. Prestained Protein Ladder (Thermo Scientific): Store at −20 °C.
15. Transfer buffer: Mix 100 mL (10×) Running buffer, 200 mL methanol, and 700 mL distilled water.
16. Polyvinylidene difluoride (PVDF) membranes (Millipore).
17. Blocking solution: 1× PBS containing 5% BSA and 0.3% Triton X-100. To prepare 10 mL blocking solution, add 30 μL Triton X-100 to 10 mL of 1× PBS and mix. Add 0.5 g BSA and mix well.
18. Primary antibody: Mouse monoclonal anti-γ-H2AX (Millipore) and rabbit monoclonal anti-H2AX antibody (Thermo Scientific). Store at −20 °C.
19. Secondary antibody: Goat anti-mouse or anti-rabbit horseradish peroxidase (HRP) -conjugated IgG. Store at −20 °C.
20. PBS-T: 1× PBS containing 0.05% Tween 20, pH 7.4.
21. Enhanced chemiluminescent reagent (GE Healthcare).
22. Restoring western blot stripping buffer (Thermo Scientific).

2.4 Flow Cytometry

1. 12 × 75 mm polypropylene tubes.
2. 70% ethanol: Store at −20 °C.
3. 1% methanol-free formaldehyde solution: To prepare 100 mL methanol-free formaldehyde (1%, v/v) solution, add 10 mL of methanol-free formaldehyde (10% in aqueous solution, VWR) to 90 mL of 1× PBS. Mix well. Store at 4 °C for up to 2 weeks (*see* **Note 5**).
4. 1% (w/v) Bovine serum albumin (BSA) solution: Weigh 1 g BSA and dissolve in 100 mL of 1× PBS. Store at 4 °C.
5. Conjugated primary antibody: FITC-conjugated mouse anti-- γ-H2AX antibody (Biolegend). Store at 4 °C, protected from light.
6. Flow cytometer (BD Biosciences).

3 Methods

3.1 Immunofluorescence Staining of γ-H2AX

3.1.1 Preparation of Adherent Cell Samples

1. Seed 1 × 10^5 cells per well into 2-well LAB-TEK II chamber slides in complete media containing 100 U/mL penicillin, 100 μg/mL streptomycin, and 10% fetal bovine serum (FBS).
2. Incubate cells overnight in a tissue culture incubator at 37 °C with 5% CO_2.
3. Remove culture media and add fresh media containing nanoparticles. Continue to culture cells.
4. At the end of the experiment, aspirate the media and remove chamber walls.
5. Rinse the slides twice with ice-cold 1× PBS carefully.
6. Fix cells with acetone solution for 15 min at −20 °C (*see* **Note 6**).
7. Wash slides three times in 1× PBS with 5 min each time.

3.1.2 Preparation of Suspension Cell Samples

1. Seed 5 × 10^5 cells per well of a 6-well plate in complete media containing 100 U/mL penicillin, 100 μg/mL streptomycin, and 10% fetal bovine serum (FBS).
2. Treat cells with nanoparticles and incubate cells in a tissue culture incubator at 37 °C with 5% CO_2.
3. At the end of the experiment, transfer cells and culture media to 15 mL conical tubes and centrifuge at 200 × *g* for 10 min.
4. Aspirate the media carefully and resuspend cell pellets with ice-cold 1× PBS. Collect cells by centrifugation at 200 × *g* for 10 min.
5. Fix cells with 2 mL of acetone solution for 15 min at −20 °C (*see* **Note 6**).

6. Add 10 mL of 1× PBS and centrifuge at 200 × *g* for 10 min. Discard the supernatant.
7. Repeat **step 6** for one more time.
8. Add 1 mL of 1× PBS and mix gently.
9. Load 200 μL of cell suspension sample into cytospin bucket/filter/glass slide assembly and spin at 600 rpm for 3 min at room temperature by using a Cytospin® 4 Cytocentrifuge.
10. Disassemble and let slides dry completely (*see* **Note 7**).

3.1.3 Preparation of Frozen Sections

1. Prepare frozen sections (5–10 μM thick) from tissues and place sections on slides (*see* **Note 8**).
2. Air-dry sections for 30 min under airflow.
3. Fix the tissue in ice-cold acetone for 10 min at room temperature (*see* **Note 6**).
4. Wash slides three times in 1× PBS with 5 min each time.

3.1.4 Preparation of Paraffin Sections

1. Prepare tissue sections (4–5 μM thick) from formalin-fixed paraffin-embedded tissue blocks and place sections on slides.
2. Deparaffinize by placing slides in xylene twice, 5 min each time.
3. Rehydrate by placing slides in 100% ethanol twice, 95% ethanol twice, 70% ethanol once, 2 min each time.
4. Rinse briefly in distilled water.
5. Incubate the tissues in antigen retrieval buffer in a water bath at 95 °C for 60 min. Allow it to cool down to room temperature (*see* **Note 9**).
6. Wash the sections in 1× PBS for three times, 5 min each.

3.1.5 Immunostaining

1. Use a PAP pen to draw a hydrophobic ring around the section or cells.
2. Incubate cells or tissues with blocking solution in a humidity chamber at room temperature for 30 min.
3. Discard blocking solution, and incubate with a 1:100–200 dilution of mouse monoclonal anti-γ-H2AX antibody at room temperature for 2 h or 4 °C overnight.
4. Rinse the slides in 1× PBS three times with 5 min each time.
5. Incubate in the dark with rhodamine-conjugated goat anti-mouse IgG (H + L) (1:500) in a humidified chamber at room temperature for 1 h.
6. Discard the solution, and rinse the slides three times in 1× PBS for 5 min each in the dark.
7. Add one drop of Prolong Diamond Antifade Mountant with DAPI on each slide and cover with glass coverslip. Store in the dark at −20 °C or 4 °C if not viewed immediately.

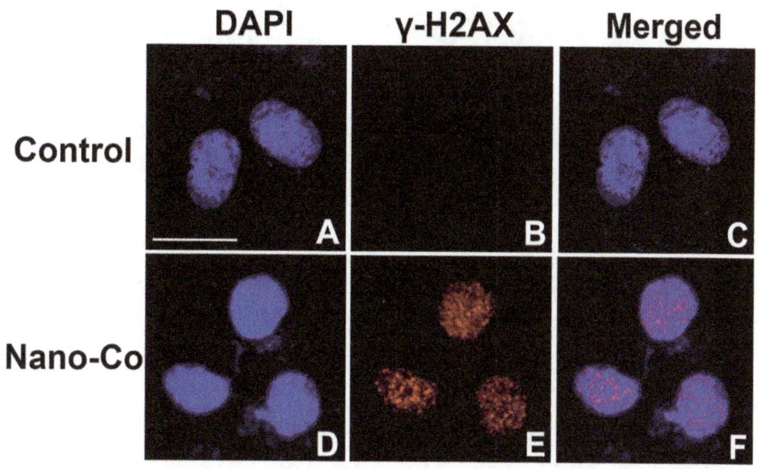

Fig. 1 Increased γ-H2AX foci formation in BEAS-2B cells exposed to Nano-Co. Normal human bronchial epithelial BEAS-2B cells were exposed to 2.5 μg/mL of Nano-Co for 24 h (**d-f**). Cells without treatment were used as control (**a-c**). Cell nuclei were stained with DAPI (blue) (**a** and **d**), and the red γ-H2AX foci (**e**) reproduced as pink in the merged image (**f**). Scale bar in (**a**) represents 20 μm for all panels

8. View the slides under a fluorescence microscope or a confocal microscope (Fig. 1).
9. Count γ-H2AX foci in 100 cells. The slide that goes through all steps and all reagents except the primary antibody is used as the negative control.

3.2 Immunohistochemical Staining for γ-H2AX

3.2.1 Preparation of Adherent Cell Samples

Follow Subheading 3.1.1.

3.2.2 Preparation of Suspension Cell Samples

Follow Subheading 3.1.2.

3.2.3 Preparation of Frozen Sections

Follow Subheading 3.1.3.

3.2.4 Preparation of Paraffin Sections

Follow Subheading 3.1.4.

3.2.5 Immunohistochemical Staining

1. Immerse the slides in methanol with 0.3% H_2O_2 for 30 min to quench endogenous peroxidase activity.
2. Rinse briefly in 1× PBS.
3. Use a PAP pen to draw a hydrophobic ring around the section or cells.

4. Incubate with blocking solution in a humidity chamber for 30 min at room temperature to block unspecific binding of the antibodies.
5. Aspirate excess blocking solution, and incubate with a 1:100–200 dilution of mouse anti-γ-H2AX antibody at room temperature for 2 h or at 4 °C overnight.
6. Wash with 1× PBS for three times, 5 min each time.
7. Incubate with diluted biotinylated secondary antibody for 30 min at room temperature.
8. Wash with 1× PBS for three times, 5 min each time.
9. Prepare VECTASTAIN® ABC working solution and allow it to stand for about 30 min before use. Incubate with VECTASTAIN® ABC working solution for 30 min at room temperature.
10. Wash in buffer for three times, 5 min each time.
11. Incubate in DAB peroxidase substrate solution until desired stain intensity develops (usually 1–2 min).
12. Counterstain with hematoxylin for 1 min.
13. Dehydrate by place slides in 70% ethanol once, 95% ethanol twice, and 100% ethanol twice, 2 min each time.
14. Clear in xylene twice, 5 min each time.
15. Mount coverslips with Permount.
16. The slide that goes through all steps and all reagents except the primary antibody is used as the negative control.
17. Examine under a light microscope, and calculate the percentage of immunostaining positive cells (*see* **Note 10**).

3.3 Immunoblotting for γ-H2AX

3.3.1 Extraction of Nuclear Protein from Cells

1. For adherent cells, harvest with trypsin-EDTA and centrifuge at 200 × *g* for 10 min at 4 °C. For suspension cells, harvest by centrifuging at 200 × *g* for 10 min at 4 °C.
2. Wash the cells twice with ice-cold 1× PBS.
3. Use a pipette to carefully remove the supernatant as more as possible.
4. Add ice-cold CER I (lysis buffer containing protease inhibitors) to the cell pellet by using NE-PER Nuclear and Cytoplasmic Extraction Reagent kit according to the manufacturer's instruction, using the reagent volumes indicated in Table 1.
5. Vortex vigorously for 15 s to fully suspend the cell pellet. Incubate on ice for 10 min.
6. Add ice-cold CER II to the tube and vortex vigorously for 5 s. Then incubate on ice for 1 min.

Table 1
Reagent volumes for different packed cell volumes

Packed cell volume (μL)	CER I (μL)	CER II (μL)	NER (μL)
10	100	5.5	50
20	200	11	100
50	500	27.5	250
100	1000	55	500

7. Vortex the tube vigorously for 5 s and centrifuge at 12,000 × *g* for 15 min at 4 °C.
8. Immediately transfer the supernatant (cytoplasmic extract) to a clean prechilled tube. Place this tube on ice until other use or storage.
9. Suspend the insoluble (pellet) fraction produced in **step** 7, which contains nuclei, in ice-cold NER.
10. Vortex the tube vigorously for 15 s. Place the sample on ice. Vortex for 15 s every 10 min, for a total of 40 min.
11. Centrifuge the tube at 12,000 × *g* for 10 min at 4 °C.
12. Immediately transfer the supernatant (nuclear extract) fraction to a clean prechilled tube and place it on ice.
13. Measure protein concentration by using Bio-Rad protein assay.

3.3.2 Extraction of Nuclear Protein from Tissues

1. Weigh the tissue (~20 mg). Cut the tissue into small pieces and place in a microcentrifuge tube (*see* **Note 11**).
2. Wash tissue with 1× PBS and centrifuge at 300 × *g* for 10 min.
3. Using a pipette, carefully remove and discard the supernatant, collect the pellet.
4. Homogenize tissue using a homogenizer in the appropriate volume of ice-cold CER I (Table 2).
5. Proceed to Cytoplasmic and Nuclear Protein Extraction following Subheading 3.3.1, **steps 5–13**, using the reagent volumes indicated in Table 2.

3.3.3 SDS–Polyacrylamide Gel Electrophoresis

Preparation of 15% SDS–Polyacrylamide Gel

1. Prepare two 15% separating gels by mixing the reagents in Table 3.
2. Carefully overlay the separating gel with 1 mL of 0.1% SDS. Let the gel polymerize for at least 40 min at room temperature.
3. Discard the overlay of 0.1% SDS solution from the separating gel.
4. Prepare stacking gel according to Table 3.

Table 2
Reagent volumes for different tissue amounts

Tissue weight (mg)	CER I (μL)	CER II (μL)	NER (μL)
20	200	11	100
40	400	22	200
80	800	44	400
100	1000	55	500

Table 3
Preparation of SDS polyacrylamide gel

	Separating gel (15%)	Stacking gel
1.5 M Tris–HCI, pH 8.8	4 mL	
1.0 M Tris–HCI, pH 6.8		0.75 mL
30% Acrylamide/Bis-acrylamide	8 mL	1.0 mL
H_2O	3.67 mL	4.1 mL
10% SDS	160 μL	60 μL
10% AP	160 μL	60 μL
TEMED	10 μL	6 μL
Total (for 2 gels)	~16 mL	~6 mL

5. Insert the combs into the liquid stacking gel immediately. Let the stacking gel polymerize at room temperature for at least 40 min.

Gel Running

1. Gently pull out the comb from the stacking gel. Fill the buffer chambers with 1× running buffer.
2. Add 5× Loading buffer to nuclear extracts.
3. Boil the mixture at 95–100 °C for 5 min, then cool on ice.
4. Briefly spin down the mixture at room temperature.
5. Load the samples and protein standard marker.
6. Electrophorese the SDS-polyacrylamide gel at 40 V until the bromophenol blue tracking dye runs into the separating gel.
7. Increase the electric voltage to 100 V and run until the bromophenol blue tracking dye reaches about ¾ of the separating gel.

3.3.4 Western Blotting

1. After gel running, cut and discard the stacking gel.
2. Place the separating gel in prechilled transfer buffer for 15 min at room temperature.
3. Wet PVDF membrane in methanol briefly, then place in prechilled transfer buffer for 15 min to equilibrate. Also wet sponges and filter papers for transfer cassette.
4. Set up the "sandwich" of transfer cassette in the following order: sponge on the black side of transfer cassette followed by wet filter paper, gel, PVDF membrane, wet filter paper, and sponge, ensuring that no bubbles are present in the sandwich.
5. Electrotransfer proteins to PVDF membrane at 100 V for 1 h or at 100 mA overnight at 4 °C. Be sure to use cooling unit to cool down the transfer system during the electrophoretic transfer.
6. Disassemble the transfer cassette and briefly rinse the PVDF membrane with distilled water.
7. Incubate PVDF membrane in 10 mL blocking solution for 1 h at room temperature. Gently agitate using a rocker platform.
8. Transfer membrane to a tray containing mouse anti-γ-H2AX antibody diluted 1:1000 in 10 mL blocking solution (10 μL of antibody diluted into 10 mL blocking solution). Incubate the membrane with gentle agitation at 4 °C overnight.
9. Wash membrane with gentle agitation in a tray containing 20 mL of PBS-T three times, 5 min each time.
10. Incubate membrane in a tray containing goat anti-mouse horseradish peroxidase (HRP)-conjugated IgG diluted 1:1000 in 10 mL blocking solution for 1 h at room temperature with gentle agitation.
11. Wash membrane with PBS-T three times, 5 min each time.
12. Mix Enhanced Chemiluminescent Reagents (GE Healthcare) 1 and 2 at a 1:1 ratio and add it to the membrane. Incubate membrane for 1 min. Drain membrane of excess developing solution (do not let it dry). Cover membrane with a clear plastic wrap.
13. Expose membrane to X-ray film.
14. After detection of γ-H2AX, wash membrane with PBS-T twice, 5 min each time.
15. Strip the membrane with restoring western blot stripping buffer according to the manufacturer's instruction.
16. Reprobe with rabbit monoclonal anti-H2AX antibody (as a loading control) diluted 1:2000 in 10 mL blocking solution. Repeat the probing and development steps as above. Use goat anti-rabbit horseradish peroxidase (HRP)-conjugated IgG as the secondary antibody (1:1000).

17. Perform densitometric analyses to quantify immunoblotting signals using NIH Image J software or other software. Use H2AX as a loading control.

3.4 Flow Cytometry for γ-H2AX

The assessment of *γ-H2*AX using flow cytometry is a high-throughput genotoxicity screening assay to predict the outcome of in vitro mammalian cell genotoxicity.

1. Seed 4 × 10^6 cells (for suspension cells) in each cell culture dish (100 mm). Incubate cells with complete media overnight.
2. Treat cells with appropriate nanoparticles and continue to grow in complete media.
3. Harvest cells by centrifugation at 200 × *g* for 10 min at 4 °C and resuspend cell pellet with ice-cold 1× PBS carefully in 15 mL conical tube.
4. Collect cells by centrifugation at 200 × *g* for 10 min at 4 °C.
5. Discard the supernatant and vortex briefly to loosen cell pellet.
6. Fix cells with 5 mL of 1% methanol-free formaldehyde for 15 min at 4 °C.
7. Centrifuge at 200 × *g* for 10 min at 4 °C and discard the supernatant.
8. Add 1 mL ice-cold 70% ethanol drop by drop. Vortex while adding 70% ethanol. Incubate at −20 °C for 1 h. The sample can be stored at −20 °C for more than 2 weeks.
9. Collect cell pellets by centrifugation at 200 × *g* for 10 min.
10. Wash cells twice with 1× PBS. Centrifuge at 200 × *g* for 10 min.
11. Incubate cells with 500 μL of 1% BSA solution in 1× PBS for 2 h and centrifuge at 200 × *g* for 10 min.
12. Discard the supernatant. Add FITC-conjugated anti-γ-H2AX antibody (Biolegend) diluted 1:200 in 100 μL of 1% BSA/PBS solution. Incubate in dark for 2 h at room temperature.
13. Wash cells with 1× PBS and centrifuge at 200 × *g* for 10 min.
14. Resuspend cells in 500 μL ice-cold 1× PBS and keep it in the dark on ice (*see* **Note 12**).
15. Measure γ-H2AX fluorescence values in 10^4 cells by using flow cytometer (BD Biosciences) with standard emission filters.

4 Notes

1. Unpolymerized acrylamide is a neurotoxin and can be absorbed via skin or respiratory mucosa. Face mask must be worn when weighing acrylamide and bis-acrylamide.

The 30% acrylamide–bis-acrylamide solution can be stored at 4 °C for up to 1 month. It is better to make the acrylamide–bis-acrylamide solution fresh about every month since acrylamide hydrolyzes to acrylic acid.

2. 10% ammonium persulfate can be prepared, aliquoted, and stored at −20 °C for later use. Remove only the required amount for each use.
3. Wear a face mask to avoid inhalation of SDS dust during preparation of the solution.
4. Do not store SDS solution at 4 °C, as SDS will precipitate at temperature below 15 °C. If there is any precipitate, redissolve it by warming (68 °C for 10 min). Do not autoclave 10% SDS solution.
5. Formaldehyde is carcinogenic and has irritant vapor. Preparation of solution must be carried out in a fume hood while wearing face mask.
6. Place acetone solution in −20 °C freezer overnight to cool down the solution. Acetone will also permeabilize. No further permeabilization step is required. Ethanol and methanol will also permeabilize.
7. It requires a wait of at least 10 min after removing the bucket and the filter paper.
8. Store frozen sections at −80 °C if not used immediately. For best result, use immediately.
9. In general, antigen retrieval process is not necessary for frozen sections. As antibody binding epitopes can be masked in formaldehyde-based fixation due to cross-linking of amino groups on adjacent molecules, antigen retrieval is required.
10. Combinative semiquantitative scoring is the most common method to analyze the IHC result. The values of the relative percentage of immunostaining positive cells to the total number of target cells can be recorded as numerical scores as follow: 1(0%~25%); 2(26%~50%); 3(51%~75%); 4(≧76%). The intensity of the immunostaining of cells is evaluated and commonly scored from 0 to 3 (0, negative; 1+, weak positive; 2+, moderate positive; and 3+, strong positive). The final immunoscore is calculated by adding or multiplying each score [19, 20].
11. The tissues need to be processed or frozen in liquid N_2 immediately after removing from the animal to prevent proteins from degradation.
12. For the best results, cells need to be analyzed by flow cytometer as soon as possible. In general, a total of 10^7 cells are required.

Acknowledgment

This work was partly supported by the National Natural Science Foundation of China (81473009), and an Intramural Research Development Grant from Fujian Medical University (JS14001) to Dr. Rong Wan; and NIESH/NIH (ES023693 and ES028911), KSEF-148-502-16-381, Kentucky Lung Cancer Research Program, and an Intramural Research Incentive Grants (50992) from UofL to Dr. Qunwei Zhang.

References

1. Moore JD, Krebs JE (2004) Histone modifications and DNA double-strand break repair. Biochem Cell Biol 82(4):446–452
2. Khanna KK, Jackson SP (2001) DNA double-strand breaks: signaling, repair and the cancer connection. Nat Genet 27(3):247–254
3. Rogakou EP, Pilch DR, Orr AH, Ivanova VS, Bonner WM (1998) DNA double-stranded breaks induce histone H2AX phosphorylation on serine 139. J Biol Chem 273 (10):5858–5868
4. Paull TT, Rogakou EP, Yamazaki V, Kirchgessner CU, Gellert M, Bonner WM (2000) A critical role for Histone H2AX in recruitment of repair factors to nuclear foci after DNA damage. Curr Biol 10:886–895
5. Burma S, Chen BP, Murphy M, Kurimasa A, Chen DJ (2001) ATM phosphorylates histone H2AX in response to DNA double-strand breaks. J Biol Chem 276(45):42462–42467
6. Ward IM, Chen J (2001) Histone H2AX is phosphorylated in an ATR-dependent manner in response to replicational stress. J Biol Chem 276:47759–47762
7. Bassing CH, Chua KF, Sekiguchi J, Suh H, Whitlow SR, Fleming JC, Monroe BC, Ciccone DN, Yan C, Vlasakova K, Livingston DM, Ferguson DO, Scully R, Alt FW (2002) Increased ionizing radiation sensitivity and genomic instability in the absence of histone H2AX. Proc Natl Acad Sci U S A 99 (12):8173–8178
8. Celeste A, Petersen S, Romanienko PJ, Fernandez-Capetillo O et al (2002) Genomic instability in mice lacking histone H2AX. Science 296(5569):922–927
9. Sedelnikova OA, Rogakou EP, Panyutin IG, Bonner WM (2002) Quantitative detection of (125)IdU-induced DNA double strand breaks with γ-H2AX antibody. Radiat Res 158 (4):486–492
10. Nikolova T, Dvorak M, Jung F, Adam I, Krämer E, Gerhold-Ay A, Kaina B (2014) The γH2AX assay for genotoxic and nongenotoxic agents: comparison of H2AX phosphorylation with cell death response. Toxicol Sci 140 (1):103–117
11. Watters GP, Smart DJ, Harvey JS, Austin CA (2009) H2AX phosphorylation as a genotoxicity endpoint. Mutat Res 679(1–2):50–58
12. Gonzaleza L, Lisonb D, Krisch-Volders M (2008) Genotoxicity of engineered nanomaterials: a critical review. Nanotoxicology 2 (4):252–273
13. Landsiedel R, Kapp MD, Schulz M, Wiench K, Oesch F (2009) Genotoxicity investigation on nanomaterials: methods, preparation and characterization of test material, potential artifacts and limitations-many questions, some answers. Mutat Res 681(2–3):241–258
14. Yousuke T, Tatsushi T, Yuko I (2012) Flow cytometric evaluation of nanoparticles using side-scattered light and reactive oxygen species-mediated fluorescence-correlation with genotoxicity. Environ Sci Technol 46 (14):7629–7636
15. Zhao X, Takabayashi F, Yuko I (2016) Coexposure to silver nanoparticles and ultraviolet A synergistically enhances the phosphorylation of histone H2AX. J Photochem Photobiol B 162:213–222
16. Åkerlund E, Cappellini F, Di Bucchianico S, Islam S, Skoglund S, Derr R, Odnevall Wallinder I, Hendriks G, Karlsson HL (2018) Genotoxic and mutagenic properties of Ni and NiO nanoparticles investigated by comet assay, γ-H2AX staining, Hprt mutation assay and ToxTracker reporter cell lines. Environ Mol Mutagen 59(3):211–222. https://doi.org/10.1002/em.22163
17. Wan R, Mo Y, Feng L, Chien S, Tollerud DJ, Zhang Q (2012) DNA damage caused by metal nanoparticles: involvement of oxidative

stress and activation of ATM. Chem Res Toxicol 25(7):1402–1411

18. Wan R, Mo Y, Zhang Z, Jiang M, Tang S, Zhang Q (2017) Cobalt nanoparticles induce lung injury, DNA damage and mutations in mice. Part Fibre Toxicol 14(1):1–15. https://doi.org/10.1186/s12989-017-0219-z

19. Kim SW, Roh J, Park CS (2016) Immunohistochemistry for pathologists: protocols, pitfalls, and tips. J Pathol Transl Med 50:411–418

20. Cynthia S, Gerald L, Jeffrey W, Carlin O, Ronald H (2002) Qualitative and quantitative analysis of nonneoplastic lesions in toxicology studies. Toxicol Pathol 30(1):93–96

Chapter 10

Analysis of Nanomaterial Toxicity by Western Blot

Gao Long, Yiqun Mo, Qunwei Zhang, and Mizu Jiang

Abstract

Western blot is a routine biochemical technique for the immunodetection of proteins in cells and tissues exposed to nanomaterials (NMs). It is a sensitive method for protein analysis that involves the solubilization and separation of proteins by sodium dodecyl sulfate–polyacrylamide gel electrophoresis (SDS-PAGE), transferring and immobilizing proteins onto a solid support, and targeted immunoprobing of a specific antigen. As a convenient and reliable research tool, the western blot plays an irreplaceable role in the era of proteomics together with mass spectrometry and protein chip. In this chapter we describe the detailed protocol for the entire process from sample preparation to quantitative measurement of target proteins.

Key words Nanomaterials, Electrophoresis, SDS-PAGE, Electroblotting, Nitrocellulose, PVDF, Antibody, Chemiluminescence

1 Introduction

The past decades have witnessed accelerating fast growth in the field of nanotechnology. Nanomaterials (NMs) exhibit physical, chemical, and biological properties associated with the unique physicochemical nanostructure [1]. They enter the cells by means of endocytosis and interact with intracellular compartments which leads to variable biological responses [2]. Endocytosis and biokinetics depend largely on NM surface chemistry, in vivo surface modifications, and size [3, 4]. Size is the key influence factor for cell modification [4]. Studies have indicated that smaller-sized particles possess the greater surface area per mass of particles, which renders NMs more active biologically [3, 5]. The mechanisms behind the toxic effects of NMs involve inflammatory response, oxidative stress, autophagy induction, lipid peroxidation, DNA damage, membrane damage, lysosomal dysfunction, mitochondrial dysfunction (in case of eukaryotic cells), apoptosis, etc. [6–8]. As a biochemical analysis technique, western blot reflects cellular functional changes that occur after the cells are exposed to

Qunwei Zhang (ed.), *Nanotoxicity: Methods and Protocols*, Methods in Molecular Biology, vol. 1894,
https://doi.org/10.1007/978-1-4939-8916-4_10,

NMs. Moreover, such changes connect the physicochemical properties of NMs to the underlying adverse biological outcomes, which make it easier to predict risk [9].

2 Materials

All solutions must be prepared with Milli-Q-purified, ultrapure, or double-distilled water and using analytical grade reagents.

2.1 Sample Preparation

1. Radioimmunoprecipitation assay (RIPA) buffer: 25 mM Tris–HCl, pH 8.0, 150 mM NaCl, 1% Nonidet P-40, 0.5–1% sodium deoxycholate, 0.1% SDS. It is the most commonly used buffer to obtain the whole cell lysate. Omit 0.1% SDS if only cytosolic proteins are needed.
2. Protease inhibitors: 1 mM phenylmethylsulfonyl fluoride (PMSF, Thermo Fisher SCIENTIFIC). Add PMSF into the RIPA buffer in a ratio of 100:1 just before use.
3. 5× SDS sample buffer: 10% (w/v) SDS, 10 mM dithiothreitol (DTT) or beta-mercaptoethanol, 20% (v/v) glycerol, 200 mM Tris–HCl, pH 6.8, 0.05% (w/v) bromophenol blue. The sample buffer must be completely dissolved before use.

2.2 SDS-PAGE and Electrotransfer

1. Polyacrylamide gel: 30% acrylamide–bis-acrylamide solution (29:1), 1 M Tris–HCl, pH 8.8, 1 M Tris–HCl, pH 6.8, 10% SDS, 10% ammonium peroxydisulfate (AP), tetramethylethylenediamine (TEMED). All solutions can be obtained from some companies such as Beyotime. Prepare polyacrylamide gel according to Table 1.
2. Prestained molecular-weight (MW) marker: Purchase a marker based on the MW of the target protein, for example, double color protein maker (10–250 kDa) from Bio-Rad.
3. 1× SDS sample buffer: Mix 200 μL of 5× SDS sample buffer with 800 μL water to make 1 mL of 1× SDS sample buffer. The sample buffer must be completely mixed and dissolved before use.
4. 10× electrophoresis buffer: Dissolve 30.3 g Tris base, 144 g glycine, and 10 g SDS in 1 L water (pH 8.3). Make sure that all powders are completely dissolved and mixed fully before use. Store at room temperature.
5. 1× electrophoresis buffer: Dilute 10× electrophoresis buffer tenfold with water. Add 100 mL of 10× electrophoresis buffer into 900 mL water. Mix fully before use. Store at room temperature.
6. Buffer dam: If only one gel is run.

Table 1
Recipe for preparation of separating and stacking gels

	Separating gel					Stacking gel
Solutions	**6%**	**8%**	**10%**	**12%**	**15%**	**5%**
H_2O (mL)	4.0	3.3	2.7	2.0	1.0	2.7
30% Acr–Bis (29:1) (mL)	2.0	2.7	3.3	4.0	5.0	0.67
1 M Tris–HCl, pH 8.8 (mL)	3.8	3.8	3.8	3.8	3.8	–
1 M Tris–HCl, pH 6.8 (mL)	–	–	–	–	–	0.5
10% SDS (μL)	100	100	100	100	100	40
10% AP (μL)	100	100	100	100	100	40
TEMED (μL)	8	6	4	4	4	4
Total volume (mL)	10	10	10	10	10	4

This recipe applies to two gels for Bio-Rad Mini-PROTEAN Tetra Cell System using spacer plates with 1.0 mm thickness integrated spacer. Adjust the solution volumes in accordance with the manufacturer's instruction if a different system is used

7. The electrophoresis system: Bio-Rad Mini-PROTEAN Tetra System.
8. Basic power supply (Bio-Rad).
9. 10× transfer buffer: Dissolve 30.3 g Tris base and 144 g glycine in 1 L water (pH 8.3). Make sure that all powders are completely dissolved and mixed fully before use. Store at room temperature.
10. 1× transfer buffer: Mix 100 mL of 10× transfer buffer, 200 mL methanol, and 700 mL water. Store at 4°C.
11. Membrane/adsorbent filter paper: Nitrocellulose/polyvinylidene difluoride (PVDF) membranes, adsorbent filter papers.
12. Methanol.

2.3 Immunodetection

1. 10× TBS: Dissolve 12.1 g Tris base and 87.66 g NaCl in 1 L water. Adjust pH to 7.6 with HCl. Make sure that all powders are completely dissolved and mixed fully before use.
2. 1× TBST: Mix 100 mL 10× TBS, 900 mL water, and 1 mL Tween 20 (final 0.1%) (*see* **Note 1**). Mix well.
3. Blocking solution: 5% nonfat milk or 1% BSA in 1× TBST. Prepare fresh before use.
4. Primary antibody.
5. Secondary antibody: Horseradish peroxidase (HRP)-conjugated IgG generated against host species of primary antibody.

6. Forceps for handling membranes, shaker, X-ray film, and dark room.
7. Chemiluminescence reagent: For example, ECL™ Western Blotting Detection Reagents (Sigma-Aldrich).

3 Methods

The effects of NMs can be assessed in both in vitro and in vivo settings. Since this chapter focuses on the basic technique of western blot, here we only chose adherent cells as a model for NM exposure and protein extraction.

3.1 Exposure of Cells to NMs

1. The NMs are weighed, prepared in normal saline, autoclaved, and stored at −20 °C as a stock solution. For working solution, NM stock solutions are sonicated at room temperature for 10 min, vortexed, and diluted in culture media (e.g., DMEM) to the desired working concentrations (*see* **Note 2**).
2. Sonicate and vortex NM working solutions just before use (*see* **Note 3**).
3. Add the NM dispersions to the culture plate and incubate the cells in a humid incubator at 37 °C and 95% air–5% CO_2 for scheduled time (*see* **Note 4**).

3.2 Sample Preparation for Electrophoresis

1. Add PMSF in protein lysis buffer (e.g., RIPA buffer) just before use to ward off proteolysis (*see* **Note 5**). If phosphorylated proteins are to be detected, also add phosphatase inhibitors.
2. Remove the medium and rinse twice with ice-cold phosphate buffered saline (1× PBS).
3. Discard the 1× PBS and add the lysis buffer to the culture plate.
4. Scrape down the adherent cells. Gently transfer the cell suspension into an ice-cold centrifuge tube.
5. Lyse for half an hour on the ice.
6. Centrifuge the samples at 4 °C and 10,000 × g for 15 min. Transfer the supernatant to a new ice-cold centrifuge tube and discard the cell debris.
7. Determine the protein concentrations of the samples by BCA protein measuring kit or Bradford assay (*see* **Note 6**).
8. Mix the protein samples with 5× SDS sample buffer in a 4:1 ratio. Vortex and heat at 100 °C for 10 min (*see* **Note 7**). Centrifuge the samples briefly to bring down the sediment.

3.3 SDS-PAGE

1. Prepare the separating gel solution according to Table 1 (*see* **Note 8**).
2. Pour the gel solution into the interspace of two glass plates until the height of the solution reaches three-fourths of the small glass plate (*see* **Note 9**).
3. Seal with H_2O or 0.1% SDS to accelerate the polymerization. Be careful not to disturb the surface of the solution.
4. After polymerizing for at least 40 min (*see* **Note 10**). Discard the liquid at the top of the gel (*see* **Note 11**).
5. Prepare the stacking gel solution according to Table 1 and pour immediately into the interspace until full. Insert a gel comb immediately without introducing air bubbles (*see* **Note 12**).
6. Wait for the stacking gel to polymerize for at least 40 min.
7. Install the electrophoresis apparatus by placing the gels into the cassette clamp with the short plate facing the inside of the upper tank reservoir. Ensure a compaction fix to prevent leakage (*see* **Note 13**). If one gel is used, insert a buffer dam.
8. Insert the electrophoresis apparatus into tank.
9. Fill the cassette clamp with 1× electrophoresis buffer. Gently extract comb from the stacking gel and rinse each well several times with the 1× electrophoresis buffer.
10. Add the 1× electrophoresis buffer to the tank.
11. Load the samples and markers in the wells. Ensure equal volume or equivalent mass across multiple samples while loading. Load an equal volume of 1× SDS sample buffer into those needless wells (*see* **Note 14**).
12. Cover the tank lid and connect the apparatus to the power supply (*see* **Note 15**).
13. Run gels at 40 V of constant voltage until the bromophenol blue dye runs into the separating gel, then at 90 V of constant voltage until the dye reaches the bottom or a desirable resolution is attained (*see* **Note 16**).
14. Shut power supply off and remove the clamp frame (*see* **Note 17**).
15. Rinse the gel with running water several times. Open the clamp and cut off the stacking gel carefully.
16. Shear a small notch at the lower left corner of the marker protein position in the gel to orient the order of loading samples.
17. Transfer the separating gel gently to the container filled with blot transfer buffer (*see* **Note 18**).

3.4 Electrotransfer

1. Cut a nitrocellulose/PVDF membrane and two pieces of filter paper with the same size as a separating gel.
2. Prewet the PVDF membrane in methanol for 15 s before immersing in 1× transfer buffer for at least 10 min (This procedure is no need for nitrocellulose membrane). Soak the membrane, filter papers, and foam sponges (in case of wet blotting) in 1× transfer buffer (*see* **Note 18**).
3. Pave the blotting sandwich in sequence of the dark side of the plastic transfer cassette, dark foam sponge, filter paper, polyacrylamide gel, membrane, filter paper, white foam sponge, and the white side of the cassette. Ensure to get rid of any air bubbles between the gel and the membrane (*see* **Note 19**).
4. Close the clip. Insert the cassette into the tank by facing the gel toward the cathode. Put the cooled ice pack in the tank next to the side of the transfer cassette.
5. Fill the tank completely with precooled 1× transfer buffer to cover the transfer cassette.
6. Set the power supply at 350 mA of constant current for 60 min or 100 mA overnight and start running.
7. When finished, stop the power supply and take out the membrane.
8. Shear a small notch at the upper left corner of the marker protein position in the membrane to orient the protein surface of membrane and the order of loading samples. The face of the membrane and top will always be oriented with the notch on the upper left (*see* **Note 20**).
9. Briefly rinse the membrane with 1× TBST.

3.5 Immunodetection

1. Incubate the membrane with blocking solution for 1 h at room temperature with gentle rocking.
2. Discard the blocking solution and add the primary antibody solution (*see* **Note 21**). Incubate at least 2 h at room temperature or at 4 °C overnight with gentle rocking.
3. Discard the primary antibody solution and wash the membrane with 1× TBST three times, 10 min each time.
4. Incubate the membrane with HRP-conjugated secondary antibody for one hour at room temperature with gentle rocking (*see* **Note 21**).
5. Discard the secondary antibody solution and wash the membrane with 1× TBST three times, 10 min each time.
6. Prepare the chemiluminescence reagent (e.g., ECL) by mixing A and B solutions at a 1:1 ratio just before use (*see* **Note 22**).
7. Drain off 1× TBST solution as much as possible and cover the membrane with the chemiluminescent reagent solution.

8. After 1–2 min of incubation, drain off the excess solution and wrap the membrane with a plastic wrap.
9. Move to the digital imaging device system. Close the device door and adjust to the optimum focus point.
10. After automatic exposure, save the image as TIFF file and annotate in detail (*see* **Note 23**).
11. Analyze the results by using a software such as ImageJ.

4 Notes

1. Tween 20 is sticky. Avoid using a micropipette to pipet. Mix well by using a stirrer.
2. The working concentrations of NMs to treat cells vary in different types of NMs and cells. Pretest to find the appropriate concentrations to treat cells.
3. Vibrate dispersions vigorously with hands to ensure homogeneity before adding.
4. Incubation time varies according to the purpose of the experiment.
5. Choose a suitable lysate for extraction of proteins according to the purpose of the experiment. RIPA buffer is commonly used to extract proteins from cells for electrophoresis. The proportion of the lysis buffer and PMSF is 100:1.
6. Avoid using Bradford method if detergent such as SDS is contained in the sample.
7. After boiling, the samples can be stored at −20 °C for about 1 week. Avoid repeated freeze–thaw cycles.
8. Choose the appropriate gel concentration according to the molecular weight of the target protein (Table 2). Add AP and TEMED at last and use immediately. Precast gels of various polyacrylamide concentrations, gradient gels (e.g., 4–12%),

Table 2
The optimal separation range of separating gel with different concentrations

Polyacrylamide concentration	Separation range
6%	50–150 kDa
8%	30–90 kDa
10%	20–80 kDa
12%	12–60 kDa
15%	10–40 kDa

formats, and thickness with up to 1 year shelf life at 4 °C are commercially available. The number of wells and thickness of the gel determine the maximum loading volume of each well.

9. Unpolymerized acrylamide is poisonous. A mask and gloves should be worn when handling the acrylamide and avoid direct skin contact.
10. If the gel cannot polymerize within 40 min, AP and/or TEMED may need to be replaced with fresh reagents.
11. Remove H_2O or 0.1% SDS as much as possible. Remaining liquid may cause the stacking gel to shrink.
12. If there are air bubbles under the comb, remove the comb, rinse the wells with stacking gel solution to remove bubbles, and insert the comb again.
13. Fill the cassette clamp with 1× electrophoresis buffer and lay aside for a few minutes. If there is a leakage, reassemble the system.
14. Normalize the volume using 1× SDS sample buffer if necessary.
15. Ensure that the red wire (positive electrode) of the electrophoresis apparatus is plugged into the red port of the power supply, while black wire (negative electrode) is plugged into the black port of the power supply.
16. Take care not to run the target protein off the gel.
17. After stopping the electrophoresis, the gel should be transferred immediately.
18. Precooling the 1× transfer buffer leads to a better blotting effect.
19. Air bubbles will prevent the transfer of protein. Remove any bubbles by rolling over the membrane with a roller. Handle the gel and the nitrocellulose membrane gently in the transfer buffer because they are brittle. Make sure that the blotting sandwich is always immersed in the transfer buffer.
20. Mark the membrane with a ball-point pen at one corner for identification of the membrane if you have two or more membranes.
21. The optimal concentration of antibody needs to be determined through experimentation. Place the protein side of the membrane upward while incubating with the antibody.
22. Be careful not to cross-contaminate the solutions A and B.
23. If necessary, the blot can be stripped and reprobed with a primary antibody against a different antigen. Note that the membrane cannot be dry during the whole blotting and detection procedure.

Acknowledgment

This work was partly supported by the Public Welfare Project of Science Technology, Department of Zhejiang Province (2016C33152) to Dr. Mizu Jiang.

References

1. Ema M, Gamo M, Honda K (2016) A review of toxicity studies of single-walled carbon nanotubes in laboratory animals. Regul Toxicol Pharmacol 74:42–63
2. Gliga AR, Skoglund S, Wallinder IO, Fadeel B, Karlsson HL (2014) Size-dependent cytotoxicity of silver nanoparticles in human lung cells: the role of cellular uptake, agglomeration and Ag release. Part Fibre Toxicol 11:11
3. Oberdörster G, Oberdörster E, Oberdörster J (2005) Nanotoxicology: an emerging discipline evolving from studies of ultrafine particles. Environ Health Perspect 113:823–839
4. Mahmood M, Casciano DA, Mocan T, Iancu C, Xu Y, Mocan L, Iancu DT, Dervishi E, Li Z, Abdalmuhsen M, Biris AR, Ali N, Howard P, Biris AS (2010) Cytotoxicity and biological effects of functional nanomaterials delivered to various cell lines. J Appl Toxicol 30:74–83
5. Poon WL, Alenius H, Ndika J, Fortino V, Kolhinen V, Meščeriakovas A, Wang M, Greco D, Lähde A, Jokiniemi J, Lee JC, El-Nezami H, Karisola P (2017) Nano-sized zinc oxide and silver, but not titanium dioxide, induce innate and adaptive immunity and antiviral response in differentiated THP-1 cells. Nanotoxicology 11:936–951
6. Ivask A, Juganson K, Bondarenko O, Mortimer M, Aruoja V, Kasemets K, Blinova I, Heinlaan M, Slaveykova V, Kahru A (2014) Mechanisms of toxic action of Ag, ZnO and CuO nanoparticles to selected ecotoxicological test organisms and mammalian cells in vitro: a comparative review. Nanotoxicology 8 Suppl 1:57–71
7. Tuli HS, Kashyap D, Bedi SK, Kumar P, Kumar G, Sandhu SS (2015) Molecular aspects of metal oxide nanoparticle (MO-NPs) mediated pharmacological effects. Life Sci 143:71–79
8. Chevallet M, Veronesi G, Fuchs A, Mintz E, Michaud-Soret I, Deniaud A (2017) Impact of labile metal nanoparticles on cellular homeostasis. Biochim Biophys Acta 1861:1566–1577
9. Hendren CO, Lowry GV, Unrine JM, Wiesner MR (2015) A functional assay-based strategy for nanomaterial risk forecasting. Sci Total Environ 536:1029–1037

Chapter 11

Quantification of Mitochondrial Genome Transcription in Male Reproductive Cells by Real-Time PCR

Cheng Xu, Qian Liu, Jin Xu, and Aihua Gu

Abstract

Mitochondria are organelles that play a key role in the regulation of cell energy metabolism, biosynthesis, and cell death. Mitochondria are also involved in important physiological processes, such as the three-carboxylic acid cycle, the oxidation of fatty acids and amino acids, and calcium ion homeostasis. The energy demands of male germ cells during mitosis and meiosis are higher than those of somatic cells, suggesting that mitochondria play a critical role in sperm. Mitochondria are nanotoxicity targets in male germ cells. The level of mitochondrial genome transcription is reflective of mitochondrial function and can therefore be used as a quantitative index for evaluating nanotoxicity. This study describes how to use real-time PCR to evaluate the effects of nanomaterials on mitochondrial genome transcription in male reproductive cells.

Key words Mitochondria, Nanotoxicity, Real-time PCR, Transcription, Germ cell

1 Introduction

The mitochondrion, an important organelle, plays many important roles during normal physiological processes, including regulation of iron–sulfur cluster biogenesis [1], apoptosis [2], and calcium homeostasis [3]; its most important role is the production of cellular ATP via oxidative phosphorylation. Sequencing experiments reveal that the mitochondrial genome consists of only 37 genes: 13 structural genes involved in oxidative phosphorylation, 2 mitochondrial rRNA genes (12S and 16S), and 22 mitochondrial tRNAs (Fig. 1). These genes primarily constitute the mitochondrial electron respiratory chain complex, lending them a physiological function.

Cell culture methods permit the observation and investigation of live cell activity in vitro. Cells in culture are unaffected by the complex internal environment of the body, allowing researchers to control the environment of the cells. Compared with animal models, cell culture systems are low-cost, easy to operate, and beneficial for animal welfare.

Qunwei Zhang (ed.), *Nanotoxicity: Methods and Protocols*, Methods in Molecular Biology, vol. 1894,
https://doi.org/10.1007/978-1-4939-8916-4_11,

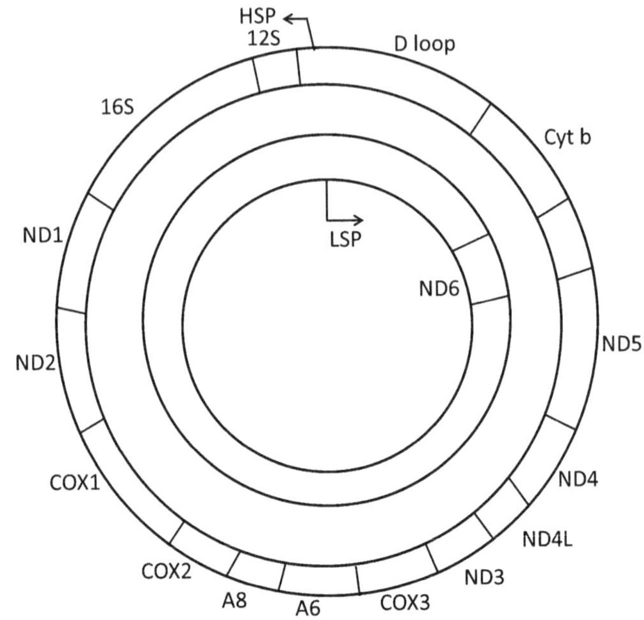

Fig. 1 The mitochondrial genome diagram. The selected 15 mitochondrial DNA encoded genes include seven subunits of complex I (ND1, 2, 3, 4, 4 L, 5, and 6), one subunit of complex III (cytochrome b (Cyt b)), three subunits of complex IV (Cyt c oxidase (COX) I, II, and III), two subunits of complex V (A6 and A8), and two rRNAs (12S and 16S). *HSP* heavy-strand promoter, *LSP* light-strand promoter

Table 1
A summary of cell culture conditions used to maintain commonly used male reproductive cell lines

Cell line	GC-1 spg	GC-2 spd	TM4	MLTC-1
Culture medium	DMEM+ 10% FBS	DMEM+ 10% FBS	DMEM+ 10% FBS	RPMI 1640+ 10% FBS
Growth conditions	Adherent	Adherent	Adherent	Adherent
Organism	*Mus musculus* (mouse)	*Mus musculus* (mouse)	*Mus musculus* (mouse)	*Mus musculus* (mouse)
Cell type	Transformed with Psv3-Neo	Spermatocyte	Sertoli cell	Leydig cell
Medium renewal	1–2 times per week	2–3 times a week	Every 3–4 days	Every 3–4 days

FBS fetal bovine serum

Depending on function and morphology, cells in the male reproductive system can be classified as Sertoli cells, Leydig cells, spermatogonia, spermatocytes, or differentiated haploid spermatocytes. The male reproductive cell lines used in this study were obtained from the ATCC cell bank; specific names, characteristics, and culture conditions of these cell lines are provided in Table 1.

Apart from several conventional assays (e.g., apoptosis, proliferation, viability, and cell cycle assays), the evaluation of nanomaterial toxicity on mitochondria has not been characterized. The real-time PCR method requires minimal DNA input and is a highly accurate measure of gene expression. In the present study, the real-time PCR method is used to evaluate the nanotoxic effects of several materials on mitochondrial organelles in male germ cells.

2 Materials

All reagents are analytical grade. Deionized water is used to prepare the solutions if not specified in the text.

2.1 General Equipment

1. Cell incubator.
2. Microplate reader.
3. Centrifugal machine.
4. Nanodrop-2000 spectrophotometer.
5. Applied Biosystems 7900HT.
6. Vortex instrument.

2.2 Reagents

1. Dulbecco's Modified Eagle's Medium (DMEM): 4 mM L-glutamine, 4500 mg/L glucose, 1 mM sodium pyruvate, and 1500 mg/L sodium bicarbonate. Weight 292.3 mg L-glutamine, 2250 mg glucose, 55 mg sodium pyruvate, and 750 mg sodium bicarbonate. Add water to a volume of 400 mL. Mix and make up to 0.5 L with water. Store at 4 °C.
2. RPMI-1640 medium: 2 mM L-glutamine, 10 mM HEPES, 1 mM sodium pyruvate, 4500 mg/L glucose, and 1500 mg/L sodium bicarbonate. Weight 146.15 mg L-glutamine, 2250 mg glucose, and 750 mg sodium bicarbonate. Add water to a volume of 400 mL. Mix and make up to 0.5 L with water. Store at 4 °C.
3. Phosphate buffered solution (PBS): Weigh 8.0 g NaCl, 0.2964 g $NaH_2PO_4{\cdot}2H_2O$, and 2.9 g $Na_2HPO_4{\cdot}12H_2O$ and dissolve in 900 mL double distilled water. Adjust pH to 7.4 with double distilled water. Add double distilled water to bring the volume to 1 L. Store at room temperature.
4. RNA reverse transcription reaction mixture: For 10 μL mixture, mix 2 μL $MgCl_2$ (25 mM), 1 μL 10× reverse transcription buffer (100 mM Tris–HCl [pH 8.3], 500 mM KCl), 3.75 μL RNase-free H_2O, 1 μL dNTP mixture (10 nM per 10 μL), 0.25 μL RNase inhibitor (40 U/μL), 0.5 μL AMV reverse transcriptase (5 U/μL), 0.5 μL random primers (50 pmol/μL), and 1 μL RNA (<500 ng per 10 μL).

5. Real-time polymerase chain reaction mixture: For 20 μL mixture, mix 1 μL forward primer (10 μM), 1 μL reverse primer (10 μM), 10 μL SYBR green (50 U/μL), 7 μL RNase-free H_2O, and 1 μL cDNA (<100 ng per 20 μL).
6. 0.25% trypsin (w/v), 10% fetal bovine serum (v/v), 0.1% penicillin (w/v), and 0.1% streptomycin (w/v). Store at −20 °C.
7. TRIzol reagent: Store at 4 °C.
8. Chloroform, isopropanol, ethyl alcohol, and water (DEPC treated): Store at room temperature.
9. Primers:
   Primers are small segments of single stranded DNA or RNA. Primers can be used as binding sites for DNA polymerase at the beginning of DNA replication. Under extracellular conditions, DNA can initiate replication only using primers. The primers listed here are synthetic two-segment oligonucleotide sequences. One primer is complementary to one DNA template chain at one end of the region of interest, and the other primer is complementary to another DNA template chain at the other end of the region of interest. The primers used in this study are detailed in Table 2.

Table 2
Primer sequences used for amplification

	Forward primer (5′–3′)	Reverse primer (5′–3′)
mt-Nd1	TCCGAGCATCTTATCCACGC	GTATGGTGGTACTCCCGCTG
mt-Nd2	ATCCTCCTGGCCATCGTACT	ATCAGAAGTGGAATGGGGCG
mt-Nd3	TTGCATTCTGACTCCCCCAA	GACGTGCAGAGCTTGTAGGG
mt-Nd4	TAATCGCACATGGCCTCACA	GCTGTGGATCCGTTCGTAGT
mt-Nd4l	TGCCATCTACCTTCTTCAACC	TGGAGCTTATGGAGTTGGAGTT
mt-Nd5	TAACCGCATCGGAGACATCG	GTGGAGGCCAAATTGTGCTG
mt-Nd6	GGATTGGGGTAGCGGCAATA	CCGCAAACAAAGATCACCCA
mt-Cytb	ACGCAAACGGAGCCTCAATA	CCTCATGGAAGGACGTAGCC
mt-Col	GCTAGCCGCAGGCATTACTA	CTCCTCCAGCGGGATCAAAG
mt-Co2	AACCGAGTCGTTCTGCCAAT	CTAGGGAGGGGACTGCTCAT
mt-Co3	AGCCTTTTCAG CCCTCCTTC	GTGGCCTTGGTAGGTTCCTT
mt-Atp6	GCAGTCCGGCTTACAGCTAA	GGTAGCTGTTGGTGGGCTAA
mt-Atp8	ACAAACATTCCCACTGGCAC	TTGGGGTAATGAATGAGGCAA
mt-Rnrl	CCACCGCGGTCATACGATTA	TTGGGTCTTAGCTGTCGTGT
mt-Rnr2	GTTCAGACCGGAGCAATCCA	GCGCTTATTTGTAAGGTGGCT

3 Methods

3.1 Cell Culture and Nanomaterial Exposure

Use DMEM and RPMI 1640 media for the culture of applicable cell lines. The media are supplemented with 10% fetal bovine serum and a 0.1% antibiotic mixture (penicillin and streptomycin, 1:1) prior to use.

1. Take preserved cell lines out of liquid nitrogen storage and rapidly thaw at 37 °C. When thawed, the cell suspension is added to the prepared cell culture medium.
2. Rock the cell culture dishes gently to disperse the cells in the culture medium; the cells are then placed in an incubator.
3. After a minimum of 6 h, remove the cell culture dishes from the incubator and change the medium (the old cell culture medium is discarded, the cells are washed with PBS, and new cell culture medium is added); the dishes are returned to the incubator.
4. When the cell density reaches 90% confluence, use 0.25% trypsin (w/v) to digest the monolayer at 37 °C for 1 min. The cell culture medium supernatant solution is centrifuged and resuspended, then is seeded into 24-well plates (cell density is about 50%). The cells are placed in a CO_2 Incubators for 6 h such that the cells completely adhere to the wall.
5. Add different concentrations of the nanomaterials to the 24-well plates, then place the plates in cell incubators at 37 °C with 5% CO_2 for 24 or 48 h. The cells are then used for RNA extraction.

3.2 RNA Extraction

The main components of TRIzol reagent are guanidinium isothiocyanate and phenol. Guanidinium isothiocyanate promotes cell lysis, ribosome dissociation, RNA and protein separation, and RNA release. Chloroform is an organic solvent with a large molecular weight. When chloroform is added to the reaction, it extracts acidic phenol, which maintains RNA in an aqueous state. After centrifugation, this solution forms an aqueous phase and organic layer, such that RNA, protein and DNA remain in the aqueous phase. In addition, chloroform can be used as a solvent to dissolve the fat-soluble impurities (e.g., fat and fat-soluble pigments) present in the extraction. The addition of isopropanol protects the hydrophilic groups in the RNA chain through the hydrophobic action of the –OH group. The water layer (clear) consists mainly of RNA, and the organic layer (yellow) contains mainly DNA and protein (*see* **Notes 1–5**).

1. In 24-well plates, add 500 μL TRIzol to each well (*see* **Notes 6** and **7**).

2. Transfer the sample to 2 mL RNase-free Eppendorf tubes and incubate for 5 min at room temperature to completely separate the nucleic acid/protein complex.
3. Combine reagents at a ratio of 1 mL TRIzol to 160 μL chloroform; place the mixture on a vortex for 30 s and incubate on ice for 15 min (*see* **Note 8**).
4. Centrifuge the sample at 4 °C and 10,000 × *g* for 15 min, causing the sample to separate into three layers: the bottom organic phase (yellow), the upper layer lucid aqueous phase containing the RNA, and an intermediate organic phase.
5. Transfer the aqueous phase to a new 2 mL RNase-free Eppendorf tube and the add same volume of isopropanol at room temperature for 10 min to precipitate RNA in the aqueous phase. The tubes are stored overnight at −20 °C.
6. The next day, centrifuge the samples at 4 °C and 10,000 × *g* for 15 min to pellet the RNA.
7. Add 1 mL 75% ethanol to wash the precipitated RNA in a 2-mL tube. The sample is centrifuged at 4 °C and 7500 × *g* for 10 min the supernatant is removed (*see* **Note 9**).
8. Dry the precipitated RNA at room temperature until transparent or translucent in appearance, then add 100 μL DEPC water to the samples at 4 °C for 2 h to fully dissolve the RNA; at this time, the RNA concentration is determined by Nanodrop-2000 spectrophotometer and the sample is stored at −70 °C.

3.3 RNA Reverse Transcription

Reverse transcription is the process of synthesizing DNA from an RNA template. Reverse transcription is thus named because the direction of nucleic acid synthesis (RNA to DNA) occurs contrary to the direction of the flow of genetic information (DNA to RNA). The reverse transcription process is catalyzed by the enzyme reverse transcriptase—also known as RNA-dependent DNA polymerase—which catalyzes the synthesis of DNA chains with RNA as a template. The synthesized DNA molecule is called complementary DNA (cDNA). The reverse transcription reaction is a key step in the quantification of RNA levels and requires that the RNA template is complete and without impurities such as DNA and protein (*see* **Note 10**).

1. We input a small amount of RNA to the reverse transcriptase system and mix the samples by centrifugation to initiate reverse transcription.
2. Each reverse transcription reaction includes the following reagents: $MgCl_2$ (2 μL), 10× RT Buffer (1 μL), RNase-free H_2O (3.75 μL), dNTP mixture (10 nM per reaction; 1 μL), RNase inhibitor (0.25 μL), AMV reverse transcriptase (0.5 μL), random 9mers (0.5 μL), and RNA (1 μL), add in sequence.

The total volume per reaction is 10 μL. The mixture is kept on ice at all times.

3. Incubate the samples at 37 °C for 15 min and at 85 °C for 5 s to terminate the reverse transcription reaction; after this step, the sample is placed on ice.
4. The product of the reverse transcription reaction is a cDNA sample (*see* **Note 11**).

3.4 Real-Time Polymerase Chain Reaction

During real-time PCR, a computer detects the fluorescence generated by DNA synthesis to monitor the PCR reaction in real time. One of the most important parameters involved is the cycle threshold (CT) value, which is the reaction cycle at which the fluorescence signal of the PCR reaction crosses a threshold level exceeding background. There is an inverse relationship between the CT value and the initial template copy number, such that the smaller the starting copy number is, the larger the value of CT is. Its mathematical relation involves the intensity of the signal at the N cycle of PCR equaling the product of the sum of the background signal intensity, the sum of the light intensity of each molecule and the number of molecules. Therefore, according to the corresponding relationship between the number of emitted light groups, appropriate light intensity and appropriate PCR products appear; if there is the fluorescence signal "real-time" detection and access to unknown samples of CT, we can analyze the absolute or relative quantity of initial template copy number according to the standard curve or the reference value of CT (*see* **Notes 12** and **13**).

1. We mix the cDNA and PCR reaction components and then add them into 384-well plates to be measured by 7900ABI thermocycler instrument. The PCR reaction contains 1 μL forward primer, 1 μL reverse primer, 10 μL SYBR green mix, ddH_2O 7 μL and 1 μL cDNA. The total volume is 20 μL per well.
2. Set up the 384-well plate on the Applied Biosystems 7900HT machine, and set the program as follows: select "Relative Quantification"; for container option, select "384-well plate"; and other step settings are set as default.

3.5 Calculation and Analysis

1. The CT value of each well is detected, transferred, and copied to a computer by 7900 ABI.
2. The following formula is used: $\Delta Ct = Ct_{\text{target gene}} - Ct_{\text{reference gene}}$, and $\Delta\Delta Ct = \Delta Ct_{\text{treatment group}} - \Delta Ct_{\text{control group}}$. The fold change is calculated as $2^{(-\Delta\Delta Ct)}$. Changes in gene expression between the control group and the treatment group are calculated.

4 Notes

1. RNA extraction must be conducted in an RNase-free environment to prevent the degradation of RNA by RNases. The materials and instruments used in the RNA extraction process must also be sterile to prevent contamination with RNA enzymes. When possible, DEPC water should be used to soak the instruments prior to use [4]. In addition, the use of non-RNA glassware or plastic utensils is required. To sterilize, glassware can be baked in an oven at 150 °C for 4 h. Plastic containers can be soaked in a 0.5 M NaOH solution for 10 min, then rinsed thoroughly with water and autoclaved.
2. RNA extraction and reverse transcription should be performed on ice to reduce the possibility of RNA degradation.
3. Because the primers used for reverse transcription are specific to the mitochondrial genome, there is no need to remove nuclear DNA from the sample.
4. Wear disposable gloves throughout the procedure. Skin is often host to bacteria and mold, which may contaminate the extracted RNA and act as a source of RNases. The cultivation of sound molecular biology practices helps to prevent microbial contamination.
5. Use sterilized, disposable plastic utensils and an autopipette to extract RNA and to avoid cross-contamination with RNases present on reusable instruments.
6. Wear gloves when extracting RNA with TRIzol. Avoid contact with skin and clothes. Complete the procedure in a chemical ventilator. Avoid inhalation of the chemicals. Without exception, all reactions should be set up at 15–30 °C, and the reagents should be stored at 15–30 °C.
7. TRIzol can be directly added to a cellular monolayer in a 3.5 cm culture plate with a pipette to generate a cell lysate. The area of the plate (rather than the number of cells) determines the amount of TRIzol required (10 cm^2 plus 1 mL). If the amount of TRIzol is insufficient, the DNA contamination will be present in the extracted RNA.
8. After homogenization and before chloroform extraction, the samples can be stored at −70 °C for at least 1 month. RNA precipitated in 75% ethanol can be preserved at 2–8 °C for at least 1 week and at −20 °C for at least 1 year.
9. Prepare 75% ethanol for sterilization (add DEPC water to an RNase-free glass bottle to 0.01% (v/v) and autoclave).

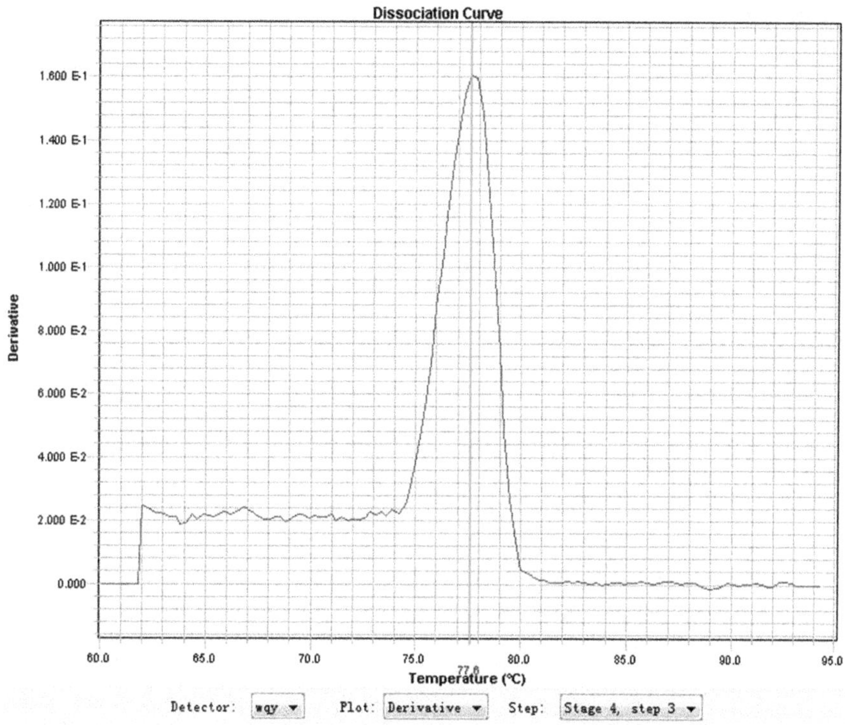

Fig. 2 The schematic diagram of the dissolution curve of a selected primer

10. Reverse transcription should be performed immediately following RNA extraction; RNA cannot be stored long-term due to its instability [5].
11. The process of reverse transcription generates cDNA from mRNA. cDNA must be stored at −20 °C or −80 °C when not in use. Furthermore, cDNA should not be repeatedly freeze-thawed. If possible, cDNA should be aliquoted and stored.
12. The CT value obtained for cDNA is considered acceptable within 15–30 of the general range. A larger CT value indicates a low concentration of cDNA, whereas a lower value indicates a high concentration of cDNA.
13. A dissolution (melting) curve can be added to the PCR program to determine the specificity of products and whether there are double peaks. Generally, for specific products, only one peak is observed in the curve (Fig. 2).

Acknowledgment

This study was supported by the National Science Foundation of China (Grant No. 81573174) and the National Science Fund for Outstanding Young Scholars (81722040).

References

1. Stehling O, Lill R (2013) The role of mitochondria in cellular iron-sulfur protein biogenesis: mechanisms, connected processes, and diseases. Cold Spring Harb Perspect Biol 5(8):a011312. https://doi.org/10.1101/cshperspect.a011312
2. Wang C, Youle RJ (2009) The role of mitochondria in apoptosis. Annu Rev Genet 43:95–118. https://doi.org/10.1146/annurev-genet-102108-134850
3. Hopper RK, Carroll S, Aponte AM, Johnson DT, French S, Shen RF, Witzmann FA, Harris RA, Balaban RS (2006) Mitochondrial matrix phosphoproteome: effect of extra mitochondrial calcium. Biochemistry 45(8):2524–2536. https://doi.org/10.1021/bi052475e
4. Huang YH, Leblanc P, Apostolou V, Stewart B, Moreland RB (1995) Comparison of Milli-Q PF Plus water to DEPC-treated water in the preparation and analysis of RNA. BioTechniques 19 (4):656–661
5. Barlow JH, Nussenzweig A (2014) Replication initiation and genome instability: a crossroads for DNA and RNA synthesis. Cell Mol Life Sci 71(23):4545–4559. https://doi.org/10.1007/s00018-014-1721-1

Chapter 12

DNA Methylation Analysis

Lingfang Feng and Jianlin Lou

Abstract

DNA methylation is a process by which methyl groups are added to cytosine or adenine. DNA methylation can change the activity of the DNA molecule without changing the sequence. Methylation of 5-methylcytosine (5mC) is widespread in both eukaryotes and prokaryotes, and it is a very important epigenetic modification event, which can regulate gene activity and influence a number of key processes such as genomic imprinting, cell differentiation, transcriptional regulation, and chromatin remodeling. Profiling DNA methylation across the genome is critical to understanding the influence of methylation in normal biology and diseases including cancer. Recent discoveries of 5-methylcytosine (5mC) oxidation derivatives including 5-hydroxymethylcytosine (5hmC), 5-formylcytsine (5fC), and 5-carboxycytosine (5caC) in mammalian genome further expand our understanding of the methylation regulation. Genome-wide analyses such as microarrays and next-generation sequencing technologies have been used to assess large fractions of the methylome. A number of different quantitative approaches have also been established to map the DNA epigenomes with single-base resolution, as represented by the bisulfite-based methods, such as classical bisulfite sequencing, pyrosequencing etc. These methods have been used to generate base-resolution maps of 5mC and its oxidation derivatives in genomic samples. The focus of this chapter is to provide the methodologies that have been developed to detect the cytosine derivatives in the genomic DNA.

Key words DNA methylation, Whole-genome bisulfite sequencing (WGBS), Reduced representation bisulfite sequencing (RRBS), Methyl-binding domain capture sequencing (MBDCap-Seq), Methylated DNA immunoprecipitation-sequencing (MeDIP-Seq), Methylation-sensitive restriction enzyme followed by sequencing (MRE-Seq), Infinium Methylation450 BeadChips (450K), Bisulfite sequencing (BS), Pyrosequencing, Methylation-specific PCR (MSP)/quantitative methylation-specific PCR (QMSP), Single molecule real-time bisulfite sequencing (SMRT-BS), Targeted bisulfite sequencing (TBS)

1 Introduction

The role of cytosine methylation is essential to gene regulation which has profound implications in developmental processes, normal biology, and disease conditions in many eukaryotic organisms. The underlying biology of DNA methylation remains largely unknown, particularly the mechanism by which it is altered in pathological diseased states, such as cancer where a disruption of

Qunwei Zhang (ed.), *Nanotoxicity: Methods and Protocols*, Methods in Molecular Biology, vol. 1894,
https://doi.org/10.1007/978-1-4939-8916-4_12,

global DNA methylation patterns is typically associated [1–5]. Many methods and approaches exist for its identification, quantification, and mapping within the genome, contributing to our comprehension of the role of DNA methylation in both development and disease states [6, 7].

Detection of DNA methylation is based on the ability to distinguish cytosine from 5mC in the DNA sequence. Different methods of analyzing methylation status are all based on three different principles: (1) digestion of DNA with methylation-sensitive restriction enzymes, (2) enrichment of methylated genomic DNA fragments using anti-methylcytosine antibody or methyl-binding domain (MBD) proteins, and (3) sequencing of bisulfite-converted DNA [8]. Recently, these principles have been scaled with high-throughput analytical platforms such as microarray and next-generation sequencing platforms, bringing us closer to unveil the whole methylome.

Here, we focus on six prominent genome-wide approaches: whole-genome bisulfite sequencing (WGBS) [6, 8], reduced representation bisulfite sequencing (RRBS) [9–11], methyl-binding domain capture sequencing (MBDCap-Seq) [12–14], methylated DNA immunoprecipitation-sequencing (MeDIP-Seq) [15–17], methylation-sensitive restriction enzyme followed by sequencing (MRE-Seq) [18, 19], and Infinium Methylation450 BeadChips (450K, Illumina) [20–22].

We introduce methods for quantitative mapping of 5mC in genomic DNA at single nucleotide resolution, which identify the context and levels of methylation at each site, including bisulfite sequencing (BS) [23, 24], pyrosequencing [25, 26], methylation-specific PCR (MSP) [27, 28], quantitative methylation-specific PCR (QMSP) [29, 30], and single molecule real-time bisulfite sequencing (SMRT-BS) [31].

In this chapter, we describe a detailed protocol of the approaches mentioned above, providing a more comprehensive map of DNA methylome.

2 Materials

2.1 Whole-Genome Bisulfite Sequencing (WGBS)

1. Qiagen DNeasy Blood and Tissue Kit (Qiagen).
2. Lambda DNA (Promega).
3. QIAquick PCR Purification Kit (Qiagen, includes Buffer EB).
4. T4 DNA Ligase (400 U/mL) and 10× buffer (NEB).
5. T4 DNA Polymerase (NEB).
6. T4 Polynucleotide Kinase (NEB).
7. Klenow DNA Polymerase (NEB).
8. Deoxynucleotide (dNTP) Solution Set (NEB, 25 μM each).

9. Klenow fragment (3′–5′ -exo) (NEB) and NEBuffer 2 ilAdap Methyl PE1 (IDT: ACACTCTTTCCCTACACGACGCTCTT CCGATC*T; all C's are methylated, *=phosphorothioate bond) ilAdap Methyl PE2 (IDT: GATCGGAAGAGCGGTT CAGCAGGAATGCCGA*G; all C's are methylated, 5′ phosphate, *=phosphorothioate bond).
10. 100 bp DNA Ladder (NEB).
11. EZ DNA Methylation Gold Kit (ZymoResearch).
12. iPCR PE1 (IDT: AAT GAT ACG GCG ACC ACC GAG ATC TAC ACT CTT TCC CTA CAC GAC GCT CTT CCG ATC* T; *=phosphorothioate bond).
13. iPCR PE2 (IDT: CAA GCA GAA GAC GGC ATA CGA GAT CGG TCT CGG CAT TCC TGC TGA ACC GCT CTT CCG ATC* T; *=phosphorothioate bond).
14. E-Gel SizeSelect Agarose Gels.
15. Platinum Taq DNA Polymerase 5 U/mL (Invitrogen, sold with 10× PCR Buffer and 50 mM magnesium chloride).
16. 5 M Betaine (Sigma).
17. Agencourt AMPure XP—PCR Purification (BeckmanCoulter).

2.2 Reduced Representation Bisulfite Sequencing (RRBS)

QIAamp® DNA Mini Kit (Qiagen)

1. Phosphate buffered saline, PBS: 137 mM NaCl, 2.7 mM KCl, 10 mM Na_2HPO_4, 1.8 mM KH_2PO_4, pH 7.4.
2. Absolute ethanol.
3. TE buffer: 10 mM Tris, 1 mM EDTA, pH 8.0.
4. *Msp* I: 20 U/μL, with compatible restriction buffer.
5. Distilled, deionized purified water.
6. QIAquick and MinElute PCR purification kits (Qiagen).
7. TruSeq Nano DNA sample preparation kit (Illumina).
8. XC loading dye 6×: 0.25% (w/v) xylene cyanol, 40% (w/v) sucrose.
9. NuSieve GTG agarose.
10. TAE buffer 0.5×: 20 mM Tris–acetate, 0.5 mM EDTA with 0.0024% ethidium bromide.
11. Mupid-exU electrophoresis tank.
12. 25-bp DNA ladder: 0.1 μg/μL.
13. QIAquick gel extraction kit (Qiagen).
14. 100% isopropanol, analytical grade.
15. EZ DNA methylation kit (Zymo Research).
16. PfuTurbo Cx Hotstart DNA polymerase (Agilent Technologies).

17. PCR-grade dNTPs: each at 2.5 mM.
18. Precast TBE 4–20% gradient gels and electrophoresis tank (Criterion, Bio-Rad).
19. TBE buffer: 45 mM Tris–borate, 1 mM EDTA.
20. SYBR green nucleic acid gel stain (Life Technologies).
21. 2100 Bioanalyzer and high sensitivity DNA kit (Agilent Technologies).

2.3 Methyl-Binding Domain Capture Sequencing (MBDCap-Seq)

1. Methylminer DNA Enrichment Kit (Invitrogen).
2. Dynabeads M-280 streptavidin (Invitrogen).
3. 3 M sodium acetate, pH 5.2 (Sigma).
4. Adapter primers (Bioo Scientific).
5. PCR master mix (KAPA Scientific).
6. EB buffer (Qiagen).

2.4 Methylated DNA Immunoprecipitation-Sequencing (MeDIP-Seq)

1. QIAquick Gel Extraktion Kit (Qiagen).
2. Orange dye (Sigma-Aldrich).
3. T4 polynucleotide kinase, 10 U/μL (NEB).
4. T4 DNA polymerase, 3 U/μL (NEB).
5. Polymerase I, large (Klenow) Fragment, 5 U/μL (NEB).
6. T4 DNA ligase reaction buffer 10× (NEB).
7. 25 mM dNTP Mix (GE Healthcare).
8. 1 mM dATP (GE Healthcare).
9. MinElute PCR Purification Kit (Qiagen).
10. Adapters included in the Genomic Adapter oligo mix for single reads or paired-reads (Illumina).
11. Quick Ligation Kit (NEB) containing Quick T4 DNA Ligase and Quick Ligation Reaction Buffer (2×).
12. 5-Methylcytidine antibody, mouse monoclonal (Eurogentec). A 5-methylcytidine antibody supplied by Diagenode works comparably well. Aliquot the antibody and store at −20 °C, avoid freeze–thaw cycles.
13. Dynabeads M-280 Sheep anti-Mouse IgG (Invitrogen).
14. Albumin, bovine serum, Fraction V, and BSA (Sigma-Aldrich).
15. 0.5% BSA/PBS (w/v).
16. 100 mM sodium phosphate, buffer solution pH 7.0 for HPCE (Sigma-Aldrich).
17. 7.5 M NaCl.
18. Triton X-100 (Sigma-Aldrich).

19. 2× Immunoprecipitation buffer (280 mM NaCl, 20 mM sodium phosphate buffer pH 7.0, 0.5% Triton X-100).
20. SDS elution buffer (50 mM Tris, pH 8.0; 10 mM EDTA, pH 8.0; 1% SDS).
21. Proteinase K (Roche Applied Science), dissolve in H_2O to 20 mg/mL, aliquot, and store at −20 °C, do not refreeze a thawed proteinase K aliquot.
22. 1× TE (10 mM Tris, pH 8.0, 1 mM EDTA).
23. 2 mL Phase Lock Gel Heavy tubes.
24. Phenol–$CHCl_3$–isoamyl alcohol, 25:24:1 (Sigma-Aldrich).
25. 10 mM Tris, pH 8.5.
26. Primers included in the Genomic Adapter oligo mix for single reads or paired-reads (Illumina).
27. Phusion High-Fidelity PCR Master Mix with HF Buffer (NEB).
28. 0.2 mL thin-walled PCR tubes.
29. Ultralow range agarose.
30. Clean scalpels for excision of the gel fragment.
31. SYBR Green PCR Master Mix (Applied Biosystems).
32. Quant-iT ssDNA kit (Invitrogen) for quantification after MeDIP.
33. Quant-iT dsHSDNA kit (Invitrogen) for quantification of the size-selected amplified library DNA.

2.5 Methylation-Sensitive Restriction Enzyme Followed by Sequencing (MRE-Seq)

1. Nuclease-free water.
2. CTAB lysis buffer: 140 mM Sorbitol, 220 mM Tris pH 8.0, 22 mM EDTA, 880 mM NaCl, 1% Sarcosyl, and 0.8% CTAB.
3. Phenol–chloroform–isoamyl alcohol: 25:24:1 saturated with 10 mM Tris, pH 8.0, 1 mM EDTA.
4. Chloroform–isoamyl alcohol: 24:1 mixture of chloroform and isoamyl alcohol.
5. Isopropyl alcohol.
6. 70% EtOH, ethanol diluted by distilled water.
7. Absolute EtOH, 100% ethanol.
8. Liquid N_2.
9. 10% SDS, sodium dodecyl sulfate dissolved in distilled water.
10. 3.0 M NaOAc pH 5.2, 3 M sodium acetate, pH adjusted with acetic acid.
11. 5 mM Tris pH 8.0, Tris dissolved in distilled water, pH adjusted with NaOH.
12. 10 mM Tris pH 8.0.

13. (10×) restriction enzyme buffer.
14. PCR buffer (10×).
15. $MgCl_2$ (25 mM), magnesium chloride dissolved in distilled water.
16. dNTP (20 μM), Mixture of the four deoxynucleotide triphosphates.
17. BSA, bovine serum albumin.
18. 20 mM EGTA.
19. T4 DNA ligase (5 U/μL) and buffer.
20. HotStar Taq DNA Polymerase.
21. RNase A: 100 mg/mL diluted in water.
22. Proteinase K: 20 mg/mL purchased as liquid.

2.6 Infinium Methylation450 BeadChips (450 K, Illumina)

1. QIAamp DNA Mini Kit (Qiagen).
2. DNeasy Blood and Tissue Kit (Qiagen).
3. Zymo EZ DNA Methylation Kit™ (Zymo Research).
4. ZR-96 DNA Clean & Concentrator-5 kit (Zymo Research).
5. Infinium Human Methylation 450 BeadChip (Illumina).

2.7 Bisulfite Sequencing (BS)

1. Agarose.
2. SYBR-Safe dye with compatible blue light transilluminator.
3. Optional: lambda phage DNA.
4. DNA loading buffer.
5. 1 kb DNA marker.
6. Purification kit for PCR product.
7. Purification kit for DNA extraction from agarose gel.
8. DNA End Repair kit (NEB).
9. 10× T4 ligase buffer with ATP (e.g., from Enzymatics or NEB).
10. 10 mM dNTP w/o dCTP (10 mM each dATP, dGTP, and dTTP).
11. Magnetic stand for 0.2 mL PCR tubes.
12. AMPure XP purification beads.
13. 80% EtOH.
14. 10× T4 ligase buffer with ATP.
15. 10 mM dATP.
16. Klenow 3′–5′ exo- (NEB).
17. Magnetic stand for 0.2 mL PCR tubes.
18. AMPure XP purification beads.

19. 80% EtOH.
20. 25 μM TruSeq 5mC double-stranded adapter.
21. 2× ligase buffer with ATP and PEG.
22. T4 Ligase HC (high concentration, NEB).
23. Magnetic stand for 0.2 mL PCR tubes.
24. AMPure XP purification beads.
25. 80% EtOH.
26. TE buffer: 10 mM Tris, 1 mM EDTA.
27. Fluorescent dye (Promega QuantiFluor dsDNA Dye).
28. Bisulfite conversion kit (ZYMO EZ DNA Methylation-Gold Kit).
29. 100% EtOH.
30. Nuclease-free water.
31. DNA polymerase (KAPA HiFi Uracilþ).
32. TruSeq Adapter and index PCR primers.
33. Magnetic stand for 0.2 mL PCR tubes.
34. AMPure XP purification beads.
35. 80% EtOH.
36. Nuclease-free water.

2.8 Pyrosequencing

1. CpG Methyltransferase (M.SssI), reaction buffer, and *S*-adenosylmethionine (SAM) (New England Biolabs).
2. CpGenome™ Universal Methylated DNA (Millipore).
3. CpGenome™ human nonmethylated DNA (Millipore).
4. Human genomic DNA from human blood (buffy coat) (Roche).
5. Whole genome amplification kit (GE Healthcare).
6. QIAamp DNA Mini/Micro Kit (Qiagen).
7. Ethanol (96–100%).
8. EZ DNA methylation kit (Zymo Research).
9. Ethanol (96–100%).
10. PCR primers (purification by desalting).
11. Biotinylated PCR primer (purification by desalting).
12. PyroMark® PCR kit (Qiagen).
13. TAE buffer: 40 mM Tris, 40 mM acetate, and 1 mM EDTA.
14. Agarose.
15. Ethidium Bromide.
16. DNA Ladder, range 50–500 bp.

17. PCR primers (purification by desalting).
18. Biotinylated PCR primer (purification by desalting).
19. Streptavidin Sepharose HP beads (GE Healthcare).
20. Pyrosequencing primer (purification by desalting).
21. Wash, denaturation, binding, and annealing buffers (Qiagen).
22. PyroMark Gold Q24 Reagents (Qiagen).

2.9 Methylation-Specific PCR (MSP)/Quantitative Methylation-Specific PCR (QMSP)

1. QIAamp DNA mini kit (Qiagen).
2. NaOH, 3 M.
3. Hydroquinone, 10 mM.
4. Sodium bisulfate, 3 M.
5. Wizard DNA purification resin (Promega).
6. Sodium acetate, 3 M.
7. Isopropanol.
8. Cold 75% ethanol.
9. Distilled water or TE buffer.
10. CpGenome DNA modification kit (InterGen) or EZ DNA methylation kit (Zymo Research) or CpGenome Fast DNA modification kit (Millipore).
11. CpGenome™ Universal Methylated DNA (Chemincon).
12. SYBR Premix Ex Taq (Takara).

2.10 Single Molecule Real-Time Bisulfite Sequencing (SMRT-BS)

1. Methylamp™ DNA Modification Kit (Epigentek).
2. Premix Taq DNA Polymerase Hot Start Version (Takara).
3. ASI Agarose (Alkali Scientific).
4. QIAquick PCR Purification Kit (Qiagen).
5. RNA6000 pico kit (Agilent).
6. 1 kb DNA Ladder (Thermo Fisher).
7. SMRTbell™ Template Prep Kit (Pacific Biosciences).
8. DNA/Polymerase Binding Kit (Pacific Biosciences).
9. MagBead Kit for amplicons >1 kb (Pacific Biosciences).
10. DNA Sequencing Reagent (Pacific Biosciences).
11. DNA Internal Control Complex (Pacific Biosciences).
12. AMPure® PB beads (Pacific Biosciences).

2.11 Targeted Bisulfite Sequencing (TBS)

1. EpiTect Bisulfite kit (Qiagen).
2. KAPA2G Robust Hot Start Ready Mix (KAPA).
3. Backman Agencourt AMPure XP bead (Invitrogen).
4. NEBNext® Ultra™II DNA Library Prep Kit (NEB).

3 Methods

3.1 Whole-Genome Bisulfite Sequencing (WGBS)

3.1.1 Isolate Genomic DNA (gDNA)

1. Isolate gDNA from cells or tissue with the DNeasy Blood and Tissue Kit (Qiagen) (*see* **Note 1**) following the manufacturer's instructions. Elute gDNA in 100–200 μL AE buffer (*see* **Note 2**).
2. Determine the concentration of gDNA with a Qubit fluorometer and estimate the gDNA quality using a NanoDrop spectrophotometer (*see* **Note 3**).
3. Store at −20 °C or proceed to next step.

3.1.2 Add Lambda DNA to gDNA

1. Add 10 ng (0.5%, w/w) unmethylated lambda DNA to 2 μg gDNA. If necessary, dilute lambda DNA with EB buffer.
2. Bring up solution to 50 μL with EB buffer.

3.1.3 Sonicate gDNA and Lambda DNA Mixture Using Covaris LE220 Sonicator

1. Place 50 μL genomic and lambda DNA mixture into a microTUBE AFA Fiber Crimp-Cap (6 × 16 mm).
2. Make sure that there are no air bubbles on the bottom of the tube.
3. Add samples (tubes) to entire column (need to fill up entire column) on metallic Covaris rack.
4. Sonicate gDNA on Covaris machine by setting target size at 400 bp (15% duty factor, 450 W, 200 cycles per burst, 80 s, <10 °C water temperature).
5. Make sure that water is level with the bottom half of metallic rack.

3.1.4 Purify gDNA

1. Clean up sonicated gDNA by using QIAquick PCR Purification Kit following the manufacturer's instruction.
2. Elute gDNA in 30 μL EB buffer.

3.1.5 End Repair gDNA

1. Mix the following reagents in a PCR tube on ice (a master mix can be prepared when processing more than one sample):

   30 μL recovered DNA fragments

   5 μL 10× T4 DNA ligase buffer (with 10 mM ATP)

   1 μL 25 μM dTTP

   1 μL 25 μM dGTP

   1 μL 25 μM dATP

   9 μL dH_2O

   1 μL T4 DNA polymerase

   1 μL T4 Polynucleotide Kinase

   1 μL Klenow DNA polymerase

   Total volume = 50 μL

2. Spin down briefly and incubate at 20 °C in a thermal cycler for 30 min.
3. Purify DNA with the QIAquick PCR Purification Kit and elute with 30 μL EB buffer prewarmed to 55 °C. Allow EB buffer to sit on the filter in the column for 1 min before spinning for 1 min.

3.1.6 Add dATP to gDNA

1. Be sure to use correct Klenow enzyme (3′–5′ exo-).
2. Mix the following reagents in a PCR tube on ice:

   30 μL end-repaired DNA fragments

   10 μL 1 μM dATP

   5 μL 10× NE buffer

   2 μL dH_2O

   3 μL Klenow fragment (3′–5′ exo-)

   Total volume = 50 μL
3. Spin down briefly and incubate at 37 °C in a thermal cycler for 30 min.
4. Purify DNA with the QIAquick PCR Purification Kit and elute with 10 μL EB buffer prewarmed to 55 °C. Allow EB buffer to sit on the filter in the column for 1 min before spinning for 1 min.

3.1.7 Ligate Methylated Illumina PE Adapters

1. Prepare 40 μM annealed methylated Illumina paired-end sequencing adapter oligonucleotides:
   (a) Set up the following reaction in a PCR tube:

   5 μL 10× T4 DNA ligase buffer

   20 μL 100 μM ilAdap Methyl PE1

   20 μL 100 μM ilAdap Methyl PE2

   5 μL dH_2O

   Total volume = 50 μL

   (b) Incubate in a thermal cycler with the following program:

   5 min 95 °C

   1 min 70 °C

   1 min 60 °C

   1 min 50 °C

   1 min 40 °C

   1 min 30 °C

   Hold 25 °C

   (c) Store the annealed adapters at −30 °C

2. Mix the following reagents in a PCR tube on ice:

   10 μL end-repaired DNA fragments

   2 μL 10× T4 DNA ligase buffer

   1 μL T4 DNA ligase (400 U/μL)

   3 μL 40 μM Methyl Index Adapter Mix (prepared above)

   4 μL dH_2O

   Total volume = 20 μL

3. Incubate in a thermal cycler at 20 °C for 30 min, hold at 4 °C.

3.1.8 Size-Select gDNA with a 2% Agarose E-Gel

1. Dilute 1 μL of 100 bp ladder DNA marker in 39 μL dH_2O and load 20 μL into the first lane of the E-Gel.
2. Load 20 μL of the gDNA sample into each lane of the E-Gel.
3. Load 20 μL dH_2O into any empty wells across the top of the gel.
4. Load 20 μL dH_2O into the bottom wells.
5. Start a 20 min run and monitor the gel every ~5 min. Since water may evaporate from the bottom wells as the gel runs, fill the wells with dH_2O as needed.
6. When the 400 bp DNA marker band migrates into the bottom well, stop the run and pipette out each sample (more dH_2O may be added to the wells before pipetting the samples out if water has evaporated).
7. Store gDNA at −30 °C.

3.1.9 Bisulfite (BS) Convert gDNA

1. Thaw 20 μL gDNA sample on ice.
2. Bisulfite convert gDNA by using EZ DNA Methylation-Gold Kit according to the manufacturer's instruction.
3. Elute converted gDNA in 10 μL M-Elution buffer.

3.1.10 Amplify BS-Converted gDNA

1. Mix the following reagents in a PCR tube on ice:

   10 μL BS converted DNA

   5 μL 10× PCR buffer (no $MgCl_2$)

   2 μL $MgCl_2$ (50 mM)

   0.25 μL Index PCR PE1 (100 μM)

   0.25 μL Index PCR PE2 (100 μM)

   μL dNTPs (12.5 μM each)

   24.5 μL dH_2O

   5.0 μL Betaine (5 M)

   1 μL Platinum Taq DNA polymerase

   Total volume = 50 μL

2. Amplify as follows:
   (a) 1 min 98 °C × 1 cycle
   (b) 30 s 95 °C
   (c) 3 min 62 °C
   (d) Return to **step 2** for 14 cycles
   (e) Hold at 4 °C

3.1.11 Final Cleanup of BS-Converted gDNA

1. Follow the Agencourt AMPure XP manufacturer's instruction to final cleanup of BS-converted gDNA with the following exceptions.
2. Use 90 μL of beads for 50 μL gDNA and 72 μL of beads for 40 μL gDNA (1.8 volume of gDNA).
3. Resuspend gDNA in 15 μL EB buffer at the final step (*see* **Note 4**). The library DNA is now ready for sequencing (Illumina HiSeq DNA sequencing platform).

3.2 Reduced Representation Bisulfite Sequencing (RRBS)

3.2.1 gDNA Isolation

Isolate gDNA using DNeasy Blood and Tissue Kit (Qiagen) according to the method described in Subheading 3.1.1.

3.2.2 MspI Digestion

1. In a PCR tube, add the following for each sample and mix:
   (a) 2.0 μg of gDNA (*see* **Note 5**)
   (b) 160 U of Msp I restriction endonuclease
   (c) 4 μL of 10× NEB Buffer
   (d) Milli-Q H_2O to 40 μL final volume
2. Incubate overnight (~16 h) at 37 °C in a thermocycler.
3. Clean gDNA by using the QIAquick PCR purification kit according to the manufacturer's instructions. Elute in 60 μL TE buffer.

3.2.3 End Repair

1. In a PCR tube, add 40 μL TruSeq End Repair mix 2 (ERP2) in the TruSeq DNA sample preparation kit to the digested gDNA (from Subheading 3.2.2) and mix.
2. Incubate for 30 min at 30 °C in a PCR thermocycler.
3. Use the MinElute PCR purification kit according to the manufacturer's instruction. Elute in 17.5 μL TE buffer.

3.2.4 A-Tailing

1. In a PCR tube, add 12.5 μL TruSeq A-Tailing mix (ATL) in TruSeq DNA sample preparation kit to the end-repaired gDNA (from Subheading 3.2.3) and mix.
2. Incubate in a thermocycler as follows:
   (a) 30 min at 37 °C

   (b) 5 min at 70 °C
   (c) 5 min at 4 °C
3. Immediately proceed to the next step.

3.2.5 Adapter Ligation

1. In the same PCR tube (from Subheading 3.2.4), add the following and mix:
   (a) 2.5 μL TE buffer.
   (b) 2.5 μL TruSeq Adapter Index (choosing a single barcoded adapter from the 24 available adapters, *see* **Note 6**)
   (c) 2.5 μL TruSeq DNA Ligase mix 2 (LIG2)
2. Incubate for 10 min at 30 °C in a thermocycler.
3. Immediately after incubation, add 5 μL of Stop Ligase mix (STL) and mix.
4. Use the minElute PCR purification kit according to the manufacturer's instruction. Elute in 18 μL TE buffer.
5. Add 2 μL of XC loading dye.

3.2.6 Agarose Gel Size Selection

1. Prepare 3% (w/v) NuSieve GTG agarose gel in 0.5× TAE buffer with 0.0024% ethidium bromide according to the manufacturer's instruction (*see* **Note 7**). Pour molten gel into a gel tray with a comb and let it solidify for 30–60 min.
2. Carefully remove the comb and transfer the tray with gel into an electrophoresis tank. Pour fresh 0.5× TAE running buffer into the tank so that the gel is fully submerged (~1 cm). Load 6 μL of 25 bp DNA ladder into the first lane and 20 μL of the first DNA sample (from Subheading 3.2.5) into the third lane. Leave a lane empty between multiple samples. Run the gel at 50 V for ~90 min (*see* **Note 8**).
3. Immediately after electrophoresis, carefully transfer the gel onto a clean surface to excise gel bands. With a clean scalpel blade, make a straight vertical cut to slice off the DNA ladder lane and transfer onto a UV gel imager alongside a plastic ruler. Visualize the DNA ladder lane under UV using the imager and determine the position (in millimeter) of the 160 and 340 bp fragments (adapter-modified sizes that correspond to 40–220 bp fragments).
4. With a new blade, make two straight vertical cuts to isolate the sample lane (should be performed in a UV light devoid environment). Align the ruler next to the excised sample lane and make a straight horizontal cut just above the calculated 340 bp mark and another straight horizontal cut just below the calculated 160 bp mark. Using the edge of the same blade, carefully transfer the excised fragment into a 2 mL plastic centrifuge tube.

5. Determine the weight of the gel fragment. Extract DNA fragment by using the QIAquick gel extraction kit according to the manufacturer's instruction without heating the gel, eluting in 40 μL TE buffer (*see* **Note 9**).

3.2.7 Bisulfite Conversion

1. Prepare EZ DNA methylation kit CT conversion reagent according to the manufacturer's instruction, mixing thoroughly until fully dissolved.
2. Add 10 μL of M-Dilution Buffer to the 40 μL DNA sample [from Subheading 3.2.6] and mix. Incubate for 15 min at 37 °C in a thermocycler.
3. Add 100 μL of the prepared CT conversion reagent to the sample and mix. Incubate for 18 h at 50 °C on a thermocycler (*see* **Note 10**).
4. After incubation, place tube on ice for 10 min and proceed with the EZ DNA methylation kit according to the manufacturer's instruction to purify the bisulfite-converted DNA, eluting in 20 μL of TE buffer.

3.2.8 Semi-quantitative PCR

1. In a PCR tube, mix the following reagents to make a total volume of 25 μL (*see* **Note 11**):
   (a) 12.3 μL of deionized (Milli-Q) water
   (b) 2.5 μL of 10× PfuTurbo Cx reaction buffer
   (c) 3 μL of 2.5 mM dNTP stock
   (d) 3 μL of TruSeq PCR Primer Cocktail
   (e) 3 μL of DNA sample (from Subheading 3.2.7)
   (f) 1.2 μL of PfuTurbo Cx Hotstart DNA Polymerase
2. Divide the above mixture into two PCR tubes (tube A and tube B, 12 μL each) and run on two different PCR thermocyclers using the following reaction conditions (tube A, $n = 15$ cycles; tube B, $n = 20$ cycles, *see* **Note 12**):
   (a) 95 °C 2 min × 1 cycle
   (b) 95 °C 30 s
   (c) 65 °C 30 s
   (d) 72 °C 45 s
   (e) Return to step 2 for n 1 cycles
   (f) 72 °C 7 min × 1 cycle
   (g) 4 °C hold
3. Following the PCR, add 2 μL of XC loading dye to each tube. Set up a 4–20% Criterion precast TBE gradient gel in electrophoresis tank according to the manufacturer's instruction. Load 6 μL of 25-bp DNA ladder into the first lane and 12 μL

of each PCR product into subsequent lanes. Run the gel at 100 V for 100 min.

4. Following the run, add 10 μL of SYBR Green stain to 100 mL of TBE buffer into a light-proof container. Carefully remove TBE gel from the plastic cassette and immerse in the SYBR Green mixture and incubate at room temperature with gentle rocking for 30 min. Visualize the gel using the UV gel imager.
5. To generate enough DNA for sequencing, the library DNA is amplified with the lowest possible number of cycles (*see* **Note 12**).
6. Assess the gel and determine the optimal cycle number carefully for large-scale PCR amplification of libraries (*see* **Note 13**).

3.2.9 Large Scale PCR Amplification and Second Size-Selection

1. In a PCR tube, mix the following reagents (125 μL total volume):
   (a) 61.5 μL of Milli-Q water.
   (b) 12.5 μL of 10× PfuTurbo Cx reaction buffer.
   (c) 15 μL of 2.5 mM dNTP stock.
   (d) 15 μL of TruSeq PCR Primer Cocktail.
   (e) 15 μL of DNA sample (from Subheading 3.2.7).
   (f) 6 μL of PfuTurbo Cx Hotstart DNA Polymerase.
2. Run the samples on a thermocycler using the reaction conditions used previously and the estimated optimal cycle number (in Subheading 3.2.8).
3. Use the minElute PCR purification kit according to the manufacturer's instructions to purify large-scale amplified libraries, eluting in 18 μL TE buffer.
4. A second round of gel size selection step is performed to remove primer contamination from the amplified libraries. Add 2 μL of XC loading dye and run on a 3% NuSieve agarose gel as before (from Subheading 3.2.6). Similarly, excise the band between 160 and 340 bp. Use the minElute gel extraction kit according to the manufacturer's instructions, eluting in 20 μL TE buffer.

3.2.10 Quantification, Quality Assessment, and Preparation for Sequencing

1. Quantify 2 μL of the final library DNA (from Subheading 3.2.9) using the Qubit fluorometer according to the manufacturer's instruction.
2. For quality assessment, run 1 μL of the final library DNA [from Subheading 3.2.9] on the 2100 Bioanalyzer using the high sensitivity DNA kit according to the manufacturer's instruction (*see* **Note 14**).
3. Dilute the library DNA to a concentration of 10 nM and store at −80 °C (*see* Subheading 3.2.11).

3.2.11 Cluster Generation for Multiplexed RRBS

1. For multiplexed sequencing runs, multiple RRBS libraries (from Subheading 3.2.10) are pooled in equimolar ratios for the cluster generation step. Each sample is diluted to 2 nM working concentration and pooled in equal volumes. For example, five RRBS libraries, 5 μL of each library DNA, are pooled, making a total volume of 25 μL.
2. 10 μL from the pooled libraries is denatured with NaOH and diluted to a concentration of 8 pM.
3. 120 μL of the final diluted sample is used in the Illumina cBot machine for the cluster generation step.

3.2.12 Multiplexed RRBS Libraries

1. Base-Calling of Multiplexed RRBS Libraries.
2. Assessing DATA Quality and Alignment.
3. Output and CpG Coverage After Alignment.
4. Visualization of DNA Methylation from RRBS Reads.
5. Tools for Detecting Differential Methylation from RRBS.

3.3 Methyl-Binding Domain Capture Sequencing (MBDCap-Seq)

3.3.1 DNA Isolation

Isolate DNA using DNeasy Blood and Tissue Kit according to the method described in Subheading 3.1.1.

3.3.2 Initial Bead Wash

1. Resuspend the stock of streptavidin beads by gently pipetting up and down to obtain a homogeneous suspension (*see* **Note 15**). Do not mix the beads by vortexing.
2. For 1 μg of input DNA, add 10 μL of beads to a tube with 90 μL of 1× Bind/Wash Buffer. Rotate for 1 min. Do not mix by vortexing.
3. Place the tube(s) on a magnetic rack for 1 min.
4. Remove the liquid with a pipette and discard the liquid.
5. Add 250 μL of 1× Bind/Wash Buffer to the beads and rotate for 1 min.
6. Repeat **steps 3** and **4** twice.

3.3.3 Coupling the MBD-Biotin Protein to the Beads

1. For 1.2 μg of input DNA, add 7 μL (3.5 μg) of MBD-biotin protein to each tube.
2. Add 93 μL of 1× Bind/Wash Buffer to the protein to make a final volume of 100 μL.
3. Mix the beads–protein mixture on a rotating mixer at RT for 1 h.

3.3.4 Fragmented DNA (Input)

1. Sonicate DNA by adding 1.2 μg of total genomic DNA in 96 μL of TE buffer and 24 μL of 5× Bind/wash buffer to make a 120 μL solution. Use 30 s power ON and 30 s power OFF during sonication, 20–25 times.
2. Run 1 μL of sonicated DNA solution using a bioanalyzer system with a commercial high sensitivity DNA kit to check the size of the fragments to be in the range of 150–350 bp according to the manufacturer's protocol.

3.3.5 Wash the MBD-Beads

1. Place the tube containing MBD-beads on a magnetic rack for 1 min.
2. Remove and discard the liquid with a pipette without touching the beads.
3. Resuspend the beads with 250 μL of 1× Bind/Wash buffer.
4. Mix the beads on a rotating mixer at RT for 5 min.
5. Repeat **steps 1–4** twice.

3.3.6 Fragmented DNA Capture Reaction (1 μg Input DNA)

1. Transfer the DNA–Buffer mixture to the tube containing the MBD-beads.
2. Mix the MBD-beads with the DNA on a rotating mixer for 1 h at RT. Alternatively, mix O/N at 4 °C.

3.3.7 Removing Noncaptured DNA from the Beads

1. After mixing the DNA and MBD-beads, place the tube on the magnetic rack for 1 min to concentrate all of the beads on the inner wall of the tube.
2. Remove the supernatant with a pipette and save it in a clean DNase-free microcentrifuge tube as nonmethylated DNA. Store this sample on ice.
3. Add 200 μL of 1× Bind/Wash buffer to the beads to wash the beads.
4. Mix the beads on a rotating mixer for 3 min.
5. Place the tube on the magnetic rack for 1 min.
6. Remove the supernatant with a pipette and save it in a microcentrifuge tube.
7. For capture reactions of $\leq$1 μg of input DNA, repeat **steps 3–6** for two more wash fractions in total.

3.3.8 Single Fraction Elution

1. Mix low-salt buffer with high-salt buffer (1:1) to get elution buffer (1 M NaCl).
2. Resuspend the beads in 200 μL of elution buffer (1 M NaCl).
3. Incubate the beads on a rotating mixer for 3 min.
4. Place the tube on the magnetic rack for 1 min.

5. With the tube in place on the magnetic rack, remove the supernatant with a pipette without touching the beads, and save it in a clean DNase-free 1.5 mL microcentrifuge tube. Store this sample on ice.
6. Repeat **steps 1–4** once, collecting the second sample in the same tube (total volume will be about 400 μL). Store the pooled sample on ice.

3.3.9 Ethanol Precipitation (DNA Cleanup)

1. To each noncaptured, wash, and elution fraction from the previous steps, add 1 μL glycogen (20 μg/μL, included in the kit), 1/10 sample volume of 3 M sodium acetate, pH 5.2 (e.g., 40 μL per 400 μL of sample) and 2 sample volumes of 100% ethanol (e.g., 800 μL per 400 μL of sample). The total volume is 1241 μL.
2. Mix well and incubate at −80 °C for at least 2 h.
3. Centrifuge the tube for 15 min at 10,000 × *g* at 4 °C.
4. Carefully discard the supernatant without disturbing the pellet.
5. Add 500 μL of cold 70% ethanol.
6. Centrifuge the tube for 5 min at 10,000 × *g* at 4 °C.
7. Carefully discard the supernatant without disturbing the pellet.
8. Repeat **steps 6** and 7 once and remove any remaining residual supernatant.
9. Air-dry the pellet for ~5 min. Do not completely dry the pellet.
10. Resuspend the DNA pellet in 37.5 μL of DNase-free water.
11. Place the DNA on ice or store the DNA at −20 °C or below until further use.
12. Check that the total amount of DNA is over 20 ng (e.g., use fluorometric quantitation system).

3.3.10 DNA Library Preparation

1. Use the DNA fragments recovered from MBDCap procedure for sequencing. For each sample to be sequenced, a total amount of 20–40 ng DNA is required for library DNA preparation.
2. For DNA-seq library DNA preparation use a fully automated library DNA construction system and follow the standard protocol supplied by the manufacturer. Select DNA fragments of size 200–400 bp for library DNA preparation (*see* **Note 16**).
3. Use adapter primers and dilute to 100× concentration. Of this, use 10 μL for each sample.
4. Following **step 2**, take out the reaction, and quantify the DNA-seq library using a fluorometric quantitation system. Set up PCR amplification procedure. The choice of PCR master mix is to improve the PCR efficiency of GC enriched region

of genome. In a PCR tube, add 15 μL DNA-seq library DNA, 25 μL PCR master mix, 2 μL PCR primer mix, and 8 μL H_2O.

5. Follow PCR recommendation from manufacturer of the PCR master mix, altering cycling times and temperatures for differing starting materials: 98 °C for 45 s, *X* cycles (8–10 cycles) of 98 °C for 15 s, 65 °C for 30 s, 72 °C for 30 s, and then 72 °C for 1 min. Hold at 4 °C. Perform enough cycles to end up with 2–10 nM of library DNA (8–10 cycles).
6. Clean up PCR reaction with 1:1 ratio of PCR purification beads according to manufacturer's instruction.
7. Elute with 20–30 μL elution buffer.
8. Barcode each sample and pool 4 samples together into one lane of a flow cell. Use the standard 50 bp single read protocol for sequencing.

3.4 Methylated DNA Immunoprecipitation Sequencing (MeDIP-Seq)

3.4.1 DNA Isolation

1. Isolate DNA using DNeasy Blood and Tissue Kit (Qiagen) according to the method described in Subheading 3.1.1.
2. The DNA has to be RNase free (*see* **Note 17**). If RNA digestion is not performed during the DNA isolation step, then perform RNase digest prior to shearing by incubating 1 μL of RNase (10 U/μL) with 4–10 μg of DNA in a 50 μL volume for 1 h at 37 °C.

3.4.2 Fragmentation of DNA

1. DNA is sheared to fragments with sizes of 100–400 bp. We use a Hielscher UTR2000 sonifier with continuous water bath cooling set to an amplitude of 1000 and a duty cycle of 0.5.
2. 4–8 μg of DNA is sheared four times for a total of 30 min in 50 μL of 10 mM Tris, pH 8.5 (or in TE) in a 0.5 mL tube.
3. After each 30 min sonication cycle, vortex the DNA and spin down the contents to collect any droplets that may have formed during sonication (*see* **Note 18**).
4. After sonication, 100 ng of the fragmented DNA is subjected to gel electrophoresis on a 2% agarose/1× TAE gel.
5. If the DNA is not sheared sufficiently, shear for an additional 30 min (*see* **Note 19**). Other shearing devices may also be used [e.g., Bioruptor (Diagenode), Covaris]. Conditions need to be adjusted for each shearing device.
6. After sonification, the sheared DNA is purified using QIAquick columns (up to 10 mg DNA can be purified using one column).

3.4.3 DNA Purification

1. Add 4 volumes of QG buffer to the sample (i.e., for 50 μL DNA sample, add 200 μL QG) and mix by vortexing.
2. Incubate for 3 min.

3. Add 1.3 volumes of isopropanol (i.e., for 50 μL DNA sample, add 65 μL of isopropanol) and vortex.
4. Transfer the solution to a QIAquick column.
5. Centrifuge for 1 min at 10,000 × *g*.
6. Change the collection tube.
7. Aspirate the QG from the inner plastic rim of the column.
8. Pipette 700 μL PE to the column and also to the lid and the outer rim of the column to remove all remaining QG since QG may inhibit subsequent enzymatic reactions.
9. Centrifuge for 1 min at 10,000 × *g*.
10. Change the collection tube.
11. Repeat **steps 8–10**.
12. Centrifuge for 1 min at 10,000 × *g*.
13. Change the collection tube.
14. Aspirate the remaining PE from the inner rim of the column.
15. Centrifuge for 2 min at 10,000 × *g*.
16. Change the collection tube.
17. Pipette 16 μL EB-buffer (10 mM Tris, pH 8.5) to the membrane.
18. Incubate for 5 min.
19. Centrifuge for 1 min at 10,000 × *g*.
20. Pipette 16 μL EB to the membrane.
21. Centrifuge for 2 min.
22. 30 μL of DNA will be obtained, since the dead volume of the column is approximately 2 μL.
    Snap-freeze your sheared DNA in liquid nitrogen and store at −20 °C or proceed with the library DNA preparation (*see* **Note 20**).

3.4.4 Library DNA Preparation

Library DNA preparation follows the protocol suggested by Illumina as described in http://molbiol.ru/wiki/Next-generation_sequencing. Use low DNA binding reaction tubes for the library DNA preparation and the immunoprecipitation.

After library DNA preparation, 100 ng of the library DNA and 100 ng of the sheared DNA may be separated on a 2% agarose/1× TAE gel in order to analyze the quality of the library DNA. The size of the library DNA should be shifted by the length of the ligated adapters (approx. 70 bp).

End Repair

1. Set up a 20 °C water bath.
2. Set up for one reaction:

50 µL	DNA (5 µg)
31.7 µL	10× T4 DNA ligase buffer
12 µL	T4 DNA polymerase (3 U/µL)
12 µL	T4 polynucleotide kinase (10 U/µL)
2.4 µL	Polymerase I, large (Klenow) Fragment (5 U/µL)
3.2 µL	dNTP Mix (25 mM)
205.7 µL	H_2O
317 µL	Total volume

3. Incubate for 30 min in a 20 °C water bath.
4. Purify using QIAquick columns and buffer QG.
5. Pipette 1270 µL QG into a 2 mL reaction tube.
6. Add end-repair DNA reaction mix.
7. Incubate for 3 min.
8. Add 412 µL isopropanol.
9. Follow the QIAquick protocol.
10. Elute in 34 µL 10 mM Tris, pH 8.5 (elute twice with 18 µL each time).

A-tailing

1. Set up a 37 °C water bath.
2. Set up for one reaction:

34 µL	End-repaired DNA
8.8 µL	NEB2 reaction buffer (10×)
17.6 µL	1 mM dATP
7.3 µL	Klenow Fragment 3′ → 5′ exo- (5 U/µL)
20.3 µL	H_2O
88 µL	Total volume

3. Incubate for 30 min in a 37 °C water bath.
4. Purify using QIAquick minElute columns and buffer QG.
5. Add 352 µL QG.
6. Incubate for 3 min.
7. Add 114 µL of isopropanol.
8. Follow the QIAquick protocol.
9. Elute in 10 µL 10 mM Tris, pH 8.5 (elute twice with 6 µL each time).

Adapter Ligation

1. Set up a 20 °C water bath.
2. Add a tenfold molar excess of adapter-oligo mix to the 10 μL A-tailed DNA fragments, for 5 μg DNA with a mean fragment size of 200 bp, add 29 μL of adapter-oligo mix.
3. Mix gently by pipetting and incubate for 5 min at RT.
4. Set up a ligase master mix, per reaction:

49 μL	2× Quick ligase buffer
10 μL	Quick T4 DNA ligase
59 μL	Total volume

5. Add 59 μL of ligase master mix to the DNA–adapter mixture and mix gently by pipetting up and down.
6. Incubate for 15 min in a 20 °C water bath. Purify using QIAquick columns and buffer QG:
   (a) Add 392 μL QG.
   (b) Incubate for 3 min.
   (c) Add 127.4 μL of isopropanol.
   (d) Follow the QIAquick protocol.
   (e) Elute in 30 μL of 10 mM Tris, pH 8.5 (elute twice with 16 μL each time).
   (f) Quantify the concentration using a NanoDrop.

3.4.5 Methylated DNA Immunoprecipitation

(A) Blocking and Coupling the Antibody to the Magnetic Beads
Note: Use 4 °C cold solutions.

1. Pipette 700 μL of 0.5% BSA/1× PBS in a 1.5 mL microcentrifuge tube. Prepare one tube per MeDIP-reaction.
2. Vortex the magnetic beads well.
3. Add 40 μL of the magnetic beads to the tube with 0.5% BSA/1× PBS and mix by inverting the tube gently several times (*see* **Note 21**).
4. Collect the magnetic beads using a magnetic rack. After the beads are trapped at the side, invert the magnetic rack to clean the lid of the tube. Aspirate and discard the supernatant.
5. Remove the magnet from the magnetic stand (or take the tube out of the magnetic stand).
6. Resuspend the magnetic beads in 700 μL of 0.5% BSA/1× PBS by inverting the tube several times.
7. Repeat **steps 4–6**.
8. Repeat **steps 4** and **5** one more time.

9. Resuspend magnetic beads in 250 μL of 1× IP-buffer by inverting the tube several times.
10. Add 10 μL of 5mC-antibody (10 μg, *see* **Note 22**).
11. Incubate overnight with rotating at 4 °C.
12. Collect the magnetic beads using a magnetic rack. After the beads are trapped, invert the magnetic rack to clean the lid. Discard supernatant.
13. Resuspend the beads in 1 mL 0.5% BSA/1× PBS solution by inverting the tube several times.
14. Collect the magnetic beads using a magnetic rack, invert the magnetic rack to clean the lid. Discard supernatant.
15. Repeat **steps 13** and **14** one more time.
16. Resuspend the beads in 1 mL 1× IP-buffer by inverting the tube several times.
17. Collect the magnetic beads using a magnetic rack, invert the magnetic rack to clean the lid. Discard supernatant.
18. Resuspend the beads in 170 μL 1× IP-buffer and place on ice for later use.

(B) Methylated DNA Immunoprecipitation

1. Dilute 4.2–4.5 μg of the library DNA to 133 ng/mL in 10 mM Tris, pH 8.5.
2. Denature library DNA in thin-walled PCR tubes for 1 min at 95 °C in a thermocycler.
3. Immediately place the tube on ice-water and let it sit for 3–5 min (*see* **Note 23**).
4. Pipette 30 μL library DNA and 30 mL ice-cold 2× IP to the magnetic beads in 170 μL of 1× IP-buffer from (A) **step 18**.
5. Incubate for 4 h at 4 °C with rotation.
6. Trap the magnetic beads in a magnetic stand and invert the magnetic rack to clean the lid. Discard supernatant.
7. Add 1 mL of ice-cold 1× IP-buffer and resuspend the beads by inverting the tubes several times.
8. Repeat **steps 6** and 7 two more times.
9. After the last washing, centrifuge for 3 min at 960 × *g* at 4 °C. Remove any residual liquid. Be careful not to disturb the beads.
10. Add 210 μL of SDS elution buffer at RT.
11. Incubate for 15 min at 65 °C with briefly vortexing every 2 min. Briefly spin the contents of the tube down.
12. Trap the magnetic beads in a magnetic stand. Pipette the supernatant in a new 1.5 mL tube. Keep the supernatant! It contains the immunoprecipitated DNA.

13. Take the tubes containing the beads out of the magnetic stand. Resuspend the beads in 200 μL TE by vortexing. Shortly spin the contents of the tube down and collect the beads with the magnetic rack.
14. Combine the supernatant with the first eluate.
15. Add 4 μL of proteinase K (20 mg/mL).
16. Incubate for 2 h at 55 °C.

(C) Phenol–$CHCl_3$ Extraction

1. Centrifuge a 2 mL PhaseLock tube for 1 min at 16,000 × *g* at RT.
2. Pipette the sample (400 μL) to the PhaseLock tube, add 400 μL phenol–chloroform–isoamyl alcohol (25:24:1), mix vigorously by shaking the tube (do not vortex).
3. Centrifuge for 5 min at 16,000 × *g* and RT. The organic phase (phenol) and the aqueous (upper) phase (DNA) are separated by a solid phase.
4. Repeat extraction two more times with 400 μL chloroform–isoamyl alcohol (24:1).
5. Pipette the aqueous phase containing the DNA into a 1.5 mL tube containing 16 μL of 5 M NaCl and 1 μL of linear polyacrylamide. Mix, add 800 μL of 100% EtOH, and precipitate overnight at −20 °C.
6. Spin for 30 min at 16,000 × *g* at 4 °C.
7. Discard the supernatant.
8. Add 800 μL of 80% EtOH, vortex, spin for 5 min at 20,000 × *g* at 4 °C.
9. Aspirate supernatant, briefly spin again and aspirate any residual liquid, air dry pellet and resuspend in 20 μL 10 mM Tris, pH 8.5.
10. Optional: quantitate the DNA using the Quant-it ssDNA kit. Since the amount of immunoprecipitated DNA is low, quantitation using a NanoDrop does not work reliable in our hands. Usually, we obtain 100–200 ng of immunoprecipitated library DNA from 4 μg of library DNA (2.5–5%).
11. Snap-freeze the sample in liquid nitrogen and store at −20 °C. Avoid repeated freeze–thaw cycles.

3.4.6 Quantitative PCR as Quality Controls

Enrichment of methylated DNA is monitored after MeDIP and after library DNA amplification by standard qPCR using control primers of known methylated and unmethylated genomic regions using SYBR-green dye. We routinely use 0.5 μL of the MeDIP sample in a 10 μL of PCR reaction (*see* **Note 24**).

The methylation status of the control regions may differ between cell types, and thus different control regions may be suitable for different cell types due to mosaic methylation patterns.

3.4.7 Amplification of the Library DNA and Size Selection

The immunoprecipitated DNA is subjected to amplification and size-selection prior to sequencing. If desired, input DNA may also be amplified and size-selected.

1. Set up for one reaction:

4 μL	MeDIP-sample (one-fifth of the MeDIP-sample or 40 ng of input library DNA)
15 μL	High-Fidelity Phusion polymerase
0.6 μL	Primer 1.1 (20 μM, Illumina)
0.6 μL	Primer 2.1 (20 μM, Illumina)
9.8 μL	H_2O
30 μL	Total volume

   For PCR cycling conditions, use a manual hot-start:

   (a) 98 °C for 30 s

   (b) 98 °C for 10 s

   (c) 65 °C for 30 s

   (d) 72 °C for 30 s

   For the amplification, six PCR cycles (repetitions of **steps 2–4**) are used, thereby keeping the risk of introducing amplification bias low.

2. Size selection is performed using a 2% Bio-Rad/1× TAE gel. We run the gel for 2 h at 100 V and use a 50 bp Marker (NEB). If a better resolution is required, 25 bp DNA ladders may be used.
3. The gel chamber is cleaned thoroughly using detergent and water. The samples and marker are loaded as follows: marker, empty well, sample, empty well, marker, empty well, sample, empty well, marker, and so on to avoid cross-contamination of the samples and to ensure a precise size-selection.
4. We excise 150–400 bp DNA fragments for later sequencing. Interestingly, the size range of an amplified MeDIP library DNA begins at about 200 bp while the size range of an amplified input library DNA starts at 150 bp, indicating a selection for larger fragment sizes by the methylated immunoprecipitation.
5. Purify the DNA using the QIAquick Gel Extraction kit and elute in about 30 μL of 10 mM Tris, pH 8.5 (elute twice with 16 μL each time).

6. Quantify the DNA using a Quant-it dsHSDNA kit. Typically, we obtain 240–300 ng of amplified library DNA.
7. Snap-freeze the library DNA and store at −20 °C until sequencing. Avoid repeat freeze–thaw cycles (*see* **Note 25**).

3.5 Methylation-Sensitive Restriction Enzyme Followed by Sequencing (MRE-Seq)

3.5.1 Preparation of Genomic DNA

Isolate DNA using DNeasy Blood and Tissue Kit (Qiagen) according to the method described in Subheading 3.1.1.

3.5.2 Adapter Preparation

1. Dissolve the lyophilized adapters and primers at 100 μM concentration in sterile PCR grade water.
2. Dilute an aliquot of both A and B (or B blunt) adapters to 10 μM concentration.
3. Mix in a 1:1 ratio.
4. Anneal in thermocycler by heating the mix to 95 °C for 5 min and subsequently cooling it stepwise by 5 °C/5 min to 25 °C.
5. Store the annealed adapters at −20 °C, aliquoted in 500 μL Eppendorf tubes (*see* **Note 26**).
6. The oligo pairs PmeI_CGWA and PmeI_CGB oligos are used for HpaII and AciI enzyme site adapters, while for Bsh1236I enzyme site PmeI_CGWA and PmeI_CGBlunt oligos are used.

3.5.3 Digestion and Ligation of Genomic DNA

1. Use a single reaction for the restriction digestion and adapter ligation of the genomic DNA. The 50 μL reaction mix contains 300 ng purified genomic DNA (*see* **Note 27**), 5 μL (10×) restriction enzyme buffer, 4 μL (10 μM) annealed adapter, 40 U of restriction enzyme, 10 U of T4 ligase, and fill up with water to 50 μL.
2. Incubate the digestion–ligation reaction overnight at 37 °C.
3. After heat inactivation at 65 °C for 20 min in a thermocycler, dilute the samples 1:1 with 50 μL PCR grade water and extract subsequently by equal volumes of phenol–chloroform–isoamyl alcohol (25:24:1), then by chloroform–isoamyl alcohol (24:1).
4. Precipitate the extracted DNA with 2.5 volumes of absolute EtOH in the presence of 0.3 M NaOAc, pH 5.2, wash with 70% EtOH. Dry and dissolve in 100 μL of 5 mM Tris, pH 8.0.

3.5.4 Amplification of the Adapter-Ligated Genomic Fragments

1. Amplification of the adapter-ligated DNA (*see* **Note 28**): Use 5 μL of digested and adapter-ligated DNA (about 15 ng) and 4 μL of 10 μM amplification primer PmeI_CG17 in a 50 μL PCR reaction containing 5 μL PCR buffer (10×), 1 μL $MgCl_2$

(25 mM), 1 μL dNTP (20 μM), 0.5 μL HotStar Polymerase (2.5 U) and add PCR grade water to 50 μL. Initialize the PCR at 95 °C for 15 min followed by 25–30 cycles of 95 °C × 30 s/ 55 °C × 40 s/72 °C × 50 s and finish by 72 °C for 5 min. The exact number of cycles has to be evaluated experimentally (*see* **Note 29**).

2. Removal of the adapter sequences: This can be achieved by PmeI digestion, because its rare cut site GTTTAAAC is present in the adapter sequence. Digest 1 μg of the PCR amplificates with PmeI (NEB) in NEB4 buffer, in two steps under the presence of 100 ng/μL BSA.
3. Perform the first digestion in a 50 μL reaction volume, containing 100 U PmeI enzyme on 37 °C for 2 h followed by a subsequent volume increase to 100 μL in 1× NEB4 buffer including additional 50 U PmeI and 2 h of incubation.
4. Finally, stop the reaction at 65 °C for 20 min.
5. Purify the samples (100 μL) with 100 μL phenol–chloroform–isoamyl alcohol (25:24:1), then twice with the same volume of chloroform–isoamyl alcohol (24:1).
6. Pipet the upper phase into a new 1.5 mL Eppendorf tube, and precipitate the DNA by adding 0.1 volume of 3.0 M NaOAc, pH 5.2 and 2.5 volumes of absolute EtOH. Incubate at −20 °C for 1 h.
7. Centrifuge the tube at 16,000 × *g* and 4 °C for 20 min, then wash with 70% EtOH. Centrifuge at 15,000 × *g* for 10 min. Discard the supernatant and let the pellet dry at room temperature.
8. Dissolve in 5 mM Tris, pH 8.0 to reach a concentration of about 200 ng/μL. Store at −20 °C. Test the effectivity of the adapter removal (*see* **Note 30**).

3.5.5 Sequencing

1. Set a 50 μL reaction containing 2 μg of PCR amplified fragments, 1× Bal31 reaction buffer, and 1 U of Bal31 enzyme. Incubate at 30 °C and take out 5 μL sample at 15, 30, 60, 120 s, etc., up to 6 min. Mix the removed sample immediately with 5 μL of 40 mM EGTA prewarmed to 65 °C and incubate for 10 min to stop the reaction.
2. To visualize the progression of the shortening, the samples are diluted 1:5 with 10 mM Tris, pH 8.0 and loaded to an Agilent Bioanalyzer. A size shift of about 30–40 bp is expected for a proper removal of the uniform parts at the fragment ends.
3. Using the results of the time-course experiment, estimate the necessary digestion time to reach this goal. The size reduction is fragment length dependent, since longer fragments are stronger affected. Therefore, we highly recommend separate

optimization for each studied set of samples/species. To prepare fragments for the sequencing set up the same reaction and use the identified time for optimal shortening.

3.6 Infinium Methylation450 BeadChips (450 K, Illumina)

3.6.1 DNA Extraction

Isolate DNA using DNeasy Blood and Tissue Kit (Qiagen) according to the method described in Subheading 3.1.1 (*see* **Note 17**).

3.6.2 Bisulfite Conversion

1. Treat the genomic DNA (800 ng) with sodium bisulfite using the Zymo EZ DNA Methylation Kit™ (Zymo Research) according to the manufacturer's instruction, with the alternative incubation conditions recommended when using the Illumina Infinium Methylation Assay.
2. Denature the cleaned DNA for 2 min at 95 °C, followed by ligation incubation at 37 °C for 1 h with RST and CMM reagents.
3. Clean the resulting DNA with ZR-96 DNA Clean & Concentrator–5 kit (Zymo Research) and elute in 10 μL of ddH_2O.

3.6.3 Infinium Methylation 450k Array Hybridization

1. Perform the methylation assay by using 4 μL bisulfite-converted genomic DNA at 50 ng/μL according to the Infinium Human Methylation Assay protocol.
2. Check the data quality with the GenomeStudio™ Methylation Module software (2010.3) and ensure that all samples pass this quality control.
3. Extract the uncorrected *b*-values with the same software. Submit raw data to the Gene Expression Omnibus (GSE29290) database.

3.7 Bisulfite Sequencing (BS)

3.7.1 DNA Extraction

Isolate DNA using DNeasy Blood and Tissue Kit (Qiagen) according to the method described in Subheading 3.1.1.

3.7.2 DNA Fragmentation and Size Selection

1. Prepare a 1% agarose gel with SYBR-Safe dye in advance.
2. Determine the concentration of the DNA sample; dilute 2 μg of DNA with ddH_2O to make a total volume of 130 μL.
3. Optional: add 2 ng of lambda phage DNA as spike–in.
4. Fragment the DNA in a sonicator. We use the Covaris M220 sonicator, and select the 300 bp fragment peak size protocol (*see* **Note 31**).
5. Transfer the sample into a snap cap microTUBE and sonicate the DNA.

6. Optional: confirm the sonication efficiency by running 50 ng of the sonicated DNA in an agarose gel.
7. Concentrate the DNA using a PCR purification kit and elute in 25 μL elution buffer.
8. Perform gel electrophoresis and recover the DNA fragments in the range between 300 and 500 bp using a gel purification kit. Elute the DNA with 25 μL water.
9. Determine the DNA concentration, around 300 ng is required.

3.7.3 End Repair

The fragmented DNA contains different types of overhangs, and these need to be blunt-ended and phosphorylated for adapter ligation. This is achieved by the combined action of the T4 DNA polymerase and the T4 polynucleotide kinase in the End Repair enzyme mix.

1. Prepare the end repair reaction in a PCR tube as follows:

Components	Volume (μL)
300–500 ng of purified DNA in water	21
10× T4 Ligase buffer with ATP	2.5
10 mM dNTP w/o dCTP (*see* **Note 32**)	0.5
End Repair Enzyme Mix	1

2. Mix by pipetting, incubate in a thermocycler at 20 °C for 30 min.
3. Add 25 μL AMPure XP beads into the end–repair reaction, mix by pipetting (at least ten times) and incubate at room temperature for 10 min.
4. Place the End–Repair reaction with AMPure XP on a magnetic stand for ~1 min or until the beads are fully attached to the magnetic side of the tube. Carefully pipette out the solution without touching the beads. Do not remove the tube from the magnet.
5. Add 150 μL of 80% EtOH without disturbing the beads and wait for 30 s, carefully remove the ethanol using the pipette.
6. Repeat the ethanol wash one more time. Do not remove the tube from the magnet throughout the process.
7. Use a new pipette tip to remove all residual ethanol from the bottom and the side of the PCR tube. Do not overdry the AMPure XP beads.
8. Add 20.5 μL of water to elute the end-repaired DNA, mix well by pipetting.

9. Place the PCR tube on the magnetic stand for ~1 min or until the beads are fully attached to the magnetic side of the tube. Carefully pipette out the end-repaired DNA to a new PCR tube without touching the beads.

3.7.4 dA Tailing

To prevent ligation between the blunt and phosphorylated DNA fragments and also self-circularization, a 3′ dA overhang is added by the Klenow Fragment (3′ exo-) of the *E. coli* DNA polymerase I.

1. Prepare the dA–tailing reaction as follows:

Components	Volume (μL)
End-repaired DNA in water	20.5
10× T4 Ligase buffer with ATP	2.5
10 mM dATP	1
Klenow 3′–5′ exo–	1

2. Place the tube in a thermocycler and incubate at 37 °C for 30 min.
3. Add 25 μL AMPure XP beads into the tube, mix by pipetting (at least ten times) and incubate at room temperature for 10 min.
4. Place the tube on a magnetic stand for ~1 min or until the beads are fully attached to the magnetic side of the tube. Carefully pipette out the solution without touching the beads. Do not remove the tube from the magnet.
5. Add 150 μL of 80% EtOH without disturbing the beads and wait for 30 s, carefully remove the ethanol using the pipette.
6. Repeat the ethanol wash one more time. Do not remove the tube from the magnet throughout the process.
7. Use a new pipette tip to remove all residual ethanol from the bottom and the side of the PCR tube. Do not overdry the AMPure XP beads.
8. Add 22 μL of water to elute the dA-tailed DNA, mix well by pipetting.
9. Place the PCR tube on the magnetic stand for ~1 min or until the beads are fully attached to the magnetic side of the tube. Carefully pipette out all the DNA to a new PCR tube without touching the beads.

3.7.5 Adapter Ligation and Double AMPure XP Cleanup

After dA-tailing, the DNA fragment with 3′ dA overhang is ready to be ligated to the Illumina adapter, which contains a complementary 3′ dT overhang. Compared to the regular Illumina adapter, the cytosines in the BS-Seq adapter are methylated, and will not be bisulfite-converted to uridine.

1. Prepare the ligation reaction as follows:

Components	Volume (μL)
dA-tailed DNA in water	22
2× Ligase buffer with ATP and PEG	25
25 μM TruSeq 5mC double-stranded adapter	2
T4 Ligase	1

2. The solution containing 2× ligase buffer is very viscous, pipet up and down at least ten times to mix after adding the T4 DNA Ligase.
3. Incubate the tube in a thermocycler at 25 °C for 15 min and hold at 4 °C for at least 1 h. Alternatively, perform the ligation overnight at 16 °C (*see* **Note 33**).
4. Add 50 μL AMPure XP beads into the tube, mix by pipetting at least ten times and incubate at room temperature for 10 min.
5. Place the tube on a magnetic stand for ~1 min or until beads are fully attached to the magnetic side of the tube. Carefully pipette out the solution without touching the beads. Do not remove the tube from the magnet.
6. Add 150 μL of 80% EtOH without disturbing the beads and wait for 30 s, carefully remove the ethanol using the pipette.
7. Repeat the ethanol wash one more time. Do not remove the tube from the magnet during the process.
8. Use a new pipette tip to remove all residual ethanol from the bottom and the side of the PCR tube. Do not overdry the AMPure XP beads.
9. Add 50 μL of TE to elute the adapter ligated DNA, mix well by pipetting.
10. Repeat the AMPure XP cleanup to achieve pure DNA. After drying the beads, add 21 μL of TE to elute the adapter ligated DNA, mix well by pipetting.
11. Place the PCR tube on the magnetic stand for ~1 min or until the beads are fully attached to the magnetic side of the tube. Carefully pipette out all the DNA to a new PCR tube without touching the beads.

3.7.6 Bisulfite Conversion

The following protocol describes a bisulfite conversion using the Invitrogen MethylCode Bisulfite Conversion Kit or QIAGEN and ZYMO conversion kits following the condition recommended by the manufacturer.

1. Use 1 μL of the library DNA for DNA concentration measurement on a Qubit fluorometer. The expected DNA amount is around 300–500 ng (*see* **Note 34**).

2. Set up the bisulfite conversion reaction as follows:

Components	Volume (μL)
Library DNA in TE	20
Freshly prepared CT conversion reagent	130

3. Mix the reaction carefully and incubate it in a thermocycler using the following cycle conditions:

Step	Time	Temp (°C)
Denature	10 min	98
Incubation	2.5 h	64
Hold	Indefinite	4

4. Purify the bisulfite-converted library DNA according to the manufacturer's instruction, except that the elution is performed using 2 × 20 μL water instead of the EB buffer, which interferes with PCR.
5. Critical step: the purified library DNA is unstable, so it should be PCR-amplified immediately. Do not store the purified libraries at −20 °C. If storage is required, it can be kept in a 4 °C refrigerator for 1 day without significant loss.

3.7.7 PCR Amplification

Archaeal DNA polymerase such as *Pfu* can recognize the uracil in the template strand and stall polymerization. Hence, uracil tolerant polymerase must be used to amplify the bisulfite-converted library DNA.

1. Prepare the PCR reaction as follows (*see* **Note 35**):

Components	Volume (μL)
BS-treated library DNA	20
2× KAPA HiFi Uracilþ ReadyMix	25
TruSeq universal primer (10 μM)	2.5
TruSeq index primer (10 μM)	2.5

2. Perform the PCR in a thermocycler using the following program.

Cycle	Denature	Anneal	Extend	Hold
1	94 °C for 1 min	–	–	–
6–8	98 °C for 10 s	65 °C for 20 s	72 °C for 30 s	–
1	–	–	72 °C for 3 min	–
1	–	–	–	4 °C

3. Purify the PCR product using 1 volume of AMPure XP as previously described (Subheading 3.7.3). The library DNA is now ready for sequencing (*see* **Note 36**).

3.8 Pyrosequencing

3.8.1 DNA Extraction

1. Isolate DNA using DNeasy Blood and Tissue Kit (Qiagen) according to the method described in Subheading 3.1.1.
2. The extracted DNA should be quantified using a spectrophotometer or other equivalent methods for the quantification of dsDNA, and the concentration should be adjusted to between 20 and 50 ng/μL depending on how much DNA to be used for sodium bisulfite conversion.

3.8.2 Sodium Bisulfite Conversion

1. For sodium bisulfite conversion we normally use the EZ DNA methylation kit (Zymo Research) or EpiTect bisulfite kit (Qiagen) according to the manufacturer's instruction.
2. Depending on the number of analyses planned for each sample between 200 ng and 1 μg DNA input should be used.
3. The final elution volume should be within a range allowing for a theoretical input of 20 ng bisulfite-converted DNA in the subsequent PCR amplification.

3.8.3 PCR Amplification

The PCR can be performed either as a standard PCR or as a real-time PCR if quantitative methylation data are needed and/or to avoid gel electrophoresis.

1. Performing a standard PCR: This kit (PyroMark PCR kit, Qiagen) contains a Master Mix with dNTPs, $MgCl_2$, PCR buffer, and a HotStarTaq DNA polymerase, and also comes with an additive, the Q-solution, which may be helpful for sufficient amplification of GC-rich regions, and a gel-tracking dye, the CoralLoad, which makes it easier to load the PCR product on a gel prior to Pyrosequencing analysis. For the reaction mixture the Master Mix is used at a final concentration of 1×. Primer concentrations should be maximum 100–200 nM of each primer (*see* **Note 37**), and for each sample 20 ng bisulfite-converted DNA is used. The final reaction volume is 25 μL (*see* **Note 38**).
   The PCR cycling protocol starts with 1 cycle of 95 °C for 15 min, followed by 45 cycles of 95 °C for 20 s and 72 °C for 20 s, and 1 cycle of 72 °C for 10 min.
2. Performing a real-time PCR: This kit (LightCycler® 480 SYBR Green I Master, Roche) contains a Master Mix with dNTPs, PCR buffer, FastStart Taq DNA Polymerase, and a dsDNA-specific dye for product detection and characterization. $MgCl_2$ is supplied separately. For the reaction mixture the Master Mix is used at a final concentration of 1×. Primer concentrations should be maximum 100–200 nM of each primer (*see* **Note 37**), and we

normally use $MgCl_2$ at a final concentration of 2.5 mM. For each sample 20 ng bisulfite-converted DNA is used. The final reaction volume is 20 μL (*see* **Note 38**). The PCR cycling protocol starts with 1 cycle of 95 °C for 10 min, followed by 45 cycles of 95 °C for 20 s and 72 °C for 20 s. Fluorescence should be acquired to the SYBR Green I channel after each extension step. Then a 10 min hold at 72 °C, a 1 min hold at 95 °C, and a 1 min hold at 40 °C are completed before performing a melting analysis from 60 to 95 °C with 20 or more acquisitions per degree Celsius. Samples that did not amplify or produce a melting profile of the expected size should not be subjected to Pyrosequencing.

3.8.4 Gel Electrophoresis

1. Prepare a 2% agarose gel with ethidium bromide.
2. Load PCR products of samples from Subheading 3.8.3, **step 1** and DNA size standard.
3. Run at 6 V/cm for 20–30 min depending on the size of the PCR product.
4. Place the gel on a UV Transilluminator or in an imaging system, and use the DNA ladder to determine if the band is of the expected size.
5. The library DNA is now ready for sequencing.

3.9 Methylation-Specific PCR (MSP)/ Quantitative Methylation-Specific PCR (QMSP)

3.9.1 DNA Extraction

Isolate DNA using DNeasy Blood and Tissue Kit (Qiagen) according to the method described in Subheading 3.1.1.

3.9.2 DNA Modification Using Sodium Bisulfite

1. Denature 1–2 μg of DNA in a volume of 50 μL by adding 3 M NaOH to final concentration of 0.3 M.
2. Incubate at 37 °C for 10 min.
3. Add 30 μL of 10 mM hydroquinone and 520 μL of 3 M sodium bisulfate at pH 5.0.
4. Mix gently and incubate under mineral oil at 50 °C for 16 h.
5. Purify modified DNA using Wizard DNA purification resin according to the manufacturer's instruction or another preferred kit.
6. Elute into 50 μL of distilled water.
7. Neutralize by adding 0.1 volume of 3 M sodium acetate and mix by vortexing.
8. Add 1 volume of isopropanol and mix gently.

9. Centrifuge at 18,000 × *g* for 30 min at 4 °C and discard the supernatant.
10. Add 500 μL of cold 75% ethanol to wash the DNA pellet.
11. Centrifuge at 18,000 × *g* for 10 min at 4 °C and discard the supernatant.
12. Air-dry the DNA pellet and dissolve in 50 μL of distilled water or TE buffer.
13. Sodium bisulfite modification kits are also commercially available such as CpGenome DNA modification kit (Intergen), Ez DNA methylation kit (Zymo Research), and CpGenome Fast DNA modification kit (Millipore).
14. CpGenome Universal Methylated DNA (Chemincon) is often used as a control DNA.

3.9.3 Primer Design

1. Prediction of CpG Islands

   For primer design of MSP, CpG islands have to be predicted with the promoter sequence of the target gene. The CpG island is a sequence at least 200 bp length in the promoter, which has a CG content exceeding 50% and an observed CpG/expected CpG ratio exceeding 0.6 (*see* **Note 39**). It is also needed for sequence conversion using bisulfate-modified DNA. The conversion can be performed in two different versions: (1) Methylation DNA: methylated cytosine of CpG dinucleotides remains intact, but cytosine of non-CpGs is converted to thymine. (2) Unmethylated DNA: all cytosines including CpG dinucleotides are converted to thymine. Two pairs of primers can be used to determine the methylated or unmethylated DNA based on the converted sequences.

   The above procedures can be performed by online software with the promoter sequence of the target gene. The websites are

   MethPrimer: http://www.urogene.org/methprimer/index1.html.

   Primo: http://www.changbioscience.com/primo/primom.html.

   BiSearch: http://bisearch.enzim.hu/.

   Also, Methylprimer Express Software 1.0 is available for free from Applied Biosystems web site.

2. CpG Island Prediction Principle

   Concerning the predicted CpG islands, several rules govern the choice of appropriative primers as target region.

   (a) If more than one island is predicted, any of them can be the target region for amplification.

   (b) If a CpG island size is smaller than the minimal product size, the primer pair should span the whole island.

(c) If a CpG island size is greater than the maximal product size, the primer pair should be within the island.

(d) If a CpG island size is between the minimal and maximal product size (*see* **Note 40**), primer pair should involve at least two-thirds of the island.

3. Primer Selection

For performing MSP/QMSP, two pairs of primers are needed. One amplifies modified and methylated DNA, and the other amplifies modified and unmethylated DNA. The following restrictions are applied to the primer selection for MSP/QMSP:

(a) Primers should include at least one CpG dinucleotide, and at least one of the last three bases in the primer should be a cytosine of CpG for maximal discrimination between methylated and unmethylated DNA.

(b) More CpG sites in the primer are preferred including CpG dinucleotide(s) at the most 3′ end.

(c) Primers for methylated DNA and for unmethylated DNA should contain the same CpG dinucleotides within their sequence. However, they may vary in length or at their start point for matching of temperature value between two sets of primers (*see* **Note 41**).

(d) Two pairs of primers having similar annealing temperature are preferred and annealing temperatures equal or higher than 55 °C is preferred.

3.9.4 PCR Amplification

1. **General PCR**

After primer design and selection, MSP is performed with general PCR conditions. For example, PCR conditions consist of 5 min at 94 °C for initial denaturation, followed by 40 cycles of 94 °C (30 s), annealing temperature of primers (30 s), and 72 °C (60 s) and a final elongation of 7 min at 72 °C. Finally, amplified products are loaded onto a 2% agarose gel and electrophoresed for 20 min at 100 V.

2. **Real-Time PCR**

QMSP is performed with real-time PCR conditions. For example, Briefly, 1 μL cDNA from each sample is mixed with 0.4 μL of 10 μM of each primer, 10 μL of SYBR *Premix Ex Taq* (Tli RNaseH Plus) (2×) (TaKaRa, Dalian, China) in a total volume of 20 μL. The PCR reaction is performed on a 7500 Fast Real-Time PCR System (Applied Biosystems, California, USA). PCR protocol consisted of four programs: (1) denaturation of the cDNA/RNA hybrid at 95 °C for 30 s; (2) amplification of cDNA for 40 cycles, each cycle using sequentially 95 °C for 3 s, 60 °C for 30 s; (3) analysis of the melting curve to confirm the single product amplification during the PCR assay; and (4) cooling the rotor and thermal chamber at 25 °C.

3.10 Single Molecule Real-Time Bisulfite Sequencing (SMRT-BS)

3.10.1 DNA Extraction

Isolate DNA using DNeasy Blood and Tissue Kit (Qiagen) according to the method described in Subheading 3.1.1.

3.10.2 Bisulfite Conversion

1. Using Methylamp™ DNA Modification Kit (Epigentek) according to the manufacturer's instruction. For each sample, add 500 ng–1 μg genomic DNA to each 1.7 mL tube (*see* **Note 42**).
2. Follow the Methylamp™ DNA Modification Kit protocol and elute the bisulfite-converted DNA with 20 μL of elution buffer.
3. (Optional) Modified DNA can be quantified by a NanoDrop 1000 (Thermo Scientific) using the ssDNA application and sized with the Agilent Bioanalyzer 2100 using the RNA6000 pico kit.

3.10.3 Primer Design

1. For the first round PCR amplification of bisulfite-converted DNA, design region-specific forward and reverse primers using MethPrimer (http://www.urogene.org/methprimer) or a comparable program capable of designing bisulfite sequencing PCR primers. Add universal oligonucleotide tags to the 5′ end of both forward and reverse primers prior to synthesis to enable the addition of barcodes through a second round PCR.
2. For the second round PCR amplification, add sample-specific barcodes to the 5′ end of the universal oligonucleotide anti-tag primers (*see* **Note 43**).

3.10.4 Bisulfite PCR Amplification

First round PCR amplifies bisulfite-converted DNA using region-specific forward and reverse primers that have 5′ universal oligonucleotide tags for subsequent barcoding.

1. Place a 96-well PCR plate on ice for PCR preparation.
2. Prepare master mix for the reaction in a 2.0 mL tube. For each 20 μL reaction, mix 11.8 μL H_2O, 2 μL 10× PCR buffer with Mg^{2+}, 3.2 μL dNTP (1.25 mM each) and 0.2 μL TaKaRa Taq HS.
3. Dispense 17.2 μL of master mix to each well.
4. Add 0.8 μL of primer mix (5 μM each) and 2 μL of bisulfite-converted DNA to each well.
5. Seal the plate with an adhesive film, vortex, and centrifuge to bring all components to the bottom of the well.
6. Place the PCR plate in a thermal cycler and set the amplification program as following: initial denaturation step at 94 °C for 2 min followed by 35 amplification cycles (94 °C for 20 s, annealing temperature for 45 s, and 65 °C for 1 min/kb + 30 s) and a final incubation at 65 °C for 5 min (*see* **Note 44**).

7. Electrophorese PCR products through a 2% agarose gel at 120 V for 40 min (or as long as needed based on the amplicon length) to confirm successful amplification (*see* **Note 45**).
8. Dilute first round PCR amplicons 1:100 by transferring 2 μL of PCR products to 98 μL H_2O in a new 96-well plate on ice. Seal the plate with an adhesive film, vortex, and centrifuge to bring all components to the bottom of the well.

3.10.5 Barcoding

Second round PCR reamplifies the first round amplicons using 50 universal oligonucleotide anti-tags that are coupled to sample-specific barcodes. Ensure that all amplicons from the same genomic DNA sample are labeled with the same barcodes.

1. Place a 96-well PCR plate on ice for PCR preparation.
2. Prepare master mix for the reaction in a 1.7 mL tube. For each 20 μL reaction, mix 16.25 μL H_2O, 2.5 μL 10× PCR buffer with Mg^{2+}, 4 μL dNTP (1.25 mM each), and 0.25 μL TaKaRa Taq HS.
3. Dispense 23 μL of master mix to each well.
4. Add 1 μL of universal primers with sample-specific barcodes (5 μM each) and 1 μL of diluted first round PCR products to each well.
5. Seal the plate with an adhesive film, vortex, and centrifuge to bring all components to the bottom of the well.
6. Place the PCR plate in a thermal cycler and set the amplification program as following: initial denaturation step at 94 °C for 2 min followed by 35 amplification cycles (94 °C for 20 s, 60 °C for 45 s, and 65 °C for 1 min/kb + 30 s) and a final incubation at 65 °C for 5 min.
7. Electrophorese PCR products through a 2% agarose gel at 120 V for 40 min (or as long as needed based on amplicon length) to confirm successful amplification.

3.10.6 Amplicon Purification and Pooling

Prior to library DNA construction and sequencing, amplicons require purification to ensure accurate quantification, which is critical to sample pooling and successful SMRT sequencing.

1. Purify PCR products using the QIAquick PCR purification kit according to the manufacturer's instruction (*see* **Note 46**).
2. Elute purified PCR products with 15 μL of elution buffer.
3. Measure the concentration of purified PCR products (2 μL) with a NanoDrop and the dsDNA application.
4. Calculate the required volume of each amplicon using the following formula:

$$V_i = \frac{M \times L_i}{n \times C_i \times \sum_{i=1}^{m} L_i}$$

where V_i is the volume of each PCR amplicon, M is the total mass of pooled PCR amplicons, L_i is the length of each amplicon, n is the total number of samples, C_i is the concentration of each amplicon, and m is the total number of amplicons.

5. Add the calculated volume of each amplicon into a new 1.7 mL tube. This pooled sample is now ready for SMRT sequencing library DNA construction.

3.10.7 SMRT Sequencing Library DNA Construction and Sequencing

SMRT sequencing libraries are constructed following the Pacific Biosciences Amplicon Template Preparation and Sequencing protocol, and SMRT sequencing performed according to the Pacific Biosciences P5-C3 protocol (*see* **Note 47**).

3.11 Targeted Bisulfite Sequencing

3.11.1 DNA Extraction

Isolate DNA using DNeasy Blood and Tissue Kit (Qiagen) according to the method described in Subheading 3.1.1.

3.11.2 Bisulfite Treatment

1. Bisufite Mix is diluted with 800 μL RNase-free water, then vortexed until the Bisulfite Mix is dissolved entirely.
2. DNA is dissolved with RNase-free water, and prepare the Bisufite reaction mix:

DNA	20 μL
Bisulfite Mix	85 μL
DNA Protect Buffer	35 μL
Total	140 μL

3. Mix the reaction reagents at the room temperature, the color of the solution would turn from green to blue after adding the DNA Protect Buffer.
4. PCRreaction: 95 °C × 5 min → 60 °C × 25 min → 95 °C × 5 min → 60 °C × 85 min → 95 °C × 5 min → 60 °C × 175 min → 20 °C hold.

3.11.3 DNA Purification

1. Centrifuge the PCR tube, and transfer the supernatant into a new 1.5 mL collecting tube.
2. Add 560 μL Buffer BL containing 10 μg/mL carrier into the 1.5 mL collecting tube, mix the solution and centrifuge.
3. Put the EpiTect Spin Columns into the 1.5 mL collecting tube, transfer the solution into the EpiTect Spin Columns, centrifuge at 15,000 × *g* for 1 min, then discard the filtrate.

4. Open the lid carefully, add 500 μL Buffer BW, centrifuge at 15,000 × *g* for 1 min, then discard the filtrate.
5. Open the lid carefully, add 500 μL Buffer BD, close the lid, incubate at the room temperature for 15 min, centrifuge at 15,000 × *g* for 1 min, then discard the filtrate.
6. Repeat **step 4** twice.
7. Transfer the EpiTect Spin Columns into a new 1.5 mL collecting tube, centrifuge at 15,000 × *g* for 1 min
8. Transfer the EpiTect Spin Columns into a new 1.5 mL collecting tube, open the lid, incubate at 56 °C for 5 min.
9. Transfer the EpiTect Spin Columns into a new 1.5 mL collecting tube, add 20 μL Buffer EB into the center of the EpiTect Spin Columns, centrifuge at 15,000 × *g* for 1 min; add 20 μL Buffer EB into the center of the EpiTect Spin Columns, centrifuge at 15,000 × *g* for 1 min.

3.11.4 Capture the Targeted Gene Region

1. Special primes are designed using Methyl Primer Express v1.0 and MethPrimer.
2. Prepare the PCR reaction solution:

KAPA2G Robust Hot Start ReadyMix	10 μL
Forward Primer	1 μL
Reverse Primer	1 μL
Bisulfite-treated genomic DNA	>5 ng
ddH_2O	up to 20 μL

3. PCR reaction:

94 °C	3 min	
94 °C	30 s	45 cycles
55 °C	30 s	45 cycles
72 °C	40 s	45 cycles
72 °C	10 min	
4 °C	Hold	

4. The PCR product are mixed with an equal volume of each targeted gene region, then purified with Beckman Agencourt AMPure XP beads.
5. DNA library is constructed using NEBNext® Ultra™II DNA Library Prep Kit for Illumina (NEB, USA) according to the manufacturer's instruction. After the completed libraries are quantified by the Agilent 2100 Bioanalyzer (Agilent

Technologies Inc., USA), sequencing is performed on the Illumina's Hiseq X ten (Illumina, USA) as 150 bp paired-end reads according to the manufacturer's instruction.

4 Notes

1. Carry out all procedures at room temperature, unless otherwise specified. Kits from other commercial companies or standard procedures such as phenol–chloroform extraction are also expected to perform well.
2. To maximize elution efficiency, carefully pipette TE buffer onto the spin column membrane and incubate at room temperature for 5 min before centrifugation. Reapply the eluate to the membrane and repeat centrifugation. This step helps to elute the remnant DNA from columns. If a small amount of eluate remains on the inside of the spin column, reapply to the membrane and centrifuge for 30 s.
3. High quality input DNA is necessary for successful RRBS library DNA preparation. NanoDrop absorbance at 260 and 280 nm ($A_{260/280}$) ratios of between 1.8 and 2.0 are indicative of relatively pure DNA, but quality assessment of samples by agarose gel electrophoresis is also recommended. NanoDrop absorbance measurements are useful as a quick estimate of DNA concentration, but fluorometric methods such as the Qubit are more accurate, especially for detecting samples with RNA contamination.
4. A 10 μL aliquot of PCR product can be viewed on a gel prior to SPRI cleanup.
5. The tubes are gently flicked to mix and briefly spun down in a minicentrifuge. Incubations are performed in a thermocycler to ensure accurate temperature control. For complete Msp I digestion, samples are incubated overnight.
6. The TruSeq DNA sample preparation kits contain either 24 single index adapters (low throughput kit) or 96 dual indices preloaded in a 96-well plate (high throughput kit). The adapters in the low throughput kit each contain a unique 6-bp index "barcode" within its 63 bp sequence. The Illumina HiSeq 2000/2500 sequencers use a red laser to sequence A/C and a green laser to sequence G/T. It is essential to maintain a balance between the color channels for each base of the index reads being sequenced, otherwise they will fail to register.
7. NuSieve GTG agarose is a low melting temperature agarose for resolving 10–1000 bp DNA fragments. It requires more delicate handling than regular agarose and it is recommended to prepare it according to the manufacturer's instruction. A 3% (w/v) NuSieve gel is relatively brittle.

8. Running a 3% NuSieve gel under higher than 50 V will cause the gel to melt.
9. To prevent degradation, we do not recommend incubating excised gel slices at 50 °C for 10 min as instructed by the QIAquick and MinElute gel extraction kits. Using gentle agitation, the gel slices will fully dissolve in ~20 min at room temperature.
10. Chatterjee et al. have achieved more consistent bisulfite conversion of size-selected libraries using the EZ DNA methylation kit with a single conversion reaction but a longer incubation of 18 h [11].
11. Chatterjee et al. have demonstrated that increasing the amount of DNA template (i.e., 3 μL DNA template in a 25 μL PCR reaction volume) yields better amplification [11] (http://www.chem.agilent.com/Library/casestudies/Public/PfuTurbo_Cx_Facilitates_High_Throughput_Methylation_Studies_5991-1927.pdf).
12. Excessive amplification of the libraries increases the prevalence of PCR errors and increases the amplification of short fragments leading to skewed CpG coverage after sequencing.
13. A PCR product with optimal cycle number will have a reasonable amount of 160–340 bp products without nonspecific amplification (a 125 bp adapter–adapter dimer band is often present, but this is removed during the second gel size selection).
14. Following the Agilent Bioanalyzer run, use the region table option on the 2100 Expert software to select the 150–325 bp region.
15. The beads are used to couple with MBD-Biotin protein, which detects DNA methylation on the genome. Beads are usually suspended in a stock solution. Use these steps to wash off this liquid.
16. The automation library DNA preparation system allows standardizing the library DNA preparation procedure and minimizing the variation across the samples due to manual preparation.
17. RNase digestion of the DNA is important since the 5 mC-antibody will also detect 5mC in the context of RNA.
18. Shearing conditions need to be adapted to each device. Also the plastic ware used (thickness of the walls) may influence shearing conditions. Cooling of the DNA during sonication is important since AT-rich regions are less stable to degradation and will be depleted from the sample.

19. Sheared DNAs within one experiment should be of equal size. MeDIP-seq is an enrichment-based method and as such it is dependent on the number of methylated CpGs within one DNA fragment. Longer fragments contain a higher number of CpGs and this will influence the enrichment.
20. Snap freezing of the DNA samples in liquid nitrogen is the best way to preserve the integrity of the sample.
21. We routinely use 4 mg of DNA library. If less DNA is used, the amount of antibody and beads needs to be adjusted.
22. Avoid repeat freeze–thaw cycles of the antibody and of your samples.
23. Ice water is better than ice alone. Immediate cooling is important to prevent renaturation of the DNA.
24. MeDIP is affected by copy number variations and especially for cancer samples, this is an important issue. In this case, sequencing of the input samples at a low coverage may be useful to identify regions of copy number variations.
25. If desired, the excised gel slices may be frozen in liquid nitrogen and stored at −20 °C.
26. Aliquot the annealed adapters in amounts, which may be used up in one ligation reaction and store at −20 °C. Use a single tube for a single restriction–ligation reaction and always discard the rest of the adapters. The annealed adapters are stable at −20 °C for at least 6 months.
27. The amount of DNA used in the reaction is dependent on the genome size of the selected species. The larger the genome the more input DNA is needed. Do not use more than 300 ng DNA per digestion ligation reaction because of the increasing possibility of partial digestion. Always use high concentration restriction enzymes.
28. In the present case using 0.8 μM primer concentration resulted in approx. 200–800 bp fragments, fulfilling the size requirements of both, the hypomethylome filtration and the Illumina HiSeq sequencing.
29. Do not overamplify the PCR. Make reactions with different cycle number to evaluate the optimal amplification. The high abundant fragments should not be showing up obtrusively on the agarose gel. We recommend parallel amplifications to get enough material for the subsequent sequencing.
30. It is important to remove as much adapter sequences from the fragments as possible before sequencing. Test the level of adapter removal with reamplification of the digested samples. Dilute the digested samples with 5 mM Tris, pH 8.0 to 100, 1000, and 10,000-fold and amplify as before.

31. Genomic DNA 1–2 μg in 130 μL is recommended as starting DNA amount. In this protocol, we choose to purify the 300 bp DNA fragment because we use HiSeq X ten for sequencing and the current read length is paired end 150 bp.
32. Due to the lack of dCTP, 5′ overhang containing guanosine cannot be filled in, and, hence, those DNA fragments cannot be converted to library DNA.
33. Although a 15 min room temperature ligation reaction is often sufficient for RNA-Seq or ChIP-Seq library DNA preparation, we found that for BS-Seq library DNA preparation, an extended ligation time at 4 °C or overnight at 16 °C will significantly improve the library DNA yield.
34. We do not recommend using more than 500 ng library DNA in each bisulfite reaction, as too much DNA can reduce conversion rate. If more DNA has to be used, the samples can be split into multiple bisulfite conversion reactions. On the other hand, too few DNA could lead to over bisulfite conversion, degradation of DNA fragments with low 5mC level and loss in the post-bisulfite column purification step. If DNA sample is limited, one could add some raw lambda DNA, which could not be PCR-amplified, to the bisulfite conversion reaction to bring the final DNA amount in the bisulfite reaction to the optimal range (300–500 ng).
35. The PCR cycle number depends on the input DNA amount, the adapter ligation efficiency and the loss during bisulfite conversion.
36. Each Illumina sequencing service provider has its preferred library format. The sequencing core facility we use requires that each library DNA be submitted in TE solution with a concentration of not <2 ng/μL and in a volume of not <10 μL. Some service providers prefer the user to ethanol precipitate 50–100 ng of library DNA with glycogen as carrier and post the library DNA in the form of a dry pellet.
37. Higher primer concentrations may give rise to background signals in the pyrosequencing reaction as excess biotinylated primer may reduce the capture of the amplification product on the streptavidin-coated beads.
38. A lower reaction volume can be used in order to spare reagents. However, at least 10 μL should be used for the Pyrosequencing reaction, and when using standard PCR we use 4 μL for gel electrophoresis.
39. The CpG count is the number of CG dinucleotides in island. The percentage of CpG is the ratio of CpG nucleotide bases (twice the CpG count) to the length.

40. When MSP is performed, PCR product size could be predicted optimal length according to specifications including minimal and maximal product size.
41. Bisulfite-modified DNA is a different sequence between methylated and unmethylated DNA. If two primer sets are made in same length and from the same start point, the pair for methylated DNA, which remains cytosine with methyl group, has higher annealing temperature than the pair for unmethylated DNA, which is converted to thymine from cytosine.
42. Examining DNA by agarose gel electrophoresis prior to bisulfite conversion is recommended as degraded genomic DNA will lead to low yield of modified DNA.
43. Paired 18-mer long barcodes for each sample is recommended so that SMRT-BS reads with only a single barcode (due to incomplete sequencing) can still be retrieved if desired. Ensure that barcodes are designed with regard to standard primer parameters such as GC content and sequence redundancy.
44. A lower extension temperature (e.g., 64–68 °C) than typical PCR (i.e., 72 °C) can lead to higher yields when amplifying A + T rich bisulfite-converted DNA.
45. Gel running times vary due to equipment used and the length of PCR amplicons.
46. PCR product purification can also be done with Agencourt AMPure XP beads. When using AMPure XP beads, ensure that the appropriate volume of beads is used for amplicons with different lengths.
47. The P6-C4 chemistry from Pacific Biosciences could also be used for SMRT-BS. In addition, please note that SMRT-BS is developed on the PacBio RS II system; however, SMRT-BS could also be run on the Sequel system.

Acknowledgment

This work was supported by grants from the National Natural Science Foundation of China (No. 81472960, 81001242, 81502794), Zhejiang Province Natural Science Foundation of China (Y13H260011), Zhejiang Provincial Program for the Cultivation of High-level Innovative Health talents (2014), and Zhejiang Medical Health Science and Technology Foundation (2015RCA007).

References

1. Feinberg AP, Tycko B (2004) The history of cancer epigenetics. Nat Rev Cancer 4 (2):143–153
2. Biswas S, Rao CM (2017) Epigenetics in cancer: fundamentals and beyond. Pharmacol Ther 173:118–134
3. Duruisseaux M, Esteller M (2018) Lung cancer epigenetics: from knowledge to applications. Semin Cancer Biol 51:116
4. Natanzon Y, Goode EL, Cunningham JM (2018) Epigenetics in ovarian cancer. Semin Cancer Biol 51:160
5. Wilkinson AW, Gozani O (2017) Cancer epigenetics: reading the future of leukaemia. Nature 543(7644):186–188
6. Skvortsova K et al (2017) Comprehensive evaluation of genome-wide 5-hydroxymethylcytosine profiling approaches in human DNA. Epigenetics Chromatin 10:16
7. Liu S et al (2017) Diagnostic role of Wnt pathway gene promoter methylation in non small cell lung cancer. Oncotarget 8 (22):36354–36367
8. Tang J et al (2015) Global DNA methylation profiling technologies and the ovarian cancer methylome. Methods Mol Biol 1238:653–675
9. Meissner A et al (2005) Reduced representation bisulfite sequencing for comparative high-resolution DNA methylation analysis. Nucleic Acids Res 33(18):5868–5877
10. Martin-Herranz DE et al (2017) cuRRBS: simple and robust evaluation of enzyme combinations for reduced representation approaches. Nucleic Acids Res 45(20):11559–11569
11. Chatterjee A et al (2017) Generating multiple base-resolution DNA methylomes using reduced representation bisulfite sequencing. Methods Mol Biol 1537:279–298
12. Rauch TA et al (2008) High-resolution mapping of DNA hypermethylation and hypomethylation in lung cancer. Proc Natl Acad Sci U S A 105(1):252–257
13. Aberg KA et al (2017) A MBD-seq protocol for large-scale methylome-wide studies with (very) low amounts of DNA. Epigenetics 12:743–750
14. Jadhav RR et al (2016) Methyl-binding DNA capture sequencing for patient tissues. J Vis Exp (116)
15. Weber M et al (2005) Chromosome-wide and promoter-specific analyses identify sites of differential DNA methylation in normal and transformed human cells. Nat Genet 37 (8):853–862
16. Beck D, Sadler-Riggleman I, Skinner MK (2017) Generational comparisons (F1 versus F3) of vinclozolin induced epigenetic transgenerational inheritance of sperm differential DNA methylation regions (epimutations) using MeDIP-Seq. Environ Epigenet 3(3): dvx016
17. Grimm C, Adjaye J (2012) Analysis of the methylome of human embryonic stem cells employing methylated DNA immunoprecipitation coupled to next-generation sequencing. Methods Mol Biol 873:281–295
18. Fouse SD, Nagarajan RO, Costello JF (2010) Genome-scale DNA methylation analysis. Epigenomics 2(1):105–117
19. Wischnitzki E et al (2016) Selecting hypomethylated genomic regions using MRE-Seq. Methods Mol Biol 1482:83–102
20. Naumov VA et al (2013) Genome-scale analysis of DNA methylation in colorectal cancer using Infinium HumanMethylation450 BeadChips. Epigenetics 8(9):921–934
21. de Ruijter T et al (2015) Formalin-fixed, paraffin-embedded (FFPE) tissue epigenomics using Infinium HumanMethylation450 BeadChip assays. Lab Invest 95(7):833–842
22. Touleimat N, Tost J (2012) Complete pipeline for Infinium((R)) Human Methylation 450K BeadChip data processing using subset quantile normalization for accurate DNA methylation estimation. Epigenomics 4(3):325–341
23. Cokus SJ et al (2008) Shotgun bisulphite sequencing of the Arabidopsis genome reveals DNA methylation patterning. Nature 452 (7184):215–219
24. Chen Y, Yu S, Zhong S (2018) Profiling DNA methylation using bisulfite sequencing (BS-Seq). Methods Mol Biol 1675:31–43
25. Kristensen L, Johansen J, Grønbæk K (2015) Allele-specific DNA methylation detection by pyrosequencing®. Methods Mol Biol 1315:271–289
26. Gao L et al (2017) Epigenetic regulation of AXL and risk of childhood asthma symptoms. Clin Epigenetics 9:121

27. Ku J, Jeon Y, Park J (2011) Methylation-specific PCR. Methods Mol Biol 791:23–32
28. Hu Y et al (2017) Candidate tumor suppressor ZNF154 suppresses invasion and metastasis in NPC by inhibiting the EMT via Wnt/β-catenin signalling. Oncotarget 8(49):85749–85758
29. Goldenberg D et al (2004) Intraoperative molecular margin analysis in head and neck cancer. Arch Otolaryngol Head Neck Surg 130(1):39–44
30. Cao Y et al (2018) Aberrant hypermethylation of the HOXD10 gene in papillary thyroid cancer with BRAFV600E mutation. Oncol Rep 39 (1):338–348
31. Yang Y, Scott S (2017) DNA Methylation profiling using long-read single molecule real-time bisulfite sequencing (SMRT-BS). Methods Mol Biol 1654:125–134

Chapter 13

Evaluation of Nrf2 with Exposure to Nanoparticles

Fuli Zheng and Huangyuan Li

Abstract

Transcription factor Nrf2, nuclear factor (erythroid-derived 2)-like 2, is considered a master regulator of redox homeostasis and plays a central role in antioxidant and anti-inflammatory defence. It has been largely reported that oxidative stress is implicated in nanoparticle-induced toxicity with the involvement of Nrf2. Several basic methods for Nrf2 evaluation with exposure to nanoparticles are described in this chapter including real-time reverse transcription-polymerase chain reaction (RT-PCR), western blotting, immunofluorescence staining, electrophoretic mobility shift assay, DNase I footprinting, dimethylsulfate footprinting, protein pulse-chase analysis, and tert-butylhydroquinone treatment.

Key words Nrf2, Nanoparticles, Antioxidant response element (ARE), EMSA, Pulse chase analysis, t-BHQ, Footprinting

1 Introduction

Nanoparticles (NPs) can cause oxidative stress through disturbance of redox homeostasis and inflammatory response, which has been widely reported [1–6]. The oxidative stress caused by NPs such as titanium dioxide (TiO_2), carbon black (CB), Ag, magnetite, cerium oxide (CeO_2), and tungsten carbide–cobalt (WCo-Co), result from an excess production of reactive oxygen species (ROS) which activate the antioxidant protection response [7–13]. Among the oxidative stress response mechanisms, nuclear factor (erythroid-derived 2)-like 2 (Nrf2) is a principal transcription factor that regulates the expression of antioxidant proteins [14, 15]. In the absence of stress, Nrf2 is bound with its repressor kelch-like associated protein 1 (Keap1) and held in the cytoplasm. Upon oxidative insult, however, thiol groups on Keap1 are oxidized, liberating Nrf2 and allowing for its nuclear translocation [16]. By binding to the antioxidant response elements (AREs) located in the promoter regions of antioxidant genes and detoxifying enzyme genes, Nrf2 facilitates the transcription of a battery of genes including heme oxygenase-1 (HO-1), superoxide dismutase-1 (SOD-1),

Qunwei Zhang (ed.), *Nanotoxicity: Methods and Protocols*, Methods in Molecular Biology, vol. 1894,
https://doi.org/10.1007/978-1-4939-8916-4_13,

and NAD(P)H:quinone oxidoreductases (NQO1) [17–19]. Although Nrf2 can regulate proteins, as a protein itself, Nrf2 protein synthesis can be inhibited by *cycloheximide (CHX)* [20, 21]. Quinone compounds, like tert-butylhydroquinone (tBHQ), may enhance Nrf2-mediated transcriptional activation and subsequent antioxidant protection [22, 23]. Previous studies have shown that various toxicants could activate Nrf2 translocation, expression, and its downstream pathways [24, 25], for example, manganese chloride can enhance the binding of Nrf2 to ARE [26, 27], and this activation is associated with ROS and ubiquitin-–proteasome pathway [28]; the pesticide deltamethrin promotes nuclear translocation of Nrf2 [29, 30]; and paraquat induces Nrf2 and HO-1 upregulation [22]. Thus, it is interesting to investigate whether NPs exposure alters Nrf2 signal pathways under pretreatment of inhibitors or activators.

In this chapter, several methods are described to evaluate Nrf2 expression with exposure to NPs, including real-time reverse transcription-polymerase chain reaction (RT-PCR) to determine the mRNA level of Nrf2 and its target genes, western blotting and immunofluorescence staining to study the nuclear translocation of Nrf2, electrophoretic mobility shift assay, DNase I footprinting and dimethylsulfate footprinting to verify Nrf2 and ARE binding activities, as well as pulse chase analysis with the help of Nrf2 inhibitor cycloheximide (CHX) and promoter tert-butylhydroquinone (tBHQ) to determine Nrf2 protein half-life and protein synthesis.

2 Materials

Prepare all solutions using ultrapure water (prepared by purifying deionized water to attain a resistivity of 18 MΩ cm at 25 °C) and analytical grade reagents. Prepare and store all reagents at room temperature (unless indicated otherwise). Diligently follow all waste disposal regulations when disposing of waste materials.

2.1 Nrf2 mRNA Expression by RT-PCR

1. RNeasy Mini Kit (QIAGEN), RNase-free DNase (QIAGEN), random primers, AMV reverse transcriptase (Roche Diagnostics), and LightCycler FastStart DNA Master SYBR Green I (Roche Diagnostics).
2. Primer sets for target genes listed in Table 1.
3. LightCycler instrument.
4. 4.0 mM $MgCl_2$.

Table 1
Primer Sequences Used for Amplification

Gene	Accession number	Forward primer	Reverse primer
GAPDH	XM_216696	AAATGGGTGATGCTGGTG	TGAGCGAGTTCTAACAGTCC
Nrf2	NM_031789	CCATTTACGGAGACCCAC	CTTATTTCAACGGCGAGT
Keapl	NM_057152	GGACGGCAACACTGATTC	TCGTCTCGATCTGGCTCATA
HO-1	NM_012580	ACAGAAGAGGCTAAGACCG	ACAGAAGAGGCTAAGACCG
Nqol	NM_017000	CAGCGGCTCCATGTACT	GACCTGGAAGCCACAGAAG
Cyplal	NM_012540.2	GTGGCCTGTATTTGCTTATG	AGCTCAGGTACGTTTTTCCT

Keapl kelch-like associated protein 1, *GAPDH* Glyceraldehydes-3 phosphate dehydrogenase, *HO-1* Heme oxygenase 1, *Nqol* NAD(P)H dehydrogenase, quinone 1, *Cyplal* cytochrome P450, family 1, subfamily a, polypeptide 1.

2.2 Nrf2 Translocation to Nucleus

2.2.1 Western Blotting (WB)

1. Nuclear and cytoplasmic extraction reagents kit (Pierce).
2. BCA protein assay.
3. Resolving gel buffer: 1.5 M Tris–HCl, pH 8.8. Add about 100 mL water to a glass beaker. Weigh 181.7 g Tris base and transfer to the beaker. Add water to a volume of 900 mL. Mix well by using a magnetic stir bar and adjust pH to 8.8 with HCl (*see* **Note 1**). Make up to 1 L with water. Store at 4 °C.
4. Stacking gel buffer: 0.5 M Tris–HCl, pH 6.8. Weigh 60.6 g Tris base and prepare a 1 L solution as the above **item 3**. Store at 4 °C.
5. 30% acrylamide/Bis-acrylamide solution (29.2:0.8): Weigh 29.2 g acrylamide monomer and 0.8 g Bis-acrylamide (cross-linker) and transfer to a 250 mL glass beaker containing about 40 mL of water. Add a spatula of AG 501-X8 (D) mixed-resin beads and mix well for about 30 min. Make up to 100 mL with water and filter through a 0.45 μm Corning filter (*see* **Note 2**). Store at 4 °C in a bottle wrapped with aluminium foil (*see* **Note 3**).
6. 10% ammonium persulfate: Weight 0.1 g ammonium persulfate and dissolve in 1 mL of water. Prepare this fresh each time.
7. TEMED: *N*,*N*,*N*,*N*′-Tetramethyl-ethylenediamine. Store at 4 °C.
8. SDS-PAGE running buffer: 0.025 M Tris–HCl, pH 8.3, 0.192 M glycine, 0.1% SDS. Prepare 10× native buffer (0.25 M Tris–HCl, 1.92 M glycine) first. Weigh 30.3 g Tris base and 144 g glycine. Dissolve in 800 mL water. Mix well and make to 1 L with water. To make 1000 mL working running buffer, mix 100 mL of 10× native buffer, 890 mL water, and 10 mL 10% SDS together (*see* **Note 4**).

9. SDS lysis buffer (5×): 0.3 M Tris–HCl (pH 6.8), 10% SDS, 25% β-mercaptoethanol, 0.1% bromophenol blue, 45% glycerol. Leave one aliquot at 4 °C for current use and store the remaining aliquots at −20 °C. Prior to use, warm lysis buffer to room temperature to solubilize SDS.
10. Bromophenol blue (BPB) solution: Dissolve 0.1 g BPB in 100 mL water. Store at −20 °C.
11. Mini-PROTEAN 3 System glass plates.
12. Medium binder clips (1¼ in.).
13. SDS-PAGE electroporator.
14. PVDF membranes.
15. Western blot transfer buffer: 0.025 M Tris–HCl, 0.192 M glycine, 20% methanol. Mix 100 mL of 10× native buffer, 700 mL water, and 200 mL methanol together to make 1000 mL working transfer buffer.
16. Transfer system.
17. Tris-buffered saline (10× TBS): 1.5 M NaCl, 0.1 M Tris–HCl, pH 7.4. Dissolve 12.11 g Tris base and 80 g NaCl in 800 mL water and mix well. Adjust pH to 7.4 with HCl. Add water to make it to 1 L.
18. TBST: 10 mmol/L Tris–HCl, 150 mmol/L NaCl, 0.1% Tween 20. Add 100 mL of 10× TBS, 900 mL water, and 1 mL Tween 20 together to make 1000 mL TBST solution. Mix well and store at room temperature.
19. 5% powdered skim milk: Dissolve 1 g of skim milk powder in 20 mL of 1× TBST solution.
20. Shaker and plastic containers.
21. Anti-Nrf2 antibody (Rabbit polyclonal to Nrf2, Abcam).
22. Horseradish peroxidase (HRP)-conjugated anti-rabbit IgG.
23. ECL developing kit.
24. Luminescence detection machine.

2.2.2 Immunofluorescence Staining

1. Slides.
2. 3% normal donkey serum in PBS.
3. Rabbit anti-Nrf2 antibody (polyclonal, Abcam).
4. Alexa Fluor 594 anti-rabbit IgG.
5. Vectashield medium containing DAPI.
6. Fluorescence microscope.

2.3 Nrf2–ARE Binding Activity

2.3.1 Electrophoretic Mobility Shift Assay (EMSA)

1. Biotin-labeled double-stranded oligonucleotides: Wt-ARE, 5′-ACTGAGGGTGACTCAGCAAAATC-3′; GC-ARE, 5′-ACTGAGGGTGACTCAatAAAATC-3′.
2. LightShift Chemiluminescent EMSA Kit (Pierce): Contains 10× binding buffer as mentioned in Subheading 3.2.1.
3. 1× TBE: 89 mM of Tris, 89 mM of boric acid, and 20 mM of EDTA·2Na (pH 8.3). Weigh 43.2 g Tris base and 22 g boric acid, add each to a 5 L beaker. Measure 160 mL of 0.5 M EDTA (pH 8.0) and add to the beaker. Add water to a final volume of 3.8 L. Adjust pH to 8.3 with HCl. Thoroughly mix the solution with a magnetic stir bar until the components are completely dissolved. Finally, make the solution up to 4 L with water. Transfer the solution to glass bottles, autoclave and store at 4 °C.
4. 10× Electrophoresis loading buffer (ThermoFisher).

2.3.2 DNase I Footprinting

1. [γ-^{32}P] ATP, T4 polynucleotide kinase, DNase I, and proteinase K.
2. DNase buffer: 5 mM $MgCl_2$, 5 mM $CaCl_2$, 200 mM KCl, 4 μg/mL sheared salmon sperm DNA. Weigh 0.48 g $MgCl_2$ and prepare 10 mL of 0.5 M $MgCl_2$ stock solution. Weigh 0.56 g $CaCl_2$ and prepare 10 mL of 0.5 M $CaCl_2$ stock solution. Weigh 3 g KCl and prepare 10 mL of 4 M KCl stock solution. Mix 100 μL $MgCl_2$ stock solution, 100 μL $CaCl_2$ stock solution, 5 mL KCl stock solution and add 4 μL of 10 mg/mL sheared salmon sperm DNA (ThermoFisher). Make the final volume to 10 mL with water. Store at −20 °C.
3. DNase I reaction stop solution: 20 mM EDTA, 1% SDS, and 0.2 M NaCl. Dissolve 0.1 g SDS and 0.12 g NaCl in 6 mL of water. Add 2.5 mL 0.5 M EDTA to the solution, and mix well. Add water to make up final volume to 10 mL.
4. 6% (w/v) polyacrylamide gel containing 8 M urea.

2.3.3 Dimethylsulfate Footprinting

1. DMS footprinting buffer: 10 mM Tris–HCl, pH 7.5, 50 mM sodium chloride, and 1.0 mM EDTA. Prepare 100 mL of 10× DMS footprinting buffer: weigh 1.21 g Tris base and 2.92 g sodium chloride. Add water to 80 mL. Add 0.2 mL of 0.5 M EDTA and adjust pH to 7.5 with HCl. Finally top up the volume to 100 mL. For usage, dilute 10× DMS footprinting buffer as required.
2. 1% and 19% vol/vol of DMS (Sigma): Add 0.1 mL of DMS to 9.9 mL of water to prepare 1% vol/vol DMS. Add 1.9 mL of DMS to 8.1 mL of water for 19% vol/vol DMS.
3. 16% native polyacrylamide DNA electrophoresis gel.

4. Elution buffer: 200 mM NaCl, 2 mM KCl. Weigh 11.7 g NaCl and 0.15 g KCl. Dissolve in 100 mL water to make 10× elution buffer. Dilute 1 mL of 10× elution buffer with 9 mL water to make final 1× elution buffer.
5. Heating blot, eletrophorator, and autoradioactive equipment.
6. 95% and 75% ethanol: Dilute 79 mL of 95% ethanol with 21 mL of water to make 100 mL of 75% ethanol.
7. Stop solution: 30% (vol/vol) β-mercaptoethanol and 0.3 M sodium acetate. Weigh 0.246 g sodium acetate and dissolve in 7 mL water. Add 3 mL β-mercaptoethanol to the mixture (*see* **Note 5**).
8. 10% piperidine.
9. A sequencing gel (Invivogen).

2.4 Downstream Target Gene Expression and Activity

1. mRNA primers: *See* Subheading 2.1 **item 2**, Table 1.
2. Anti-HO1 antibody (Abcam) and anti-NQO1 antibody (Sigma).

2.5 Regulation of Nrf2

2.5.1 Pulse-Chase Analysis of Nrf2 Protein Half-Life

1. [^{35}S]-Methionine/cysteine labeling mix.
2. Trichloroacetic acid.
3. Bovine serum albumin (BSA).
4. Ice-cold acetone.
5. 10% SDS stock solution: Dissolve 10 g SDS in 100 mL water.
6. 0.5 M EDTA: Add 14.6 g EDTA to 80 mL water. Add NaOH to fully dissolve EDTA and adjust pH to 8.0. Top up the final volume to 100 mL.
7. 100 mM PMSF: Dissolve 1.74 g PMSF in 100 mL water.
8. 1 M Tris–HCl, pH 6.8: Dissolve 12.11 g Tris base in 50 mL water. Adjust pH to 6.8 with HCl. Add water to 100 mL.
9. Antibody (to the protein of interest).
10. Protein A-agarose beads.
11. SDS-PAGE materials [31, 32].
12. Synthetic growth medium (YNB-X): 2% preferred carbon source, 0.17% yeast nitrogen base w/o amino acids and ammonium sulfate, 0.5% ammonium sulfate, 0.2% amino acid mixture, 0.01% any amino acid (except leucine) and 0.035% leucine. Weigh 1.2 g of yeast nitrogen base w/o amino acids and ammonium sulfate, 3.5 g of ammonium sulfate, 1.4 g of amino acid mixture, 70 mg of any amino acid (except leucine) and 250 mg of leucine. Add 700 mL of water and preferred carbon source to 2%. Sterilize by filtration.

13. Wash/labeling medium (YNB + essential amino acids only according to the genotype of the strain): 2% preferred carbon source, 0.17% yeast nitrogen base w/o amino acids and ammonium sulfate, 0.5% ammonium sulfate, 0.01% any amino acid (except leucine), and 0.035% leucine. Weigh 1.2 g of yeast nitrogen base w/o amino acids and ammonium sulfate, 3.5 g of ammonium sulfate, 70 mg of any amino acid (except leucine), and 250 mg of leucine. Add 700 mL of water and preferred carbon source to 2%. Sterilize by filtration (*see* **Note 6**).
14. Chase medium: YNB-X medium with 10 mM methionine and 10 mM cysteine. Prepare the medium as same as YNB-X medium, with the addition of 1.5 g methionine and 1.2 g cysteine before the addition of 700 mL water.
15. Extraction buffer: 1.85 M NaOH and 7.4% β-mercaptoethanol. Dissolve 0.74 g NaOH in 9 mL water. Add 0.74 mL β-mercaptoethanol to the mixture and fill water to 10 mL. Aliquot extraction buffer in 1 mL portions.
16. Resuspension solution: 2.5% SDS, 5 mM EDTA, 1 mM phenylmethylsulfonyl fluoride (PMSF). Mix 2.5 mL of 10% SDS, 0.1 mL of 0.5 M EDTA, and 0.1 mL of 100 mM PMSF. Add water to 10 mL.
17. Immunoprecipitation buffer (IP buffer): 1% Triton X-100, 0.15 M NaCl, 5 mM EDTA, and 50 mM Na-HEPES, pH 7.5. Weigh 6 g NaCl and 13.01 g Na-HEPES. Add 800 mL water to dissolve. Adjust pH to 7.5. Add 10 mL 0.5 M EDTA and 10 mL Triton X-100 (*see* **Note 7**). Fill the solution to 1 L.
18. 250× protease inhibitor stock: 5 mg/mL of chymostatin, pepstatin A, leupeptin, and antipain each in dimethyl sulfoxide (DMSO). Weigh 0.01 g chymostatin, 0.01 g pepstatin A, 0.01 g leupeptin, and 0.01 g antipain and dissolve in 10 mL DMSO.
19. IP wash buffer: 1× IP buffer and 0.1% SDS. Take 990 mL of IP buffer and add 10 mL of 10% SDS.
20. 2× SDS Loading buffer: 100 mM Tris–HCl, pH 6.8, 4% SDS, 20% glycerol, 0.02% bromophenol blue, and 4% β-mercaptoethanol. Mix 10 mL of 1 M Tris–HCl and 40 mL of 10% SDS. Add 20 mL glycerol, 4 mL β-mercaptoethanol, and 20 mg bromophenol blue to the mixture. Add water to 100 mL. Store short term at 4 °C or long term at −20 °C.

2.5.2 Nrf2 Expression Enhancement and Inhibition

1. Corn oil.
2. Tert-butylhydroquinone (tBHQ).
3. Cycloheximide (CHX).

3 Methods

Carry out all procedures at room temperature unless otherwise specified.

3.1 RT-PCR

1. Extract total RNA using the RNeasy Mini Kit (QIAGEN) or TRIzol (Thermo Fisher) and digest with RNase-free DNase (QIAGEN).
2. Measure absorbance of the RNA sample at 230 nm, 260 nm, and 280 nm using a NanoDrop 1000 (Thermo Fisher). Determine the A_{260}/A_{280} and the A_{260}/A_{230} ratio (*see* **Note 8**).
3. Prepare primer sets (probes) for target genes listed in Subheading 2.1, Table 1.
4. Convert total RNA (0.1 μg) into cDNA by reverse transcription using random primers and AMV reverse transcriptase, with temperature cycling conditions as follows: incubation at 30 °C for 10 min, at 42 °C for 45 min, at 90 °C for 5 min, and then at 4 °C.
5. Prepare PCR reaction mixture: 20 μL reaction consists of LightCycler FastStart DNA Master SYBR Green I, 4.0 mM of $MgCl_2$, 0.5 μM of each probe, and 2 μL template cDNA.
6. PCR amplification of cDNA using a LightCycler instrument: predenaturation at 94 °C for 10 min, 35 cycles of denaturation at 94 °C for 60 s, annealing 55 °C for 30 s, and extension at 72 °C for 60 s, and a final extension at 72 °C for 5 min.
7. Quantify relative mRNA levels in each sample according to the standard curves constructed by the LightCycler software.
8. Calculate the levels of mRNA with reference to external standard curves constructed by plotting the log number of tenfold serially diluted cDNA samples against the respective threshold cycle using the second derivative maximum method.
9. Normalize expression of mRNA levels in each sample to GAPDH mRNA levels.

3.2 Translocation of Nrf2 to Nucleus

3.2.1 Western Blotting (WB) to Determine Protein Level and Distribution of Nrf2

1. Extract nuclear and cytoplasmic proteins with nuclear and cytoplasmic extraction reagents kits (Pierce) according to the manufacturer's protocol (*see* **Note 9**).
2. Measure protein concentrations using BCA protein assay.
3. Separate proteins using 10% or 12% of sodium dodecyl sulfate–polyacrylamide gel electrophoresis (SDS-PAGE) according to standard procedure [31, 32].
4. Transfer proteins onto PVDF membranes at 150 V for 2 h using 1× transfer buffer.
5. Block the nonspecific protein on the membrane with 5% skim milk in TBS-T for 1 h at room temperature.

6. Incubate the membrane overnight with anti-Nrf2 antibody diluted in TBST at 4 °C.
7. Wash the membrane in TBS-T for three times, 10 min each time.
8. Incubate the membrane with horseradish peroxidase-conjugated anti-rabbit IgG overnight at 4 °C.
9. Wash the membrane in TBS-T for three times, 10 min each time.
10. Develop Nrf2 protein bands using ECL developing kit with an instrument that detects luminescence (Fig. 1a).
11. Analyze the optical density of bands using ImageJ software (Fig. 1b).

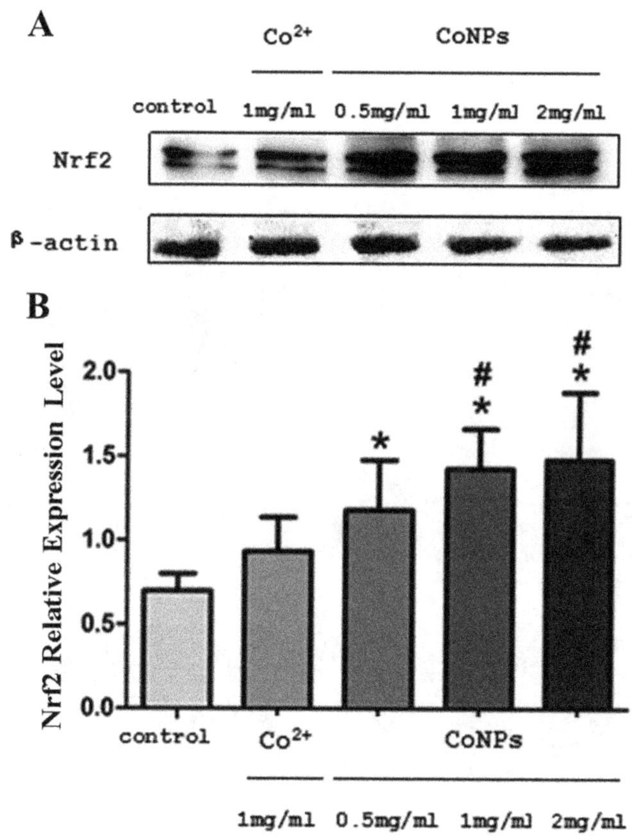

Fig. 1 Upregulation of Nrf2 protein induced by Co^{2+} and Co-NPs. Nrf2 and β-actin protein levels were measured by western blotting in rat hippocampus tissues obtained from control, 1 mg/mL of $CoCl_2$, and 0.5 mg/mL, 1 mg/mL, and 2 mg/mL of Co-NPs groups, using anti-Nrf2 antibody and anti-β-actin antibody. (**a**) Blot showing Nrf2 protein level in varying groups. (**b**) Data was analyzed by ImageJ and presented as mean ± SD. Asterisks (*) indicates significance when compared with the control group ($P < 0.05$). Pound sign (#) demonstrates significance compared with $CoCl_2$ group ($P < 0.05$)

3.2.2 Localization of Nrf2 Detected by Immunofluorescence Staining

1. Block fixed cells or tissue with 3% normal donkey serum in 1× PBS (*see* **Note 10**).
2. Incubate the slide with rabbit anti-Nrf2 antibody for 1 h at room temperature.
3. Wash the slide with 1× PBS for three times, 10 min each time.
4. Incubate the slide with Alexa Fluor 594 anti-rabbit IgG for 1 h at room temperature.
5. Wash the slide with 1× PBS for three times, 10 min each time.
6. Mount the slide with Vectashield medium containing DAPI.
7. Use fluorescence microscopy to detect the localization of Nrf2 (excitation 594 nm; emission 617 nm).
8. Determine the translocation of Nrf2 by combining the distribution of Nrf2 fluorescence and DAPI (excitation 358 nm; emission 461 nm) (Fig. 2).

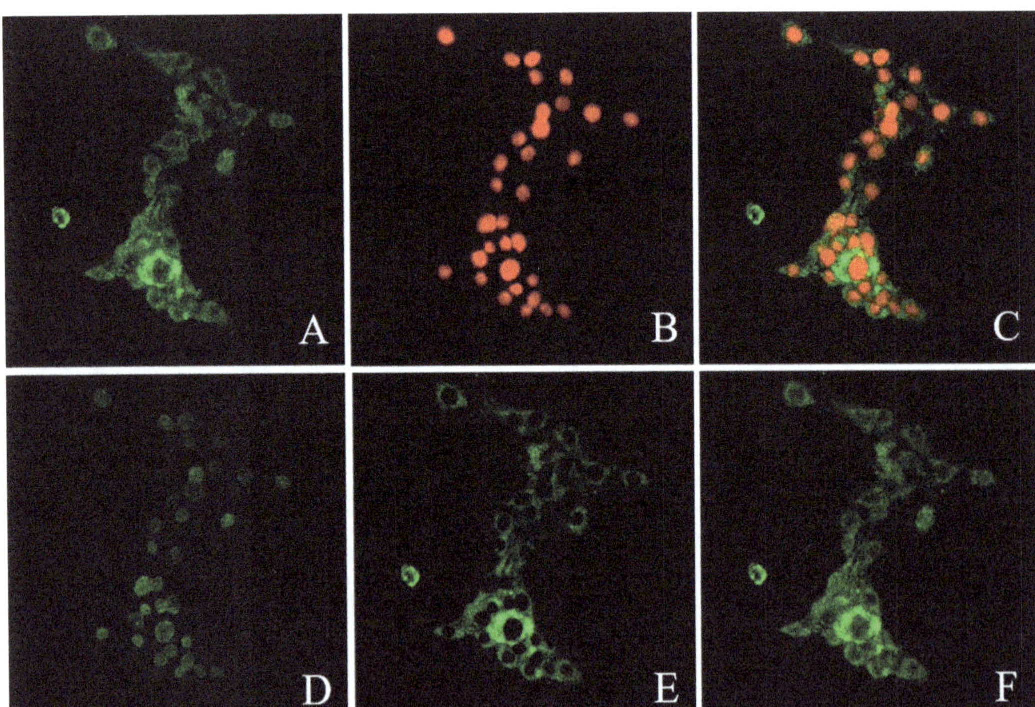

Fig. 2 Confocal micrographs of Nrf2 nuclear translocation detected by immunofluorescence staining in PC12 cells. (**a**) Nrf2 signals stained by FITC in green. (**b**) Nuclei stained by PI in red. (**c**) The signals from Nrf2 and nuclei were merged. (**d**) Nrf2 signals in nuclei. (**e**) Nrf2 signals over cytoplasm. (**f**) Nrf2 signals over the whole cell

3.3 Nrf2–ARE Binding Activity

3.3.1 Electrophoretic Mobility Shift Assays (EMSA)

1. Label a synthetic double-strand HO-1 ARE containing the Nrf2-binding domain with biotin using terminal deoxynucleotidyl transferase (TdT).
2. Pre-electrophorese a native 4% polyacrylamide gel in 0.5× TBE for 60 min (*see* **Note 11**).
3. Prepare nuclear extracts from a Pierce kit (NE-PER Nuclear and Cytoplasmic Extraction Kit), and quantify protein concentrations using BCA assay.
4. Incubate 10 μg of nuclear extracts for 15 min in 1× binding buffer.
5. Incubate the nuclear extracts with biotin-labeled double-strand oligonucleotides (sequences can be found in Subheading 2.3) for 20 min at room temperature (*see* **Note 12**).
6. Add electrophoresis loading buffer to incubation mixture, load them onto the pre-electrophoresed gel and electrophoreses at 100 V until the bromophenol blue dye migrates two-thirds to three-fourths of the length of the gel.
7. Transfer proteins in the gel to a positively charged nylon membrane in 0.5× TBE at 100 V for 30 min in a standard transfer apparatus.
8. Crosslink DNA to the membrane for 15 min using a transilluminator with a 312 nm bulb (*see* **Note 13**).
9. Determine the binding activity of Nrf2 to the probe by chemiluminescence following the protocol and using buffers provided in the kit.

3.3.2 DNase I Footprinting

1. Label DNA probes of ARE with [γ-^{32}P] ATP using T4 polynucleotide kinase.
2. Incubate the ^{32}P-labeled probe (2×10^5 c.p.m.) with or without Nrf2 proteins (500 ng) in 50 μL of binding buffer.
3. Incubate the binding mixture with 50 μL of DNase buffer and 20 ng of DNase I for 3 min at room temperature (25 °C). Terminate the reaction by the addition of 100 μL of stop solution.
4. Treat the reaction mixture with 100 μg/mL of proteinase K for 15 min.
5. Extract and analyze DNA on a 6% (w/v) polyacrylamide gel containing 8 M urea.
6. Modify and digest the guanine and adenine bases of the same probes using Maxam–Gilbert method [33] and load onto the gel (same as Subheading 3.3.1, **step 6**) as a marker ladder.

3.3.3 Dimethylsulfate Footprinting

1. Heat a 31-mer single-stranded DNA oligonucleotide corresponding to nt -198 to -168 of the NRF2 5′ UTR in dimethylsulfate (DMS) footprinting buffer at 95 °C for 10 min.
2. After cooling down to room temperature, label the oligonucleotide with [γ-^{32}P] ATP at the 5′ end and purify by alcohol precipitation.
3. Treat DNA with 1% (vol/vol) DMS for 2 min for methylation and terminate the reaction by the addition of gel loading buffer.
4. Electrophorese the DNA on a 16% native polyacrylamide gel for 3.5 h.
5. Visualize the DNA via autoradiography and excise the target band for elution.
6. Elute DNA band in elution buffer for 1 h at 65 °C.
7. Precipitate DNA with 95% ethanol and wash with 75% ethanol twice.
8. Resuspend in 20 μL of nuclease-free water.
9. Treat DNA with 19% DMS for 1 min, and stop methylation by stop solution and incubate at −20 °C for 2 h.
10. Precipitate and wash DNA according to **step** 7.
11. Air-dry DNA and treat with 10% piperidine for 5 min at 85 °C, and vacuum dry the DNA pellet.
12. Denature the DNA pellets at 90 °C for 5 min (*see* **Note 14**).
13. Electrophorese the DNA on a sequencing gel at 100–200 V (*see* **Note 15**).

3.4 Downstream Target Gene Expression and Activity

1. Prepare mRNA and protein samples for RT-PCR and Western blotting as described in Subheadings 3.1 and 3.2.1.
2. Set up standard RT-PCR reactions and western blotting for Nrf2 downstream mRNA and proteins such as HO-1 and NQO-1, and analyze results as described above (Fig. 3).

3.5 Regulation of Nrf2

3.5.1 Pulse-Chase Analysis of Nrf2 Protein Half-Life

1. Dilute cells in 10 mL of the appropriate synthetic medium to $OD_{600} = 0.15$ and grow for at least two cell doublings.
2. Collect cells in a 15-mL conical polypropylene tube, resuspend in 1 mL wash medium and transfer to a 1.5 mL microcentrifuge tube.
3. Wash the cells three times with wash medium (In each wash step, resuspend cells in 1 mL then spin down 10 s in a microcentrifuge at 6165 × *g*). Resuspend in 0.3 mL of wash medium.

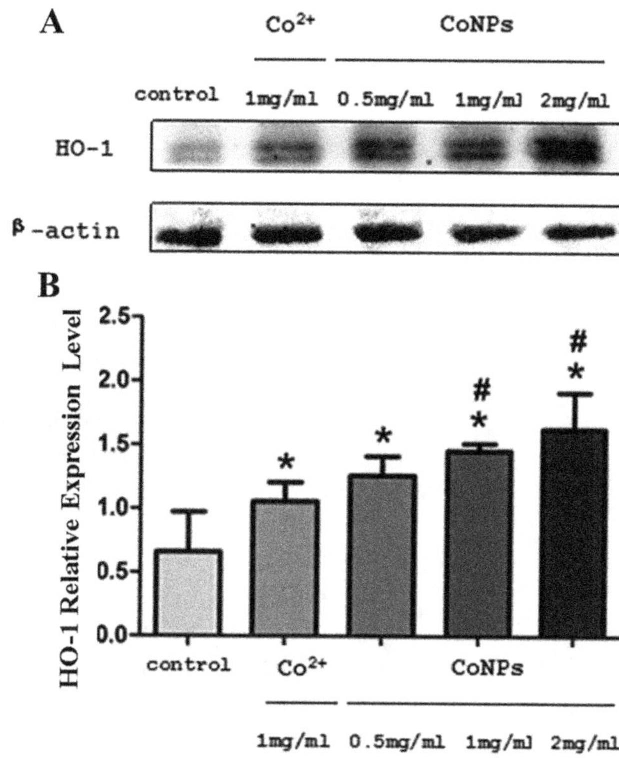

Fig. 3 Upregulation of HO-1 protein induced by Co^{2+} and Co-NPs. HO-1 and β-actin protein levels were measured by western blotting in rat hippocampus tissues in control, 1 mg/mL of $CoCl_2$, and 0.5 mg/mL, 1 mg/mL, and 2 mg/mL of Co-NPs groups, using anti-HO-1 antibody and anti-β-actin antibody. (**a**) Blot showing HO-1 protein level in varying groups. (**b**) Data was analyzed by ImageJ and presented as mean ± SD. Asterisks (*) indicate significance when compared with the control group ($P < 0.05$). Pound sign (#) demonstrates significance compared with $CoCl_2$ group ($P < 0.05$)

4. Transfer the cell suspension to a 1.5 mL screw-capped tube containing 0.5–1 mCi of [^{35}S]-methionine/cysteine labeling mix (*see* **Note 16**).
5. Incubate the tubes in a 30 °C water bath for 5 min with occasional shaking.
6. Pellet cells for 10 s at 6165 × *g*. Discard the supernatant and resuspend the cells in 2.5 mL of chase medium in an Erlenmeyer flask. Keep the flask in the shaker water bath for the duration of the experiment.
7. Remove a 0.6 mL aliquot immediately and add it to a 1.5-mL screw-capped tube containing 102 μL of extraction buffer. Place on ice. Remove additional 0.6 mL samples at appropriate times accordingly after the chase and treat in the same manner.
8. Incubate the mixture on ice for 10 min. Add 42 μL of 100% TCA to each tube.

9. Incubate for 10 min on ice (or longer), and then centrifuge the extracts at 18,880 × g at 4 °C for 5 min.
10. Wash the pellets with 1 mL of ice-cold acetone, and then dry under vacuum in a Speedvac centrifuge (*see* **Note 17**).
11. Resuspend the pellets in 0.1–0.2 mL of resuspension solution by vortexing (*see* **Note 18**).
12. Heat the samples to >90 °C for 10 min, and then clear by spinning in a microcentrifuge for 5 min.
13. Determine incorporation of [^{35}S]-methionine by counting acid-insoluble radioactivity. Add 2 μL of the extract to 20 μL of 10 mg/mL BSA, add 1 mL of 5% trichloroacetic acid, and incubate for 15 min on ice. Collect the TCA-precipitated proteins on a Whatman GF/C glass fiber filter using a filtering flask equipped with a stainless-steel holder, air-dry the filter, and measure the radioactivity on the filter by scintillation counting.
14. Add equal amounts of total incorporated radioactivity (up to 0.1 mL) to 1 mL of IP buffer containing protease inhibitors, 1 mM PMSF, and antibody.
15. Incubate samples at 4 °C for 2 h, and then add 20 μL of protein A-agarose beads (50% suspension in IP buffer) to each tube. Incubate samples for 2 h to overnight at 4 °C while rocking.
16. Wash the beads three times with 1 mL IP wash buffer, then resuspend in 20 μL of 2× SDS loading buffer.
17. Heat the samples to >90 °C for 5 min, centrifuge for 1 min at room temperature, load samples on a polyacrylamide gel, and separate proteins by SDS-PAGE.
18. Dry the gel and expose to a phosphorimager plate.
19. Scan the plate using a PhosphorImager and quantify the bands.
20. Plot the amount of protein remaining against time on a semi-logarithmic graph (*see* **Note 19**).

3.5.2 Nrf2 Expression Promotion and Inhibition

In Vivo Experiment

1. Divide animals (male Sprague-Dawley rats, approx. 4–5 weeks old, weight 60–70 g) randomly into different groups according to treatment: control (corn oil), t-BHQ, t-BHQ + nanoparticles (of varying concentrations), corn oil + nanoparticles (of varying concentrations).
2. Animals in t-BHQ and t-BHQ + nanoparticles groups receive t-BHQ dissolved in corn oil at 150 mg/kg.

In Vitro Experiment

1. Pretreat cells with 10 μg/mL of protein synthesis inhibitor cycloheximide (CHX) for 1 h.

2. Treat cells with Nrf2 inducer tert-butylhydroquinone (tBHQ) or DMSO as a control.
3. Analyze protein expression and localization using western blotting and/or immunofluorescence staining described above in Subheadings 3.2.1 and 3.2.2, respectively.

4 Notes

1. Initially use concentrated HCl (e.g., 12 N) to narrow the gap from the starting pH to the required pH. Then use a series of HCl (e.g., 6 and 1 N) with lower ionic strengths to avoid a sudden drop in pH below the required pH.
2. Wear a mask when weighing acrylamide. To avoid exposing acrylamide to coworkers, cover the weigh boat containing the weighed acrylamide with another weigh boat when transporting it to the fume hood. Transfer the weighed acrylamide to the cylinder inside the fume hood and mix on a stirrer placed inside the hood. Unpolymerized acrylamide is a neurotoxin and care should be exercised to avoid skin contact.
3. The acrylamide solution can be stored at 4 °C for 1 month. The acrylamide mixture can be prepared in large batches, frozen in aliquots (for greater day-to-day reproducibility).
4. Care should be taken to add SDS solution last, since it makes bubbles.
5. Add β-mercaptoethanol in fume hood to avoid gas exposure to coworkers.
6. The wash/labeling medium must not include methionine or cysteine.
7. Dissolving Triton X-100 in the aqueous buffer requires extensive stirring.
8. In this experiment, we used RNA samples with $A_{260/280}$ ratios greater than 1.8 and $A_{260/230}$ ratios greater than 1.5.
9. Anti-β-actin and anti-PCNA (proliferating cell nuclear antigen) antibodies are recommended for cytoplasmic and nucleus loading control. The two antibodies could also apply to nucleus (anti-β-actin) and cytoplasmic (anti-PCNA) samples, which is a convenient way to unveil potential contamination as a quality control.
10. Pinacocytes are highly recommended for this method as they are most suitable for cytoplasm–nucleus ratio measurements.
11. The process is started first to save time. For the same reason, **steps 3** and **4** of Subheading 3.3.1 could be set up in parallel.

12. Three different binding reactions are suggested for each sample: (1) labeled DNA (probe) alone, (2) probe with protein extract, and (3) probe with protein extract along with 100-fold excess of identical unlabeled DNA. The last reaction, also known as "cold competition experiment," is to show competition and specific DNA–protein binding since the unlabeled DNA should bind more protein and thus no or little shift should be detected.
13. Other equipment that can be used for crosslinking includes a UV-light cross-linker or a handheld UV lamp. Also, chemiluminescent EMSA kit and Immobilon Western Chemiluminescent HRP substrate can detect DNA–protein complex bands.
14. This step is normally processed 3–4 h before electrophoresis.
15. ChIP and reporter gene assays can also be used to determine the DNA–protein interaction (i.e., Nrf2–ARE).
16. To avoid radioactive contamination, 1.5 mL tubes with a screw cap and O-ring are used.
17. The dried pellets can be kept at −20 °C overnight, but longer storage is not recommended due to radiolysis of proteins in the pellets.
18. This step can take a while with large pellets.
19. This should yield a straight line that crosses the 50% intercept at the protein's half-life.

Acknowledgments

This work was supported by NSFC grant (No. 81573195, 81172715, and 30800936) and Fujian Provincial Key Laboratory of Environmental Factors and Cancer.

References

1. Johnston HJ, Hutchison G, Christensen FM, Peters S, Hankin S, Stone V (2010) A review of the in vivo and in vitro toxicity of silver and gold particulates: particle attributes and biological mechanisms responsible for the observed toxicity. Crit Rev Toxicol 40 (4):328–346. https://doi.org/10.3109/10408440903453074
2. Borm PJ, Robbins D, Haubold S, Kuhlbusch T, Fissan H, Donaldson K, Schins R, Stone V, Kreyling W, Lademann J, Krutmann J, Warheit D, Oberdorster E (2006) The potential risks of nanomaterials: a review carried out for ECETOC. Part Fibre Toxicol 3:11. https://doi.org/10.1186/1743-8977-3-11
3. Borm PJA, Müller-Schulte D (2006) Nanoparticles in drug delivery and environmental exposure: same size, same risks? Nanomedicine (Lond) 1(2):235–249. https://doi.org/10.2217/17435889.1.2.235
4. Borm P, Klaessig FC, Landry TD, Moudgil B, Pauluhn J, Thomas K, Trottier R, Wood S (2006) Research strategies for safety evaluation of nanomaterials, Part V: role of dissolution in biological fate and effects of nanoscale particles. Toxicol Sci 90(1):23–32. https://doi.org/10.1093/toxsci/kfj084

5. Oberdörster G (2010) Safety assessment for nanotechnology and nanomedicine: concepts of nanotoxicology. J Intern Med 267 (1):89–105. https://doi.org/10.1111/j.1365-2796.2009.02187.x
6. Oberdörster G, Oberdörster E, Oberdörster J (2005) Nanotoxicology: an emerging discipline evolving from studies of ultrafine particles. Environ Health Perspect 113(7):823–839 PMCID: PMC1257642
7. Xia T, Kovochich M, Brant J, Hotze M, Sempf J, Oberley T, Sioutas C, Yeh JI, Wiesner MR, Nel AE (2006) Comparison of the abilities of ambient and manufactured nanoparticles to induce cellular toxicity according to an oxidative stress paradigm. Nano Lett 6 (8):1794–1807. https://doi.org/10.1021/nl061025k
8. Hussain S, Boland S, Baeza-Squiban A, Hamel R, Thomassen LCJ, Martens JA, Billon-Galland MA, Fleury-Feith J, Moisan F, Pairon J-C, Marano F (2009) Oxidative stress and proinflammatory effects of carbon black and titanium dioxide nanoparticles: role of particle surface area and internalized amount. Toxicology 260(1-3):142–149. https://doi.org/10.1016/j.tox.2009.04.001
9. Eom H-J, Choi J (2009) Oxidative stress of CeO_2 nanoparticles via p38-Nrf-2 signaling pathway in human bronchial epithelial cell, Beas-2B. Toxicol Lett 187(2):77–83. https://doi.org/10.1016/J.TOXLET.2009.01.028
10. Kim S, Choi JE, Choi J, Chung KH, Park K, Yi J, Ryu DY (2009) Oxidative stress-dependent toxicity of silver nanoparticles in human hepatoma cells. Toxicol In Vitro 23 (6):1076–1084. https://doi.org/10.1016/j.tiv.2009.06.001
11. Park EJ, Yi J, Kim Y, Choi K, Park K (2010) Silver nanoparticles induce cytotoxicity by a Trojan-horse type mechanism. Toxicol In Vitro 24(3):872–878. https://doi.org/10.1016/j.tiv.2009.12.001
12. Park EJ, Yi J, Chung KH, Ryu DY, Choi J, Park K (2008) Oxidative stress and apoptosis induced by titanium dioxide nanoparticles in cultured BEAS-2B cells. Toxicol Lett 180 (3):222–229. https://doi.org/10.1016/j.toxlet.2008.06.869
13. Ding M, Kisin ER, Zhao J, Bowman L, Lu Y, Jiang B, Leonard S, Vallyathan V, Castranova V, Murray AR, Fadeel B, Shvedova AA (2009) Size-dependent effects of tungsten carbide–cobalt particles on oxygen radical production and activation of cell signaling pathways in murine epidermal cells. Toxicol Appl Pharmacol 241 (3):260–268. https://doi.org/10.1016/J.TAAP.2009.09.004
14. Nguyen T, Huang HC, Pickett CB (2000) Transcriptional regulation of the antioxidant response element. Activation by Nrf2 and repression by MafK. J Biol Chem 275 (20):15466–15473. https://doi.org/10.1074/jbc.M000361200
15. Venugopal R, Jaiswal AK (1996) Nrf1 and Nrf2 positively and c-Fos and Fra1 negatively regulate the human antioxidant response element-mediated expression of NAD(P)H: quinone oxidoreductase1 gene. Proc Natl Acad Sci U S A 93(25):14960–14965 PMCID: PMC26245
16. Traboulsi H, Guerrina N, Iu M, Maysinger D, Ariya P, Baglole CJ (2017) Inhaled pollutants: the molecular scene behind respiratory and systemic diseases associated with ultrafine particulate matter. Int J Mol Sci 18(2):243. https://doi.org/10.3390/ijms18020243
17. Kaspar JW, Niture SK, Jaiswal AK (2009) Nrf2: INrf2 (Keap1) signaling in oxidative stress. Free Radic Biol Med 47(9):1304–1309. https://doi.org/10.1016/j.freeradbiomed.2009.07.035
18. Osburn WO, Kensler TW (2008) Nrf2 signaling: an adaptive response pathway for protection against environmental toxic insults. Mutat Res 659(1-2):31–39. https://doi.org/10.1016/j.mrrev.2007.11.006
19. Aggarwal BB, Shishodia S, Sandur SK, Pandey MK, Sethi G (2006) Inflammation and cancer: how hot is the link? Biochem Pharmacol 72 (11):1605–1621. https://doi.org/10.1016/J.BCP.2006.06.029
20. Xu B, Zhang J, Strom J, Lee S, Chen QM (2014) Myocardial ischemic reperfusion induces de novo Nrf2 protein translation. Biochim Biophys Acta 1842(9):1638–1647. https://doi.org/10.1016/j.bbadis.2014.06.002
21. Lee SC, Zhang J, Strom J, Yang D, Dinh TN, Kappeler K, Chen QM (2016) G-quadruplex in Nrf2 5′ UTR regulates de novo Nrf2 protein translation under oxidative stress. Mol Cell Biol 37(1):e00122–e00116. https://doi.org/10.1128/MCB.00122-16
22. Li H, Wu S, Wang Z, Lin W, Zhang C, Huang B (2012) Neuroprotective effects of tert-butylhydroquinone on paraquat-induced dopaminergic cell degeneration in C57BL/6 mice and in PC12 cells. Arch Toxicol 86 (11):1729–1740. https://doi.org/10.1007/s00204-012-0935-y
23. Ye F, Li X, Li L, Yuan J, Chen J (2016) t-BHQ provides protection against lead neurotoxicity via Nrf2/HO-1 pathway. Oxid Med Cell Longev 2016(2016): 1–15. doi: https://doi.org/10.1155/2016/2075915

24. Li H, Wu S, Shi N (2007) Transcription factor Nrf2 activation by deltamethrin in PC12 cells: involvement of ROS. Toxicol Lett 171 (1-2):87–98. https://doi.org/10.1016/j.toxlet.2007.04.007
25. Li H, Zhong Y, Wu S, Shi N (2007) NF-E2 related factor 2 activation and heme oxygenase-1 induction by *tert* -butylhydroquinone protect against deltamethrin-mediated oxidative stress in PC12 cells. Chem Res Toxicol 20 (9):1242–1251. https://doi.org/10.1021/tx700076q
26. Li H, Wu S, Shi N, Lin W, You J, Zhou W (2011) NF-E2-related factor 2 activation in PC12 cells: its protective role in manganese-induced damage. Arch Toxicol 85 (8):901–910. https://doi.org/10.1007/s00204-010-0625-6
27. Zhang Z, Guo Z, Zhan Y, Li H, Wu S (2017) Role of histone acetylation in activation of nuclear factor erythroid 2-related factor 2/heme oxygenase 1 pathway by manganese chloride. Toxicol Appl Pharmacol 336:94–100. https://doi.org/10.1016/j.taap.2017.10.011
28. Li H, Wu S, Shi N, Lian S, Lin W (2011) Nrf2/HO-1 pathway activation by manganese is associated with reactive oxygen species and ubiquitin-proteasome pathway, not MAPKs signaling. J Appl Toxicol 31(7):690–697. https://doi.org/10.1002/jat.1654
29. Li H, Wu S, Ma Q, Shi N (2011) The pesticide deltamethrin increases free radical production and transcription factor Nrf2 in rat brain. Toxicol Ind Health 27(7):579–590. https://doi.org/10.1177/0748233710393400
30. Li H, Wu S, Chen J, Wang B, Shi N (2013) Effect of glutathione depletion on Nrf2/ARE activation by deltamethrin in PC12 cells. Arch Ind Hyg Toxicol 64(1):87–97. https://doi.org/10.2478/10004-1254-64-2013-2251
31. Laemmli UK (1970) Cleavage of structural proteins during the assembly of the head of bacteriophage T4. Nature 227:680–685
32. Brunelle JL, Green R (2014) One-dimensional SDS-polyacrylamide gel electrophoresis (1D SDS-PAGE). Methods Enzymol 541:151–159
33. Sambrook J, Fritsch EF, Maniatis Y (1989) Sequencing by the Maxam-Gilbert method: a laboratory manual. Cold Spring Harbor Laboratory Press, Cold Spring Harbor, NY, pp 13.78–13.104

Chapter 14

Application of Electron Microscopes in Nanotoxicity Assessment

Junzhe Zhang, Xiao He, and Michael T. Tseng

Abstract

In this chapter, we highlight the applications of electron microscopes (EMs) in nanotoxicity assessment. EMs can provide detailed information about the size and morphology of nanomaterials (NMs), their localization in cells and tissues, the nano-bio interactions, as well as the ultrastructural changes induced by NMs exposure. Here, we share with the readers how we prepare the tissue sample, and the different types of EMs used among the nanotoxicologists. It is possible to deploy conventional EMs along or in combination with other analytical techniques, such as electron energy loss spectroscopy (EELS), energy dispersive X-ray spectroscopy (EDS or EDX), and TEM-assisted scanning transmission X-ray microscopy (STXM), toward further elemental and chemical characterization. Appropriate images are inserted to illustrate throughout this chapter.

Key words Electron microscopes, Nanomaterials, Characterization, Tissues and cells, Ultrastructure, Localization

1 Introduction

Electron microscopes (EMs) mainly including transmission electron microscope (TEM) and scanning electron microscope (SEM) have been widely used for the size and morphological characterization of nanomaterials (NMs). They are also used for visualization of NMs in cells and tissues, since many NMs possess a better image contrast (electron density) than the soft biotissues surrounding them. A TEM can be modified into a scanning transmission electron microscope (STEM) by focusing the electron beam to a fine spot (with the typical spot size 0.05–0.2 nm) which is then scanned over the sample in a raster. New development of EMs such as the environmental scanning electron microscope can provide images of sufficient quality and resolution even when the sample is wet. Electron cryomicroscopy has also been used for visualizing the NMs, as well as the unstained biomolecules and intracellular structures.

Qunwei Zhang (ed.), *Nanotoxicity: Methods and Protocols*, Methods in Molecular Biology, vol. 1894,
https://doi.org/10.1007/978-1-4939-8916-4_14,

EMs can be used to identify the intracellular behaviors of NMs and the ultrastructural changes caused by NMs exposure (cell uptake of NMs, mitochondrial swelling, apoptosis, and so on). Autophagy is the natural, regulated, destructive mechanism of the cell that disassembles unnecessary or dysfunctional components. NMs-induced autophagy has recently become a hot topic in nanotoxicological studies. Because the presence of autophagic vacuoles is by far the most important morphological feature of cells with autophagic activity, demonstration of these structures by TEM remains the gold standard—even in recent years—to identify autophagy [1]. Wang et al. studied the biocompatibility and cell uptake of new nanocarriers called anodic alumina nanotubes (AANTs) by RAW 264.7 macrophages and MDA-MB231-TXSA breast cancer cells. TEM images proved after an overnight incubation at 100 mg/mL AANTs were internalized by both kinds of cells. Moreover, they also identified the fusion of autophagosome with autophagic vacuoles and autophagic vacuoles containing cellular debris within the TEM images (Fig. 1) [2]. Hussain et al. treated human monocytes with 10 μg/mL CeO_2 NPs for 40 h, and by TEM they observed increased formation of autophagic vesicles and mitochondrial swelling together with mitochondrial elongation (Fig. 2) [3]. With further results they demonstrated the toxic effects were mediated by both endosomes/lysosomes-related autophagy and mitochondrial-mediated apoptosis. Apoptosis is a process of programmed cell death that occurs in multicellular organisms. In an early literature, Bennett showed a serial of TEM images of a human vascular smooth muscle cell (VSMC) undergoing apoptosis in culture (Fig. 3). The author also pointed out the gold standard for detecting apoptosis was still based on morphology observed by TEM [4]. Apoptosis could be frequently found in the cells exposed to NMs. Via TEM observation, Zhang et al. found that C_{60} aggregates could induce macrophage apoptosis [5]. When MC3T3-E1 preosteoblasts were treated with 10 or 100 μg/mL TiO_2 NPs, intracellular vesicles containing endocytosed material could be found in the cytoplasm by TEM [6]. In the cells treated with 100 μg/mL TiO_2 NPs for 24 h, a number of mitochondria swelled, vacuoles appeared, and karyoplasms were found concentrated in some samples, suggesting the occurrence of apoptosis in preosteoblast cells. The endoplasmic reticulum (ER) is the cellular organelle that is critical for protein folding and secretion, calcium homeostasis, and lipid biosynthesis. Disturbance in any of these functions, which results in the disruption of the proper folding and secretory capacity of the ER and increased load of unfolded proteins in its lumen, defines a condition known as "ER stress." Chen et al. compared the TEM images of ZnO NPs treated cells with the control group, and found a significant decrease in the number of mitochondria, while more ERs showed obvious aggregation or swelling (Fig. 4) [7]. ER stress response might be used as an earlier

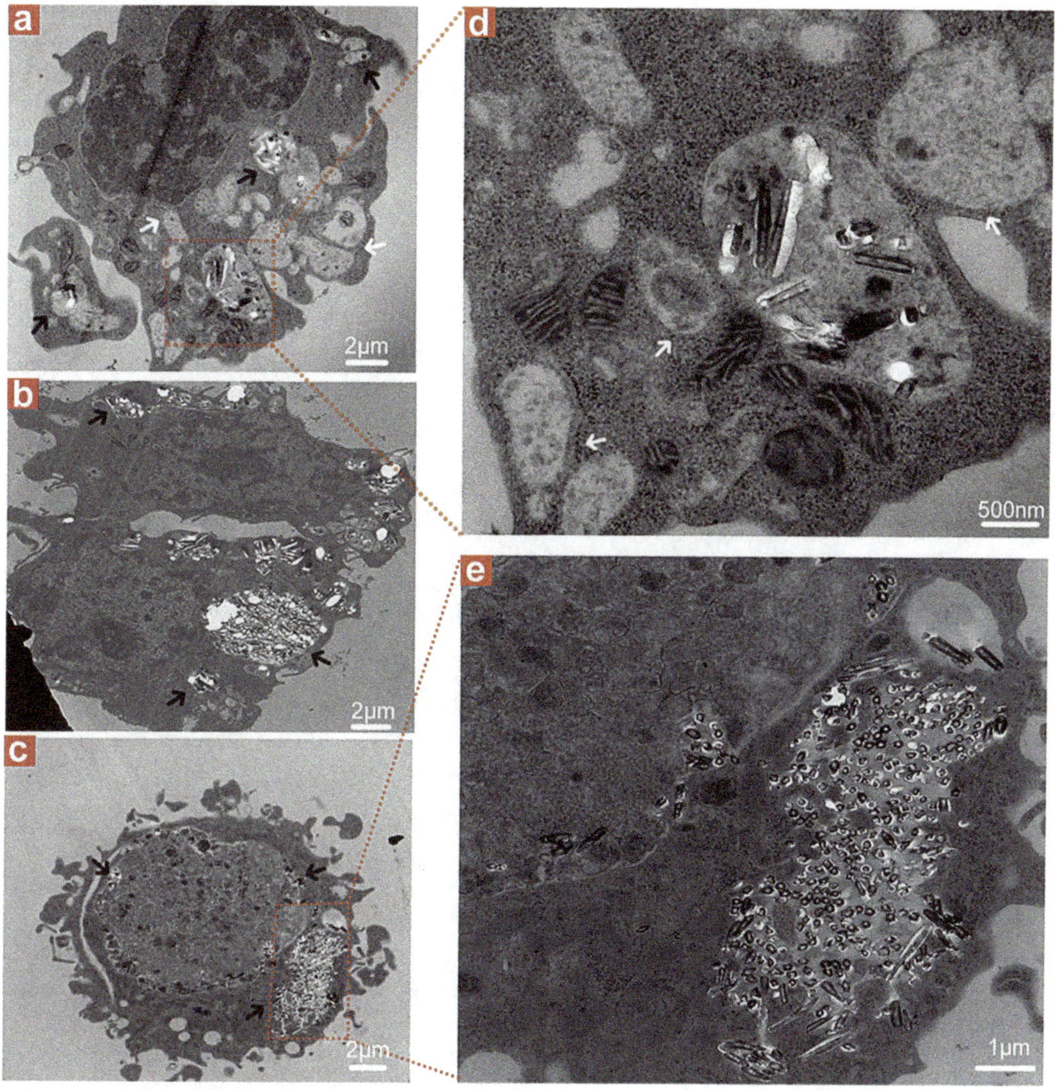

Fig. 1 TEM of AANTs internalized by RAW 264.7 macrophage cells (**a**, **b**, and **d**) and MDA-MB231-TXSA cell (**c** and **e**); (**d**) and (**e**) are magnified views of (**a**) and (**c**). The black arrows identify AANTs inside cells; white arrows indicate the fusion of autophagic vacuoles, in which cellular debris were located inside. Hussain et al. treated human monocytes with 10 μg/mL CeO_2 NPs for 40 h, and by TEM they observed increased formation of autophagic vesicles and mitochondrial swelling together with mitochondrial elongation (Fig. 2) [3]. With further results they demonstrated the toxic effects were mediated by both endosomes/lysosomes-related autophagy and mitochondrial-mediated apoptosis

and sensitive end point for nanotoxicological study. EMs also provide images for other pathologic alteration caused by NMs, for example, the hepatic granuloma induced by nanoceria infusion. Beyond the traditional use of ceria as an abrasive, the scope of nanoceria applications now extends into fuel cell manufacturing, diesel fuel additives, and for therapeutic intervention as a putative

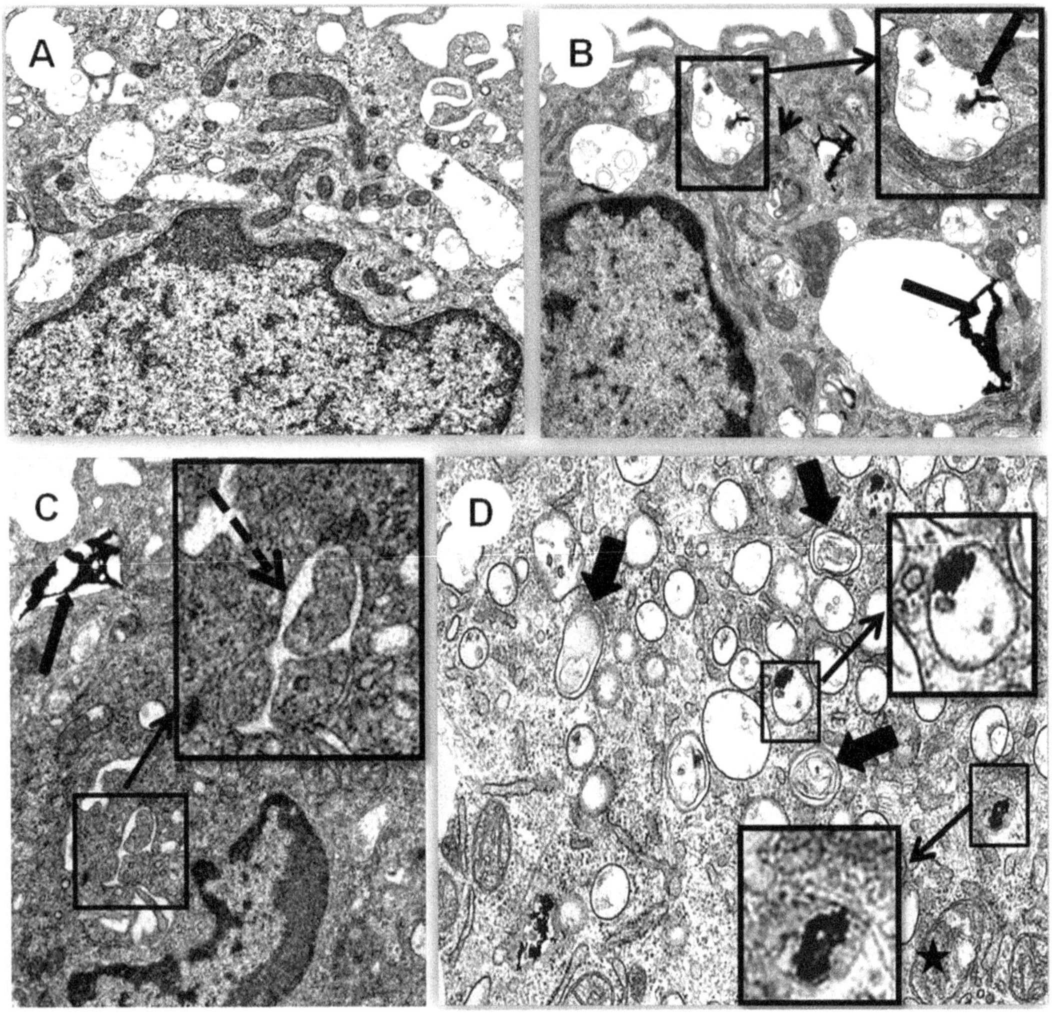

Fig. 2 TEM images of human monocytes after CeO_2 NPs exposure. Photo micrographs of control cells (**a**) and CeO_2 NPs-treated cells (**b**, **c**, and **d**). Intracellular accumulation of CeO_2 NPs in vesicles (long arrows), enlargement of mitochondria (arrowhead), autophagic vesicle formation (broken arrow), autolysosomes (thick short arrows), swollen mitochondria (asterisk). Insets present detailed structure of vesicle containing an aggregate of CeO_2 NPs (**b**), autophagic vesicle (**c**), and CeO_2 NPs inside vesicles and free in cytoplasm (**d**). (**a**, **b**, and **c**) 9900×, (**d**) 20,500×

antioxidant. However, the biological effects of nanoceria exposure have yet to be fully defined, which gave us the impetus to examine its systemic biodistribution and biological responses. The infusion of nanoceria in rodents can lead to the hepatic granuloma in the liver as reported in earlier paper. The report herein confirmed the discovery of granulomatous formation in liver and, more importantly, intracellular nanoceria was detected by EM (Fig. 5) [8].

EMs can be connected to various detectors that give more information of samples about their chemical composition and

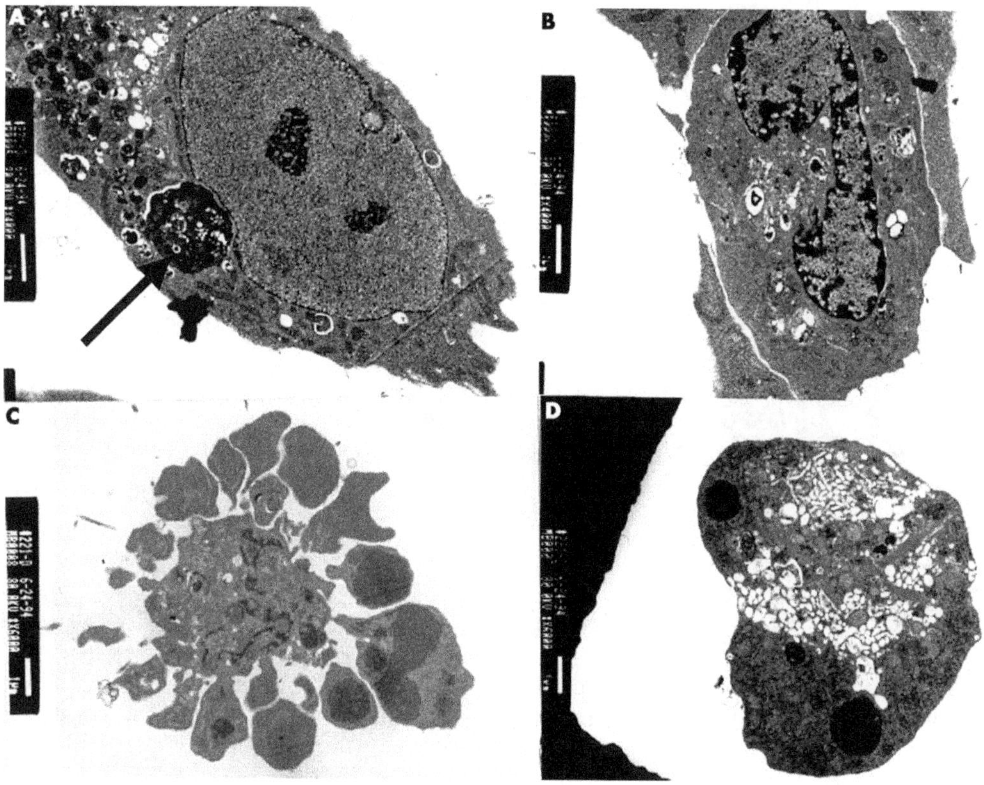

Fig. 3 TEM images of a human vascular smooth muscle cell (VSMC) undergoing apoptosis in culture. (**a**) Appearance of a normal human VSMC, which also contains an apoptotic body (arrow). (**b**) Peripheral condensation of nuclear chromatin. (**c**) Intense membrane blebbing and vesicle formation in apoptosis, with condensation of the nuclear chromatin into clumps. (**d**) An apoptotic body, the end product of apoptosis

structure. The combination of energy dispersive X-ray spectroscopy (EDS or EDX) and electron energy loss spectroscopy (EELS) with the high-resolution EM provides a powerful approach to provide detailed chemical information of NMs. EDS is a common spectroscopy technique available on many EMs, which provides most standard and reliable methods for elemental analysis. Once a high energy beam of electrons is focused into a specimen, an electron in an inner shell might be excited to a high energy level, leaving an electron hole where the electron was. An electron from an outer, higher-energy shell then fills the hole, and the difference in energy between the higher-energy shell and the lower energy shell may be released in the form of an X-ray. The characteristic X-ray corresponding to each element can be used to identify different elements through the specific peak energy, while the integrated intensity of the peak can provide each element contents in the specimen [9].

There are two mainly analysis methods for TEM/SEM-EDS, point analysis and mapping analysis. For point analysis, X-rays are

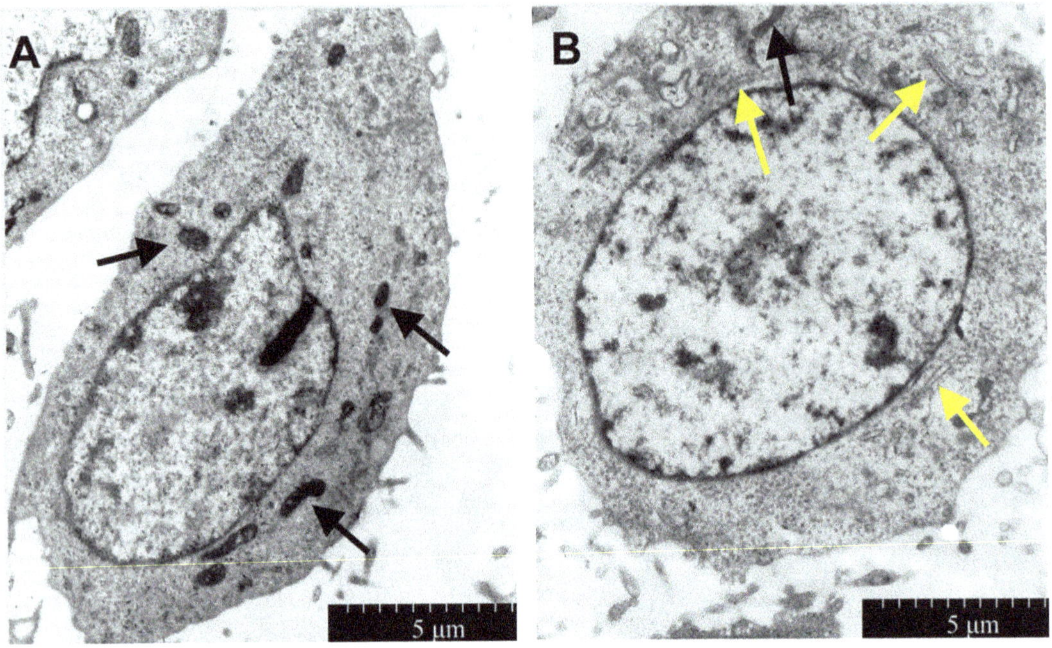

Fig. 4 TEM images of HUVECs of untreated control (**a**) and cells exposed to 120 μm ZnO NPs (**b**). Black arrows show mitochondria and yellow arrows show the apparently aggregated or swelled endoplasmic reticulum in the cytoplasm of NPs-treated cells

emitted throughout the volume of material into which the electron beam is scattered and decelerated, so the resolution is commonly 1 μm laterally and about 1–2 μm in depth. Better spatial resolution is obtainable with ultrathin (~100 nm) specimens (e.g., TEM slice). With mapping analysis, two-dimensional distribution of the constituent element can be obtained. Using routine procedures, detection limits are typically about 1000 ppm (by weight) but can be reduced by using long counting times. TEM/SEM-EDS analysis has been widely used for the characterization of NMs as well as the detection of NMs in biological samples. For example, TEM/EDS was used for the morphological and elemental classification of a variety of freshly emitted soot particles and atmospheric ultrafine particles [10]. TEM/EDS data showed distinct differences in morphological properties among the different types of fresh soot particles, such as primary particle diameter, fractal dimension, and microstructure; and the atmospheric ultrafine particles were classified based on their morphology, elemental composition, and beam sensitivity (Fig. 6). Austin et al. used TEM-EDS to identify the distribution of silver NPs in pregnant mice and developing embryos [11]. Silver NPs with an average diameter of 50 nm were intravenously injected into pregnant CD-1 mice on gestation days (GDs) 7, 8, and 9, and visceral yolk sac tissues were collected on GD 10. TEM observation found vesicle-bound electron-dense areas within

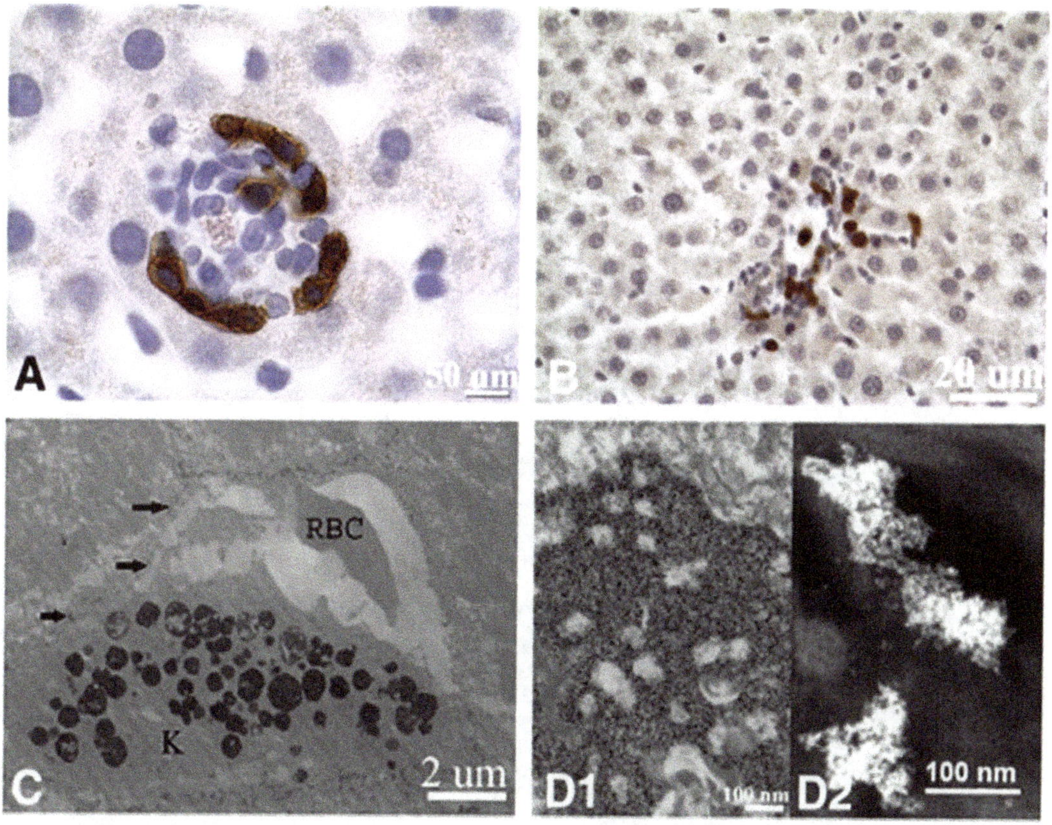

Fig. 5 Light microscopy, IHC, and TEM features of ceria-exposed liver tissue. A population of brown staining, CD3+, mononucleated cells in a granuloma (**a**). At a lower magnification, perivascular accumulation of CD3+ cells (**b**). Biodistribution of ceria appeared as large, electron-dense cytoplasmic agglomerates in a Kupffer cell (K), the presence of strands of ceria in the space of Disse (arrows), but none in an erythrocyte (RBC) (**c**). Large agglomerates punctuated by a lightly stained cytoplasmic component are illustrated by TEM (**d1**). An HR-TEM/STEM image from a similar area demonstrates heterogeneity of the ceria agglomerate (**d2**)

the endoderm layer of the visceral yolk sac. Elemental analysis using EDS confirmed that these electron-dense regions contained silver. No silver particles were detected outside of vesicles or in the mesodermal layer of the visceral yolk sac. Shim et al. treated rats with SiO_2 NPs by repeated dermal administration for 90 days to study the permeability through the blood–brain barrier (BBB), a tight physical barrier for controlling homeostasis and stopping the transmission of foreign substances into the central nervous system [12]. They observed nanosized dots in each brain region and used EDS to confirm the presence or absence of SiO_2 NPs. The EDS results indicated the dots were dye materials (with Os and Pb peaks) and grid materials (with C and Cu peaks) with the absent signal of Si elements (Fig. 7), suggesting the SiO_2 NPs could not permeate the BBB or induce significant neurotoxic effects in the brain. Ma et al. exposed cucumber roots to La_2O_3 NPs, and

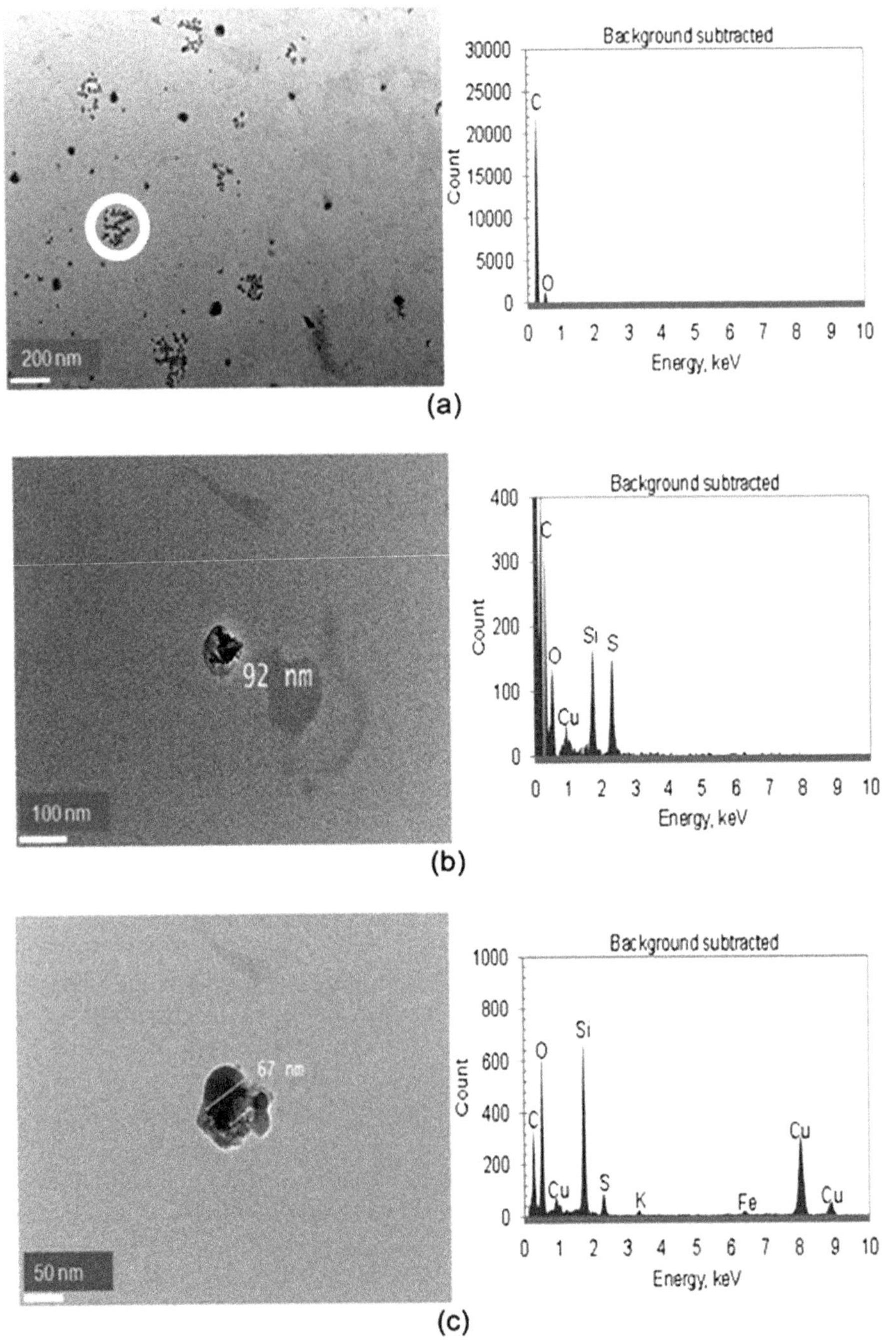

Fig. 6 TEM and EDS data of atmospheric ultrafine particles. (**a**) a fresh agglomerate with no visible coating and a major element of C in its EDS spectrum; (**b**) an aged agglomerate included in the sphere, containing multi elements (e.g., S, Si, C); (**c**) an aged agglomerate coagulated with spherical particles, showing more compact structure with additional chemical species (e.g., C, O, Si, S, K, and Fe)

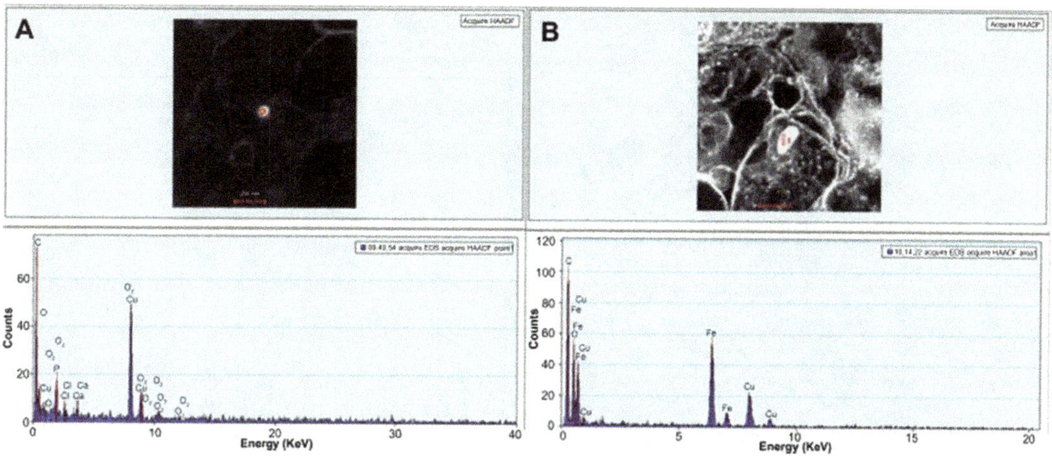

Fig. 7 The TEM and EDS results of SiO_2 NPs treated rat hippocampus via dermal administration. (**a**) and (**b**) are examples of suspected nanosized dot and TEM graph of EDS analysis

observed some needle-shaped nanoclusters in the intercellular spaces and middle lamellas of roots by TEM [13]. With EDS analysis, they found the needle-like nanoclusters contained high concentrations of La and P. The semiquantitative results of La and P were calculated by the integrated intensities of the respective peaks, and the good correlation ($R = 0.9976$) between the two elements suggested that the composition of the deposits was $LaPO_4$. Compared with the La^{3+} ion treatment, similar EDS results were obtained, indicating that the phytotoxicity of La_2O_3 NPs probably be correlated with the dissolution of the NPs. The transformation of Yb_2O_3 NPs was similarly studied by TEM-EDS analysis (Fig. 8) [14]. The semiquantitative results of Yb and P were calculated by the integrated intensities of the respective peaks, and the relative atomic ratios of Yb/P were close to 1, suggesting that the composition of the deposits was $YbPO_4$. EDS could also be used to identify the formation of nano–bio complexes as NMs dispersed in a biological solution. TEM grid was immersed into the NMs suspension for 24 h, and after the NMs settled on the surface of grid, the sample was observed with TEM [15]. Figure 9 shows the TEM elemental maps of CuO NPs dispersed in the DMEM supplemented with 10% FBS. The crystalline CuO NPs are surrounded by elements such as Ca, K, Na, Cl, and P. TEM-EDS data clearly suggest the formation of nano–bio complexes in biological environments, and the results also suggest that NPs exhibited different binding affinities for the various components of the medium. Scanning transmission electron microscope equipped with EELS is a widely used hyphenated technique for in situ chemical and morphological analysis, with high spatial (<1 nm) and energy (<0.2 eV) resolution [16]. EELS is capable of measuring atomic composition, chemical bonding, electronic properties,

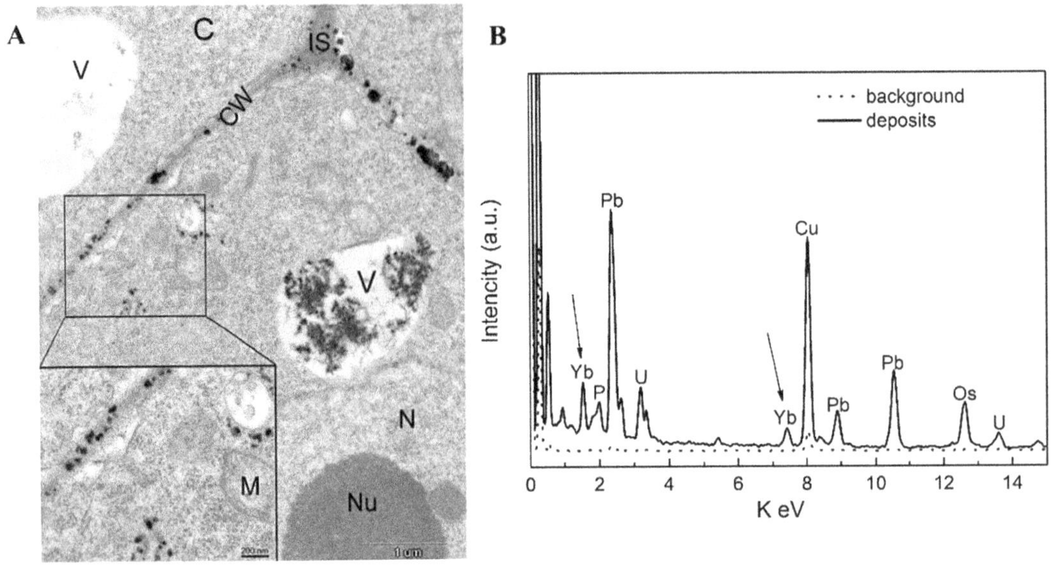

Fig. 8 TEM images of cross sections of cucumber root cells under 2000 mg/L nm-Yb_2O_3 (**a**), and representative EDS spectra of background and dense deposits in TEM images (**b**). The insets are higher magnification of the rectangle areas. Cells walls (CW), nucleus (N) with nucleolus (Nu), intercellular space (IS), mitochondria (M), and vacuole (V)

valence and conduction band, and pair-distance distribution functions. Turner et al. studied surface reduction of nanoceria with predominant {111} and {100} type surfaces using a combination of TEM and EELS [17]. The nanoceria is mapped using the fine structures of the Ce M_4 and M_5 edges as fingerprints for the valency of surface Ce. A color map overlaying the Ce^{3+} and Ce^{4+} maps (Fig. 10) shows that the surface reduction shell is present over the whole particle surface owing to the oxygen deficiency (vacancies) close to the surface. At its thinnest, the Ce^{3+} shell appears to extend over ~2 nm. Nanoceria sized below 5 nm appear to be predominantly in a reduced state. For the {111} facets and for {111} surface islands, the reduction shell is found to extend over a single fully reduced surface plane and 1–2 underlying mixed valency planes. For the {100} facets the reduction shell extends over a larger area of 5–6 oxygen vacancy-rich planes. This finding provides a plausible explanation for the higher catalytic activity of the {100} surface facets in ceria. TEM-EELS was also used to identify the reduction of nanoceria in vivo. Graham et al. demonstrated that the intravenously infused nanoceria undergo in vivo transformation after a prolonged residence time in the liver (90 days) [18]. This transformation includes a breakdown of the first-generation nanoceria and the formation of ultrafine (second-generation) nanoceria, combined with a measurable change in the valence reduction and redox activity. EELS spectra revealed a significant enrichment in Ce^{3+} always observed in surface layers whereas the core regions are

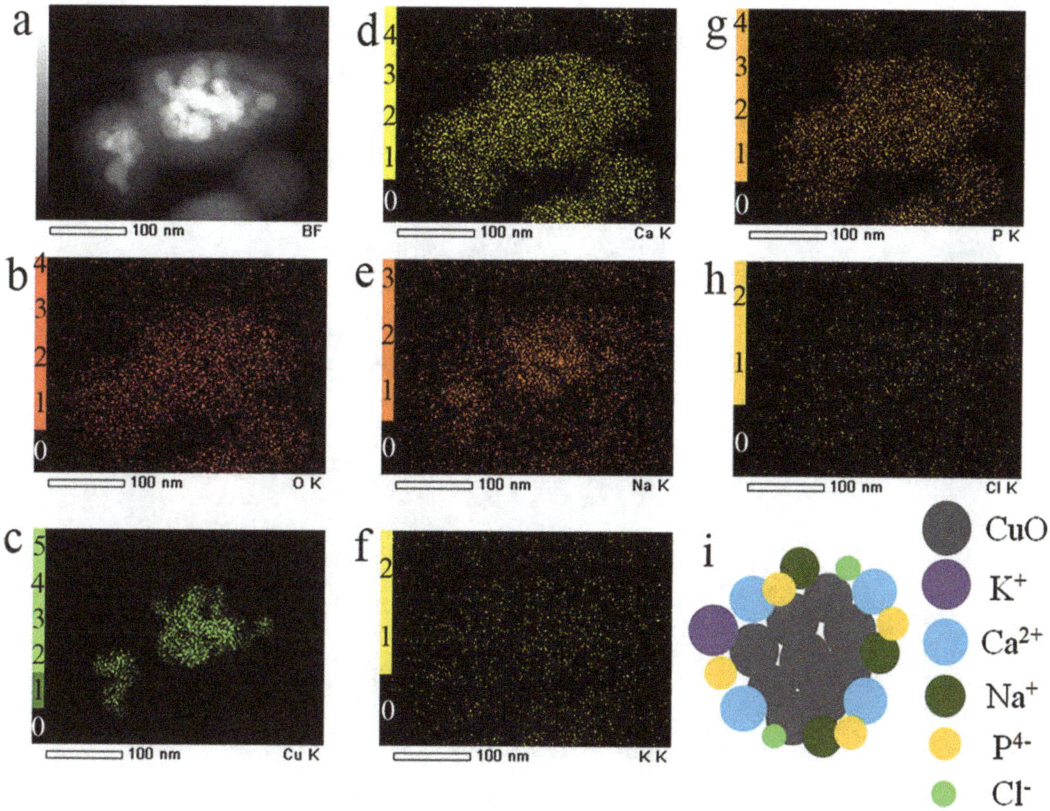

Fig. 9 Formation of CuO nanoparticle biocomplexes in medium with fetal bovine serum. (**a**) Dark-field TEM image showing where the elemental maps were obtained; (**b**) TEM-EDS O mapping; (**c**) TEM-EDS Zn mapping; (**d**) TEM-EDS Ca mapping; (**e**) TEM-EDS Na mapping; (**f**) TEM-EDS K mapping; (**g**) TEM-EDS P mapping; (**h**) TEM-EDS Cl mapping; (**i**) A simple model of CuO biocomplexes

predominantly in the Ce^{4+} state (Fig. 11). However, EELS analyses of ultrafines (≈1–3 nm) from ceria clouds had much weaker M_4 lines and lacked satellite peaks, suggesting that ceria cloud formation shifts the overall redox activity of ceria to a more reduced state and thus higher free-radical scavenging activity. This information will establish a direct linkage between cellular processes like the reversal in pro-oxidative stress in the brain and in vivo processing and transformation of nanoceria. TEM is recently used to assist the in situ chemical analysis employing scanning transmission X-ray microscopy (STXM). STXM based on synchrotron radiation is another spatial-resolved technique for detection of the in situ chemistry. The fundamental diffraction limit for X-rays makes STXM unable to match the spatial resolution of STEM-EELS. Currently the highest reported spatial resolutions in conventional STXMs are about 10 nm, and concentrations of 0.1–1% are typically detectable. On the other hand, STXM is superior to EELS with respect to the limited radiation damage caused by X-ray irradiation, and is therefore particularly suitable for the chemical

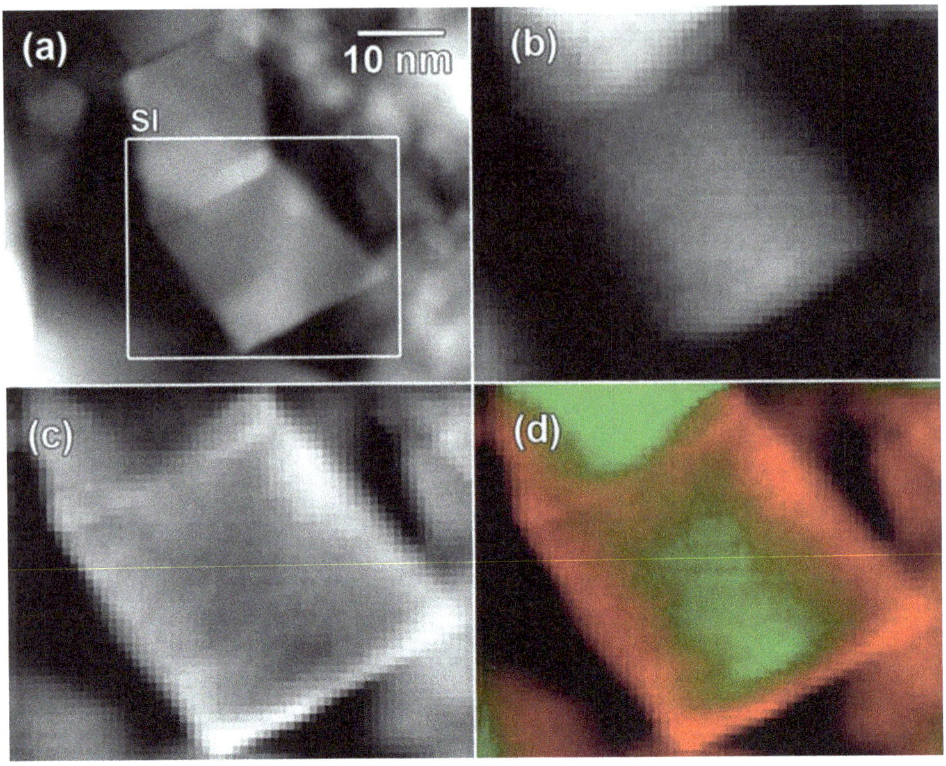

Fig. 10 Low magnification surface reduction mapping: (**a**) HAADFSTEM survey image showing the scanned particles and the 60 × 47 pixel SI scan region. (**b**) Ce^{4+} map (**c**) Ce^{3+} map (**d**) Color map with Ce^{3+} (Red) and Ce^{4+} (Green). Notice that smaller particles on the right are almost fully reduced

speciation in biological samples. The application of STXM was once considered of limited significance in nanotoxicological study because the concentrations of NMs in organisms usually range from ppb (parts-per-billion) level to hundreds of ppm (parts per million), much lower than the detection limit of STXM. But actually, the local concentration of NMs can be high enough for STXM to detect once the beam focal spot covers the exact location where NMs deposited. The real challenge is how to position the NMs in the sample slice to the focal spot of X-ray beam. Only when the NMs are close to the X-ray focal spot can a relatively clear absorption image be obtained; only with the absorption image obtained, can the focal position of X-ray beam be determined by moving the sample along the beam axis. So it will take a particularly long time to determine the proper location of the sample as well as the region of the interest (ROI) to be scanned. In some recent work, a TEM-assisted protocol has been developed to shorten the time for sample positioning in STXM analysis.

TEM-assisted STXM analysis has provided concreted evidence for the degradation of ceria NPs. Ceria NPs, with the predominant presence of Ce^{4+}, could be reduced during the interactions with

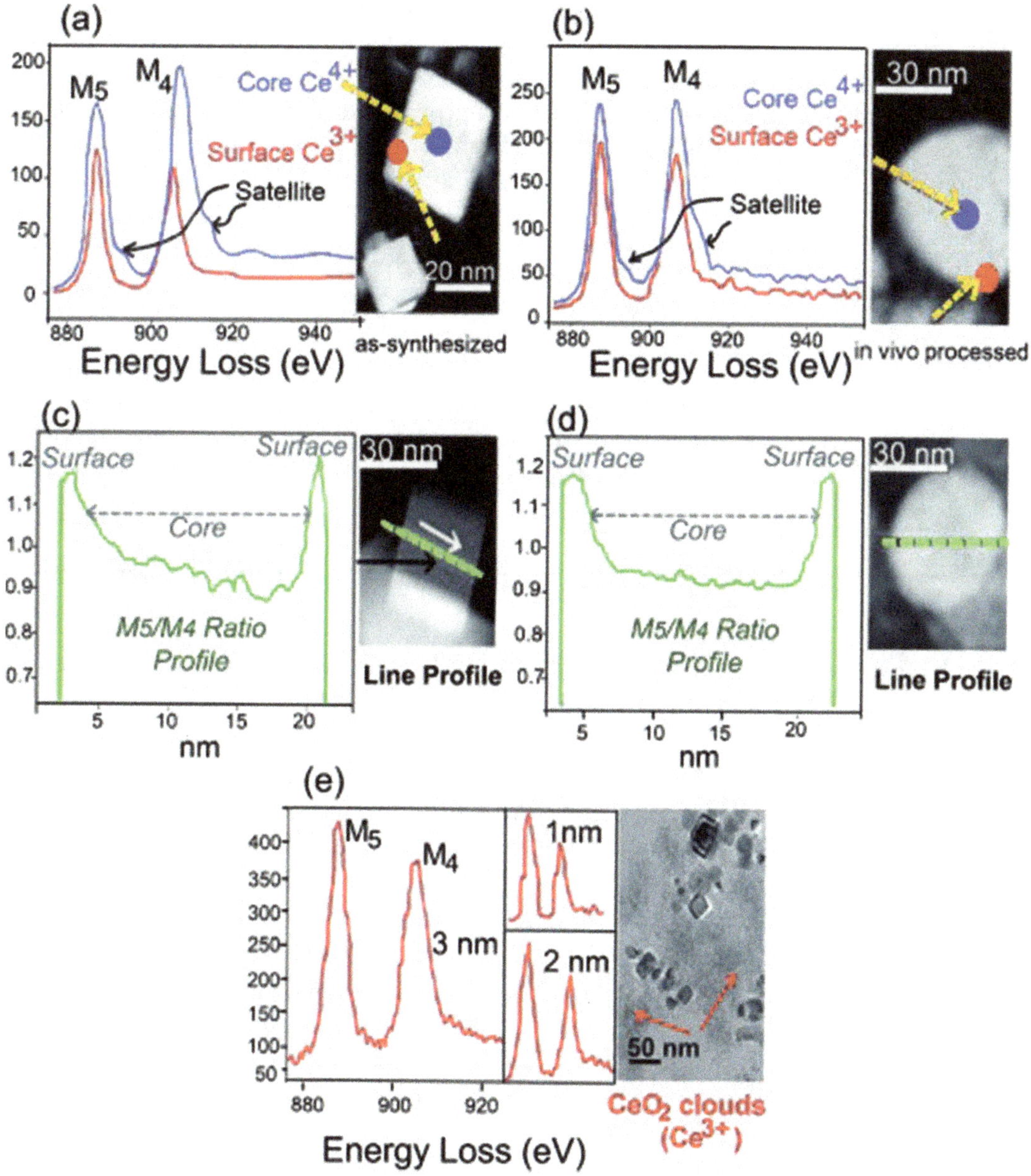

Fig. 11 EELS analysis of nanoceria: (**a**) the as-synthesized nanoceria cubes; (**b**) in vivo processed ceria after 90 days in the liver; (**c**) M_5/M_4 ratio from the line profile of as-synthesized nanoceria; (**d**) M_5/M_4 ratio from the line profile of rounded in vivo processed nanoceria; (**e**) representative M_4 and M_5 lines for individual 1, 2, and 3 nm crystallites (in ceria clouds), which indicate enhanced +3 reduction as a function of particle size

organisms. Increased percentages of Ce^{3+} have been proved by XAFS [19], EELS [18], and STXM [20]. However, it remained unclear whether the reduction of ceria NPs would result in the release of Ce^{3+} ions. Consequently, the toxicity of ceria NPs was once attributed exclusively to their particle-specific effects. By using TEM-assisted STXM analysis, Zhang et al. and Ma et al. found the separate deposition of Ce^{3+} and Ce^{4+} in plant: when cucumber root was exposed to ceria NPs in phosphorus-deficient medium, the particle surface would undergo a reduction, and the Ce^{3+} ions were released, transported, and precipitated in the intercellular spaces and vacuoles of roots, with Ce speciation exclusively in the trivalent state; the residual particulate forms outside the roots had no detectable Ce^{3+} (Fig. 12) [20, 21]. These results suggest that the reduction of ceria NPs in biosystem is followed by the release of Ce^{3+} ions, and therefore, the bioeffects of Ce^{3+} ions should also be taken into account when trying to understand the toxicity of ceria NPs.

To sum up, EMs have been widely used in the field of nanotoxicology. Their applications include the characterization of NMs, tracking the NMs in cells and tissues, visualizing the nano–bio interactions, identifying the ultrastructural changes caused by NMs exposure, and so on.

2 Materials

Prepare all solutions using Milli-Q water (18.2 MΩ cm) and analytical grade reagents. Prepare and store all reagents at room temperature unless otherwise specified.

1. 5% uranyl acetate: add 2.5 g of uranyl acetate to 50 mL of water. Cover with foil and stir overnight. Add ten drops of glacial acetic acid. Store at 4 °C. This solution is stable for at least 6 months at 4 °C. Dilute to 2% or 1% when used.
2. Phosphotungstic acid: prepare 2% stock solution (e.g., Sigma Cat. No. P4006) in water, pH 1.5. Dilute to 1% when used.
3. Ammonium molybdate: 10% ammonium molybdate (e.g., Qorpak Cat. No. Q05211-1). Dilute to 5% when used.
4. 0.1 M Phosphate buffer (PB): mix 19 mL 0.2 M NaH_2PO_4 with 81 mL 0.2 M Na_2HPO_4 to get 0.2 M PB, then dilute to 200 mL.
5. 0.2 M cacodylate buffer: 21.4 g Na cacodylate in 250 mL water. Adjust the pH to 7.4 with 1 M HCl and make up to a final volume of 500 mL.
6. 2.5% glutaraldehyde: 5 mL 50% glutaraldehyde (e.g., Sigma Cat. No. G6403), 45 mL water and 50 mL 0.2 M PB.
7. 4% Paraformaldehyde: 4% paraformaldehyde in 0.1 M PB.
8. 10% Formalin: 10 mL formaldehyde solution (e.g., Sigma Cat. No. F8775), and make up to 50 mL with water. Make up to 100 mL with 0.2 M PB.
9. 2% glutaraldehyde and 2% paraformaldehyde: (a) Add 2 g paraformaldehyde to ~35 mL water, then add approx. 0.5 mL of

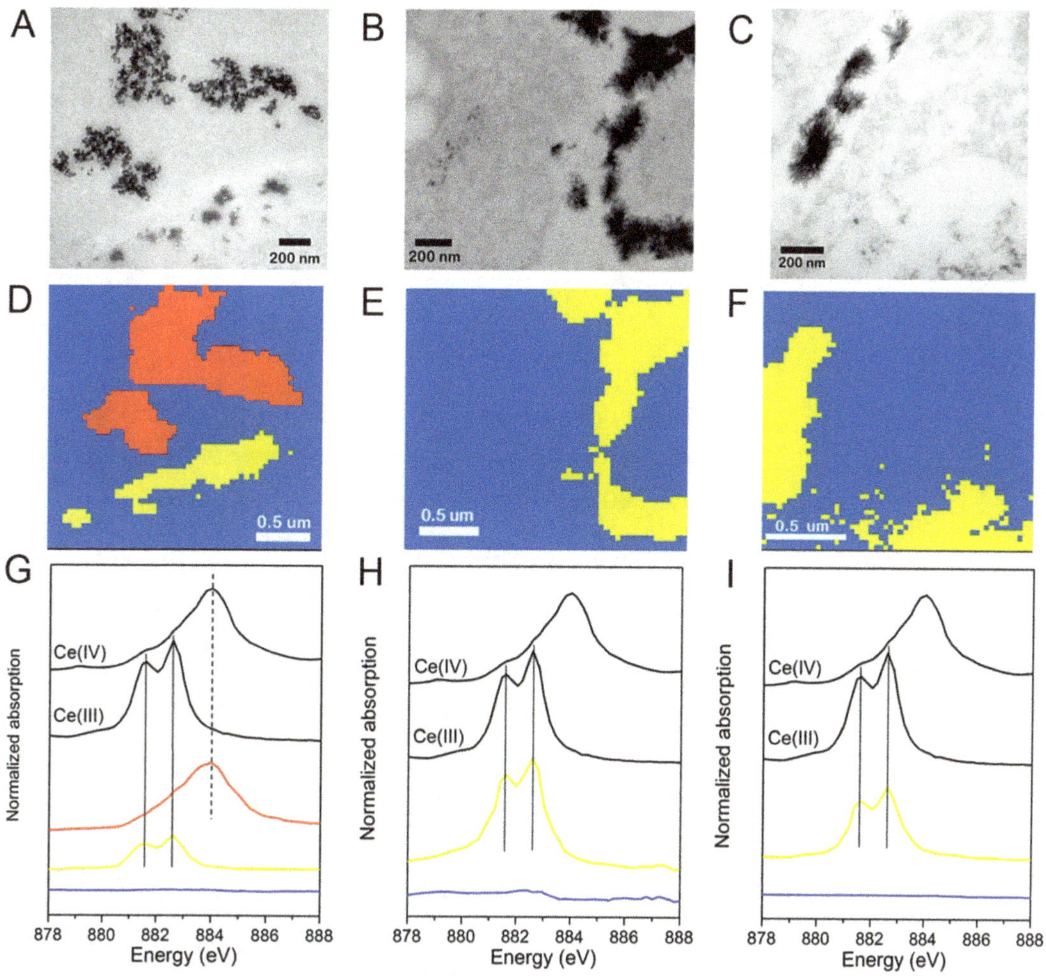

Fig. 12 TEM observations of root cross sections at the root surface (**a**), intercellular space and cytoplasm (**b**), and vacuole (**c**). STXM stack images (**d**–**f**) of Ce components in the same areas as in panels (**a**)–(**c**), and the corresponding XANES spectra (**g**–**i**) extracted from the color image sequences in panels (**d**–**f**). The above black line spectra belong to the standard compounds, and the colored spectra below belong to the samples. The solid and dashed lines indicate the absorption peaks of Ce(III) and Ce(IV), respectively. Red and blue colors represent the different Ce components. The results shown are representative of three replicates

1 M NaOH (freshly prepared just before use). (b) Heat the paraformaldehyde solution in a fume cupboard to ~60 °C until the paraformaldehyde dissolves. (c) Cool and add 8 mL of EM grade 25% glutaraldehyde. (d) Make up to 50 mL with water. (e) Make up to 100 mL with 0.2 M PB. (f) Filter before use in animals.

10. 0.5% trypsin–EDTA: 0.5% trypsin and 0.2% ETDA in water.
11. Osmium tetroxide: 4% in 0.1 M PB.
12. Ethanol for dehydration: 30%, 50%, 70%, 90%, and 100%.
13. Propylene oxide (e.g., Merck, Cat. No. S4912527).

14. Poly/Bed 812 Embedding Kit/DMP-30 (Polysciences, Cat. No. 08792-1).
15. Toluidine Blue: 0.5% Toluidine Blue and 1% sodium borate in water. Filter with 0.22 μm filter.
16. Lead citrate: 1% lead citrate in water. Add three drops of 10 M NaOH (around 0.5 mL).
17. Eppendorf tubes.
18. Droppers.
19. Syringes.
20. Centrifuge.
21. Vacuum drying oven.
22. Ultracut.
23. Grid (200 or 400 mesh), formvar/carbon-coated.
24. Gilder Reference Locater Grids (Ted Pella, Cat. No. G200F2).

3 Methods

Carry out all procedures at room temperature, unless otherwise specified.

3.1 NMs Sample Preparation

For NMs characterization, the NMs sample should be brought on an EM grid in a state of dispersion which is fit for EM analysis (*see* **Note 1**). In case that the NMs in the stock dispersion or in the administration medium are homogeneous and stable, a small drop of suspension (usually 5–10 μL) is pipetted onto a grid (drop on grid) or float a grid on a droplet of suspension (grid on drop). Allow to stand for 1–15 min (depending on the sample), then the excess of the sample is blotted with filter paper from the edge of the grid, or simply allowed to dry at room temperature (*see* **Note 2**). Powdered NMs may be more difficult to disperse finely divided particles in a liquid, therefore highlighting the importance of vortex mixing and sonication, selection of dispersion solvents, and addition of stabilization agents. After dispersing, NMs are then recovered from suspension either by grid on drop or drop on grid. In case of soft nanomaterials like liposomes, staining with heavy metals is needed for the enhancement of contrast in EM observation (*see* **Note 3**). Uranyl acetate (2%), phosphotungstic acid (1%), and ammonium molybdate (5%) are commonly used stain agents.

3.2 Tissue or Cell Fixation

1. Tissues or cells for conventional EMs analysis should be fixed and dehydrated first. There are two methods of fixation of tissues from organs: perfusion and immersion. The most commonly used method is immersion. Two widely used buffers are phosphate buffer (PBS) and cacodylate buffer; they are not compatible with each other.

2. Immersion fixation: commonly use 2.5% glutaraldehyde in 0.1 M buffer, alternatively, use 4% paraformaldehyde, or 10% formalin in PBS. Paraformaldehyde and formalin penetrate faster than glutaraldehyde, but result in poorer ultrastructure. The largest recommended size of tissues is 1 mm^3, when there is optimal penetration. Proceed to **step 5**.
3. Perfusion fixation: use 2% glutaraldehyde and 2% paraformaldehyde in 0.1 M buffer. The conditions depend upon the animal, its age, and the organs collected for EM assay.
4. For cells (bacteria) fixation: collect cells with 0.5% trypsin–EDTA in an Eppendorf tube by centrifugation, then add 0.5 mL 2.5% glutaraldehyde or 4% paraformaldehyde in 0.1 M PBS to fix cells.
5. Fix tissues or cells for at least 30 min (or store at 4 °C for 1–2 days up to 1 week before subsequent processing). Sometimes, a secondary fixation (postfixation) of the sample is needed, often using 2–4% osmium tetroxide to fixate lipids (*see* **Note 4**).

3.3 Dehydration

Dehydrate sample in ascending concentrations of ethanol (30–100%) for 5–15 min each (*see* **Note 5**). The replacement of the aqueous portion of the sample with ethanol helps the resin to efficiently penetrate into the cells.

3.4 Embedding

1. Add propylene oxide (*see* **Note 6**) or 100% ethanol to the sample and incubate for 3–15 min twice. Then, add a 50:50 resin–propylene oxide (or ethanol, correspondingly) mixture for 30–45 or longer time with Eppendorf tubes capped. The resins commonly used are Epon 812, Araldite 502, Eponate 12, Spurr's, Poly/Bed 812, or LRW resin.
2. Replace the diluted resin mixture with 100% resin and allow resin to infiltrate into the sample for 2–4 h or overnight and change out to fresh resin.
3. Polyethylene capsules are placed in a holder and numbered strips of paper are inserted. A drop of fresh resin is placed in the capsules and the specimen is transferred to the appropriate capsule and cured in 60 °C oven for a day or more.

3.5 Sectioning and Staining

1. Trimming-remove the edge of the block with embedded sample and prepare the block face, then get 1 μm thick sections with Ultracut using diamond knife. Stain the sections with 0.5% toluidine blue for light microscopy observation and screening.
2. Once the region of interest is identified, change the thickness of Ultracut to get thin sections (50–100 nm) of the selected blocks, and mount the thin sections on 200-mesh grids (3–4 sections on one grid).
3. Stain sections with 1% uranyl acetate and 1% lead citrate.

3.6 EMs Operation

Selected sections are mounted on 200-mesh copper grids and examined in a Phillips CM-10 electron microscope equipped with LaB6 cathode (Phillips Electronic Instruments Co. Eindhoven, The Netherlands) operated at 80 kV.

Here is a general operating procedure that the majority of users will apply. Login to the operating PC, load the specimen, and turn the beam on after the vacuum is established. Confirm the operating voltage is at 80 kV and is READY, then switch on the beam current. Focus and center a section, and adjust the brightness and *Z*-axis settings. Center, refocus, and screen the area of interest (*see* **Note 7**).

For high resolution microscopy (HR-TEM), sections are collected on Formvar/carbon coated copper grids (200 mesh, Ted Pella Inc. Redding, CA) without staining for analysis in STEM mode, energy-dispersive X-ray spectroscopy (EDS), and EELS analysis in a JEOL 2010 TEM operated at 200 kV.

3.7 TEM Coupled with EELS

Sample Preparation

1. The sample must be stable in a rarefied environment (e.g., vacuum), and the region around the sample is typically under vacuum so that the electron beam can pass through. Some specialized TEMs (e.g., cryo-EM) or sample holders enable higher pressure or humidity in the vicinity of the sample at the cost of reduced resolution [22, 23]. Usually, biological samples are resin-embedded before EELS analysis.
2. Sometimes, the biological samples prepared for TEM observation are used for EELS analysis. However, in order to obtain a more accurate EELS spectrum, samples should be dehydrated and prepared for resin-embedment using high-pressure freezing protocol or chemical fixing protocol as described previously (*see* **Note 8**) [24].
3. The sections are sliced and picked up on 400 mesh bare copper grid. A clean and electron transparent sample is essential for the EELS analysis. The mostly used slices are about 70–100 nm in thickness, which are equal to the mean free path for 200 kV electron. But in other cases, such as different TEM accelerating voltages or sample geometries, the sample thicknesses are various within bounds.
4. Some imperceptible changes of environmental factors could cause image drift during the analysis and affect the quality of the results. Moreover, samples themselves could also induce image drift, due to the sample charging, improper sample mounting or beam sensitivity. Thus, all of these should be taken into consideration before experiments. To ensure the stability of the sections under the electron beam, the grids supporting the slices are covered with a 5–10 nm carbon film.

TEM Setup for Analysis

5. After the sample is inserted, it would be better to clean its surface with plasma to remove some impurities introduced by synthetic operations.
6. Find the ROI and align the TEM. The alignment process is critical for the analysis quality, especially for energy-filtered TEM (EFTEM).
7. Enter the imaging filter system or EFTEM lens series to make the EELS spectrum and TEM stay at the same focus during the analysis.
8. Locate the filter field to the center of the screen, preview the filtered image and take a thickness map.
9. Select a technique (point measurement or mapping) based on the purpose of the study, such as the concentration, distribution or status of the concerned element.

EELS Spectral Analysis

10. After the beam located, the spectrometer is focused to ensure the adequate signal during the EELS analysis.
11. A low-loss spectrum of the ROI is firstly acquired by reducing the beam spot size and condenser aperture to typical values for microanalysis under diffraction mode on the TEM (*see* **Note 9**). Then the spectrometer is set with variable energy range for the experimental requirements. If two parts with independent energy are needed, dual range EELS is a recommend acquisition mode.
12. Auto exposure mode is used to obtain a high-quality spectrum by reducing the shot noise effectively.
13. After the EELS spectrum acquired, suitable energy edges for the interested elements are selected and identified using the software package provided by the equipment manufacturer. The sample thickness is also analyzed to ensure the energy range is suitable and the plural scattering is insignificant.
14. Fit, extrapolate, and subtract a background model to extract the energy edge intensities for the final spectrum.

More detailed guidance for the experimental and computational procedures of EELS could be found in the chapter written by Aronova and Leapman [24].

3.8 TEM Coupled with STXM

TEM

1. STXM analysis is based on the X-ray absorption of the interested elements, and is usually not interfered by the contaminants originating from the sample preparation (*see* **Note 10**). Therefore, tissues are fixed and dehydrated according to the

conventional protocols for TEM sample preparation without any modification.

2. After the sample is resin-embedded and sliced, the section with a thickness of 50–100 nm is put on a reference grid (as shown in Fig. 13b, also referred to as finder grid, locater grid, and pinpointer grid).
3. TEM is used to photograph the ultrastructure of sample as well as the distribution of nanomaterials.
4. The ROI, usually where the nanomaterials are stacked together, is pinpointed on the TEM image based on the coordinate system of the grid (Fig. 13a, b).

STXM

5. After TEM observation, the very section is then used for STXM imaging. Fix the reference grid on the sample holder and load into the experimental chamber of STXM. Move the ROI into the center of the beam path, determining the XY coordinates of the ROI for STXM analysis (Fig. 13c).
6. Scan the ROI along the XY direction across the stationary X-ray probe, with the transmitted X-ray absorption image collected at a single photon energy (Fig. 13d). Scan the ROI long the XZ or YZ direction to obtain the focal position (the *Z* coordinate position where the adsorption image has the highest spatial resolution).
7. Move the sample along the beam axis to the focal position. And the exact location of ROI for STXM imaging is positioned by comparing the elemental mapping image with the images taken by TEM.
8. With dual-energy ratio contrast analysis method, the in situ 2-dimensional distribution of the interested element can be mapped quantitatively from its absorption difference at selected photon energies.
9. Chemical imaging is done using image sequence (stack) scans over a range of photon energies around the relevant absorption edge of the interested element.
10. Stack images are aligned via a spatial cross-correlation analysis method, and finally, the NEXAFS spectra are extracted from groups of pixels that have similar absorption features within the ROI using the interactive data language (IDL) package aXis2000 (Fig. 13e, f).

4 Notes

1. The primary size of NMs obtained by EMs may be much smaller than the mean size of NMs aggregates in dosing

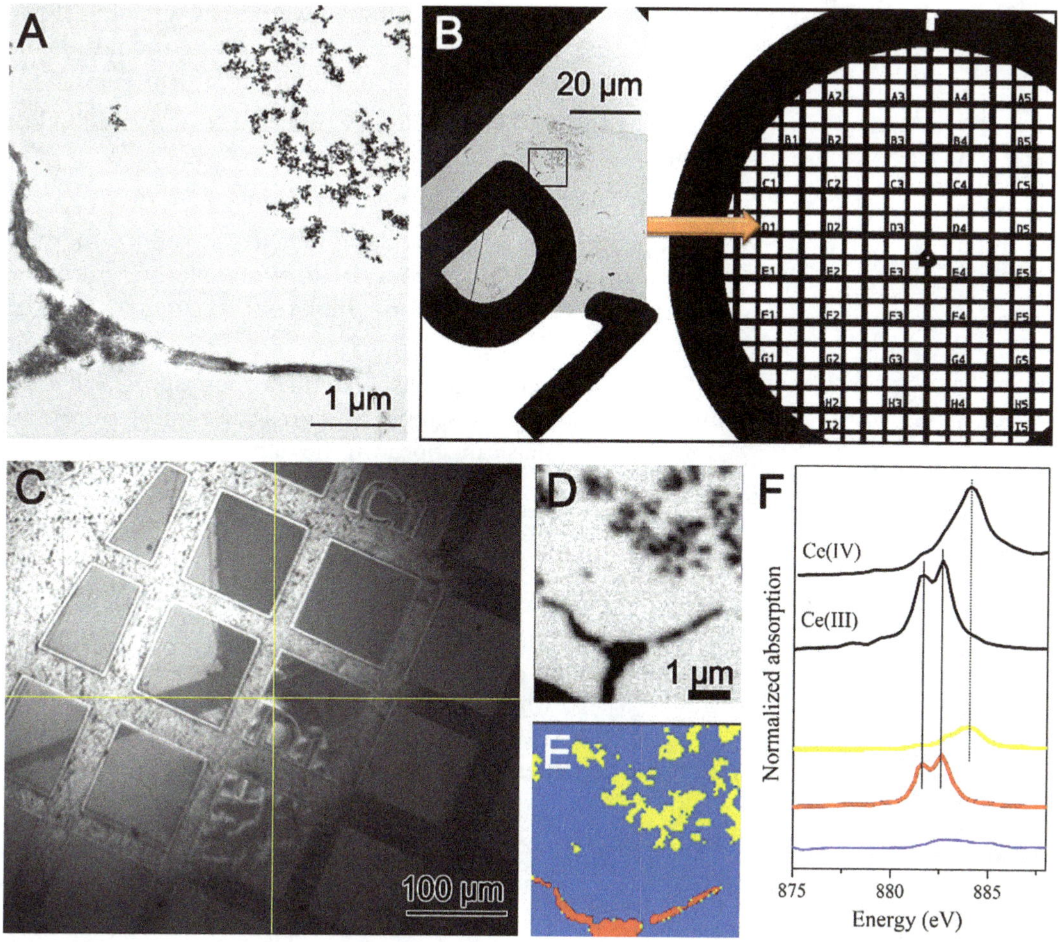

Fig. 13 Schematic illustration of the process of TEM-assisted STXM analysis. (**a**) high-magnification TEM observation to find the region of interest (ROI). (**b**) locating the position of ROI in the coordinate system under low-magnification TEM observation. (**c**) moving the ROI for STXM scanning to the center of beam path. (**d**) the adsorption image of ROI at a selected photon energy. (**e**) the STXM stack image of the ROI. (**f**) NEXAFS spectra extracted from groups of pixels that have similar absorption features within the ROI as shown in (**e**) with the corresponding colors

media, which can be examined with techniques such as dynamic light scattering.

2. If NMs are dispersed with buffer containing a lot of salts (e.g., PBS), the drop of the suspension on the grid should be blotted with filter paper to remove the excess salts. Otherwise, residual salts will form dense crystals on the supporting film of grid during drying, disturbing the subsequent EM observation of NMs.
3. EMs prefer to be used for imaging electron-dense materials (such as metal-based NMs), but not for soft materials.

4. Osmium tetroxide penetrates slower than glutaraldehyde (0.5 mm/h), for most tissues, 1 mm^3 blocks, should not be exposed to osmium for less than 0.5 or more than 1.5 h.
5. The dehydrating times should be adjusted to size and kind of tissue.
6. The propylene oxide used should be from 60 °C oven.
7. The operating settings can be modified to produce the best images of specimens. With this in mind, please return the microscope to the standard mode of operation for the next user.
8. No heavy elements such as uranium or osmium should be introduced during the sample fixation and staining, since spurious EELS signals can appear in the data.
9. EELS spectra should be collected using a low beam current and a short scanning time. Otherwise, the sample slice may be damaged by the electron irradiation, and the chemical state of the interested element may also be shifted.
10. The sample preparation process for EM may bring in contaminants, which are very similar to NMs in appearance and contrast [25]. So when EMs are used to confirm the presence or absence of NMs, the EM results should be further verified by elemental analysis by EDS/EELS or ICP-MS [26].

References

1. Martinet W, Timmermans J-P, De Meyer GRY (2014) Chapter Five - Methods to assess autophagy in situ—transmission electron microscopy versus immunohistochemistry. In: Galluzzi L, Kroemer G (eds) Methods in enzymology, vol 543. Academic Press, New York, NY, pp 89–114. https://doi.org/10.1016/B978-0-12-801329-8.00005-2
2. Wang Y, Santos A, Kaur G, Evdokiou A, Losic D (2014) Structurally engineered anodic alumina nanotubes as nano-carriers for delivery of anticancer therapeutics. Biomaterials 35 (21):5517–5526. https://doi.org/10.1016/j.biomaterials.2014.03.059
3. Hussain S, Al-Nsour F, Rice AB, Marshburn J, Yingling B, Ji Z, Zink JI, Walker NJ, Garantziotis S (2012) Cerium dioxide nanoparticles induce apoptosis and autophagy in human peripheral blood monocytes. ACS Nano 6 (7):5820–5829. https://doi.org/10.1021/nn302235u
4. Bennett MR (2002) Apoptosis in the cardiovascular system. Heart 87(5):480
5. Zhang B, Bian W, Pal A, He Y (2015) Macrophage apoptosis induced by aqueous C60 aggregates changing the mitochondrial membrane potential. Environ Toxicol Pharmacol 39 (1):237–246. https://doi.org/10.1016/j.etap.2014.11.013
6. Zhang Y, Yu W, Jiang X, Lv K, Sun S, Zhang F (2011) Analysis of the cytotoxicity of differentially sized titanium dioxide nanoparticles in murine MC3T3-E1 preosteoblasts. J Mater Sci Mater Med 22(8):1933–1945. https://doi.org/10.1007/s10856-011-4375-7
7. Chen R, Huo L, Shi X, Bai R, Zhang Z, Zhao Y, Chang Y, Chen C (2014) Endoplasmic reticulum stress induced by zinc oxide nanoparticles is an earlier biomarker for nanotoxicological evaluation. ACS Nano 8 (3):2562–2574. https://doi.org/10.1021/nn406184r
8. Tseng MT, Lu X, Duan X, Hardas SS, Sultana R, Wu P, Unrine JM, Graham U, Butterfield DA, Grulke EA, Yokel RA (2012) Alteration of hepatic structure and oxidative stress induced by intravenous nanoceria. Toxicol Appl Pharmacol 260(2):173–182. https://doi.org/10.1016/j.taap.2012.02.008

9. Shindo D, Oikawa T (2013) Analytical electron microscopy for materials science. Springer Science & Business Media, New York, NY
10. Tumolva L, Park J-Y, J-s K, Miller AL, Chow JC, Watson JG, Park K (2010) Morphological and elemental classification of freshly emitted soot particles and atmospheric ultrafine particles using the TEM/EDS. Aerosol Sci Tech 44 (3):202–215
11. Austin CA, Umbreit TH, Brown KM, Barber DS, Dair BJ, Francke-Carroll S, Feswick A, Saint-Louis MA, Hikawa H, Siebein KN (2012) Distribution of silver nanoparticles in pregnant mice and developing embryos. Nanotoxicology 6(8):912–922
12. Shim KH, Jeong K-H, Bae SO, Kang MO, Maeng EH, Choi CS, Kim Y-R, Hulme J, Lee EK, Kim M-K, An SSA (2014) Assessment of ZnO and SiO_2 nanoparticle permeability through and toxicity to the blood–brain barrier using Evans blue and TEM. Int J Nanomedicine 9(Suppl 2):225–233. https://doi.org/10.2147/IJN.S58205
13. Ma Y, He X, Zhang P, Zhang Z, Guo Z, Tai R, Xu Z, Zhang L, Ding Y, Zhao Y (2011) Phytotoxicity and biotransformation of La_2O_3 nanoparticles in a terrestrial plant cucumber (*Cucumis sativus*). Nanotoxicology 5 (4):743–753
14. Zhang P, Ma Y, Zhang Z, He X, Guo Z, Tai R, Ding Y, Zhao Y, Chai Z (2012) Comparative toxicity of nanoparticulate/bulk Yb_2O_3 and $YbCl_3$ to cucumber (*Cucumis sativus*). Environ Sci Technol 46(3):1834–1841
15. Xu M, Li J, Iwai H, Mei Q, Fujita D, Su H, Chen H, Hanagata N (2012) Formation of nano-bio-complex as nanomaterials dispersed in a biological solution for understanding nanobiological interactions. Sci Rep 2:406. https://doi.org/10.1038/srep00406 https://www.nature.com/articles/srep00406#supplementary-information
16. Goode AE, Porter AE, Ryan MP, McComb DW (2015) Correlative electron and X-ray microscopy: probing chemistry and bonding with high spatial resolution. Nanoscale 7 (5):1534–1548
17. Turner S, Lazar S, Freitag B, Egoavil R, Verbeeck J, Put S, Strauven Y, Van Tendeloo G (2011) High resolution mapping of surface reduction in ceria nanoparticles. Nanoscale 3 (8):3385–3390
18. Graham UM, Tseng MT, Jasinski JB, Yokel RA, Unrine JM, Davis BH, Dozier AK, Hardas SS, Sultana R, Grulke EA (2014) In vivo processing of ceria nanoparticles inside liver: impact on free-radical scavenging activity and oxidative stress. ChemPlusChem 79 (8):1083–1088
19. Thill A, Zeyons O, Spalla O, Chauvat F, Rose J, Auffan M, Flank A (2006) Cytotoxicity of CeO_2 nanoparticles for Escherichia coli. Physico-chemical insight of the cytotoxicity mechanism. Environ Sci Technol 40 (19):6151–6156
20. Zhang P, Ma Y, Zhang Z, He X, Zhang J, Guo Z, Tai R, Zhao Y, Chai Z (2012) Biotransformation of ceria nanoparticles in cucumber plants. ACS Nano 6(11):9943–9950
21. Ma Y, Zhang P, Zhang Z, He X, Zhang J, Ding Y, Zhang J, Zheng L, Guo Z, Zhang L (2015) Where does the transformation of precipitated ceria nanoparticles in hydroponic plants take place? Environ Sci Technol 49 (17):10667–10674
22. Dohnalkova AC, Marshall MJ, Arey BW, Williams KH, Buck EC, Fredrickson JK (2011) Imaging hydrated microbial extracellular polymers: comparative analysis by electron microscopy. Appl Environ Microbiol 77 (4):1254–1262
23. Jungjohann K, Evans J, Arslan I, Browning N (2011) Electron energy loss spectroscopy for aqueous in situ scanning transmission electron microscopy. Microsc Microanal 17(S2):778
24. Aronova MA, Leapman RD (2013) Elemental mapping by electron energy loss spectroscopy in biology. In: Sousa AA, Kruhlak MJ (eds) Nanoimaging. Springer, New York, NY, pp 209–226
25. Brandenberger C, Clift MJD, Vanhecke D, Mühlfeld C, Stone V, Gehr P, Rothen-Rutishauser B (2010) Intracellular imaging of nanoparticles: Is it an elemental mistake to believe what you see?. Particle and Fibre Toxicology 7 (1):15
26. He X, Zhang Z, Liu J, Ma Y, Zhang P, Li Y, Wu Z, Zhao Y, Chai Z (2011) Quantifying the biodistribution of nanoparticles. Nature Nanotechnology 6 (12):755–755

Chapter 15

Metabolic Fingerprinting of Bacteria Exposed to Nanomaterials, Using Online Databases, NMR, and High-Resolution Mass Spectrometry

Theodoros G. Chatzimitakos and Constantine D. Stalikas

Abstract

Nanomaterials are examined more and more for their antibacterial properties. Herein, we propose a method for assessing the bactericidal properties of nanomaterials against *Escherichia coli* and *Staphylococcus aureus*, as well as a method to investigate the metabolic alterations occurring to bacteria, induced by their exposure to nanomaterials. Bacterial metabolome is extracted and metabolic fingerprint is recorded by ^{1}H-NMR. Using metabolomic databases, the tentative metabolites in the samples are revealed, which are further confirmed by UHPLC-HRMS. Finally, conducting a pathway analysis, the metabolic network is revealed.

Key words Metabolomics, Nanomaterials, Bacteria, *Escherichia coli*, *Staphylococcus aureus*, Antibacterial properties, Metabolite extraction, ^{1}H-NMR, UHPLC-HRMS, Fingerprint

1 Introduction

Nanomaterials have come into their own as a novel and highly promising class of antimicrobial materials. Their main advantage over common antibiotics lies within the mechanisms via which the antimicrobial action is achieved, which hinder the development of resistance [1]. Their antibacterial action can be categorized into oxidative stress mechanisms, metal ion release, and nonoxidative mechanisms [1, 2]. However, the proposed modes of action are not always thoroughly examined in molecular/metabolic level, despite the fact that survivability of microorganisms depends on the metabolic processes [3]. Metabolomics can shed light upon the metabolic alterations occurring in the metabolome of an organism [2]. Conducting metabolomic studies can be a challenge due to the complexity of the results. Moreover, the experimental procedures are tricky, requiring care and skills, because even the smallest errors can significantly affect the results [4]. Therefore, well-grounded experimental protocols, combined with high-edge

Qunwei Zhang (ed.), *Nanotoxicity: Methods and Protocols*, Methods in Molecular Biology, vol. 1894, https://doi.org/10.1007/978-1-4939-8916-4_15,

analytical techniques (i.e., nuclear magnetic resonance spectroscopy and mass spectrometry) are a requisite for a reliable outcome.

Herein, we demonstrate an experimental protocol for evaluating the bactericidal properties of nanomaterials against *Escherichia coli* and *Staphylococcus aureus* (other bacteria can also be employed, with minor modifications of the procedure, as will be mentioned in Subheading 4), as well as a protocol for conducting an untargeted metabolomic fingerprint analysis of bacteria, exposed to various nanomaterials. Obtaining cell viability information with the technique used for the metabolic fingerprint is mandatory for two main reasons: firstly, to assess the optimum conditions for conducting the metabolomic fingerprinting and secondly, to correlate metabolic alterations to cell viability. The proposed protocol combines simple, yet reliable procedures for bacterial cell growth, exposure to nanoparticles and harvesting, as well as an effective metabolites extraction step (Fig. 1) along with the analysis of the resulting pooled samples using proton nuclear magnetic resonance (^{1}H-NMR) and ultra-high-pressure liquid chromatography/high resolution/high accuracy mass spectrometry (UHPLC-HRMS) (Fig. 2). Furthermore, the obtained data can be deconvoluted using online free metabolic databases (e.g., *E. coli* Metabolome Database and MetaboAnalyst) (Fig. 2) [5, 6]. Meticulous execution of the proposed protocol ensures reproducibility and thus, different batches of microorganisms can be used. Overall, with the proposed protocol, results for global metabolic fingerprint profiling can be obtained along with an evaluation of the bactericidal properties of nanomaterials [2, 7].

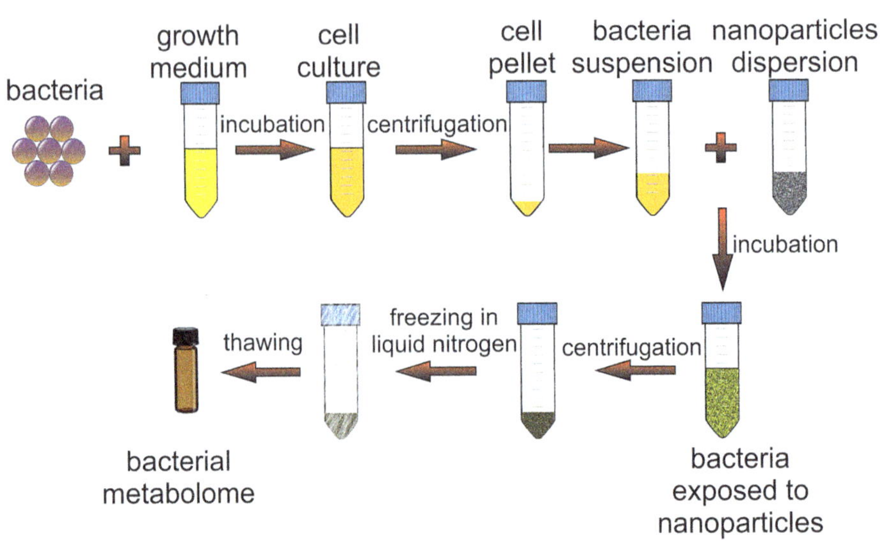

Fig. 1 Step-by-step procedure for the bacterial cell growth, exposure to nanoparticles, harvesting, and extraction of metabolites for the metabolomic fingerprinting

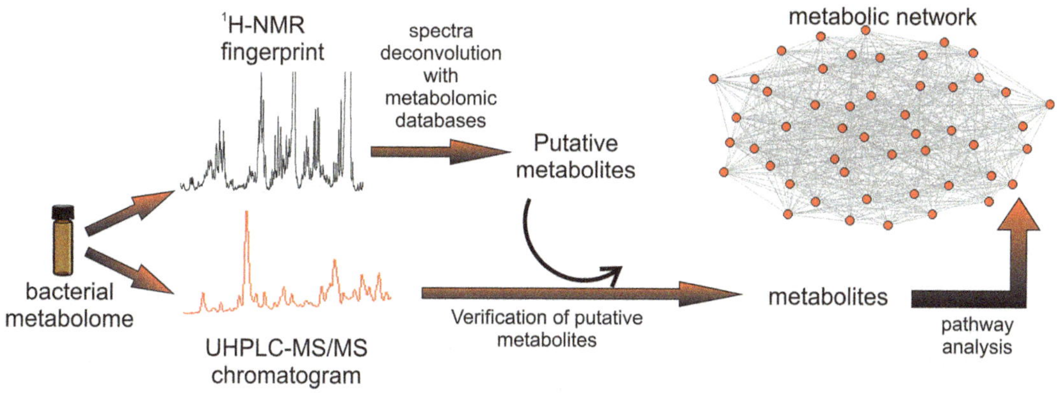

Fig. 2 Workflow to obtain untargeted metabolomic fingerprint data for exposed bacterial species using proton nuclear magnetic resonance, ultrahigh-pressure liquid chromatography/high-resolution/high-accuracy mass spectrometry and metabolic databases

2 Materials

Prepare all solutions using double distilled water or other of highest available purity, as well as analytical grade reagents. Sterilize all solutions, glassware, tips, eppendorf tubes, and everything else used, by autoclaving at 121 °C for 20 min, at 15 psi. Avoid contact of microorganisms with metal utensils, since mortality may occur. The growth medium for cell cultures was prepared as follows:

1. Lysogeny Broth (LB): Dissolve 10.0 g NaCl, 5.0 g yeast extract, and 10.0 g bacteriological peptone in about 0.95 L water (*see* **Note 1**). Adjust pH to 7.4 with NaOH 5 M (approximately 0.2 mL), at 25 °C. Add water to a volume of 1 L and mix well. Sterilize by autoclaving and store at 4 °C (*see* **Note 2**).
2. Lysogeny Broth plates: Add 15.0 g agar to 1 L LB prior to autoclaving. After sterilization, pour in petri plates the proper amount of broth and let cool. Store inverted at 4 °C in plastic bags (*see* **Note 3**).
3. Isotonic saline solution (ISS): Dissolve 9.0 g NaCl in 0.9 L water and make up to 1 L. Autoclave and store at 4 °C.

3 Methods

All experiments must be conducted in sterile conditions. Carry out experiments either in a laminar flow hood or with the use of a Bunsen burner/Fireboy™ (INTEGRA Biosciences AG, Switzerland). Disinfect the working bench thoroughly, using ethanol (*see* **Note 4**). The time needed to complete each of the following steps must be highly reproducible and strictly controlled so as to maximize the between-day reproducibility of the experiments.

3.1 Cell Cultures

1. Prepare bacterial preinocula of each bacterial species (*Escherichia coli* or *Staphylococcus aureus*) by transferring a small amount of a single clonal population of cells to a fixed amount of LB (e.g., 10 mL) (*see* **Notes 5** and **6**). Incubate at 37 °C for 10 h and 16 h for *Staphylococcus aureus* and *Escherichia coli*, respectively, at 250 rpm (*see* **Notes 7–9**).
2. Inoculate 2.0 mL of a fresh preinoculum in 200 mL of LB and incubate further, at 37 °C for 10 h and 16 h, for *Staphylococcus aureus* and *Escherichia coli*, respectively.

3.2 Cell Pellet Formation

1. Centrifuge the bacterial culture in six sterile, preweighed, falcon tubes (~35 mL of culture in each tube) at 900 × *g*, for 5 min (*see* **Note 10**).
2. Remove the supernatant and add 30 mL of ISS in the cell pellets. After mild hand mixing for 10 s, centrifuge at 900 × *g* for 5 min (*see* **Note 11**).
3. Repeat the two previous steps twice more.
4. Weigh out the falcon tubes containing the cell pellets and write down the weights. Calculate the cell pellet weight by subtracting the initial weight of the falcon tube from the total weight.

3.3 Incubation of Bacteria with Nanomaterials

1. Resuspend the previously prepared cell pellets (*see* **Note 12**) in a fixed amount (*see* **Note 13**) of ISS (*see* **Note 11**).
2. Measure the optical density of the cell suspension at 540 nm and verify that the optical density is 0.20 ± 0.01 A.U (*see* **Note 14**).
3. Add an equal volume of ISS containing twice the desired concentration of the tested nanomaterials prepared beforehand (*see* **Notes 15** and **16**).
4. Incubate at 37 °C, under stirring at 250 rpm, for the desired length of time.

3.4 Cell Viability Assessment

1. During incubation of cells with the nanomaterials (*see* **step 4** in Subheading 3.3), retract 0.1 mL of sample at a specified time and transfer into an eppendorf tube containing 0.9 mL of ISS (*see* **Notes 17** and **18**).
2. Mix well by mild hand shaking.
3. Transfer 0.1 mL of the resulting solution into a new eppendorf containing 0.9 mL of ISS and mix well by hand shaking.
4. Repeat the above step until the desired dilution is achieved (*see* **Notes 19** and **20**).
5. Take 0.1 mL from the solution with the desired dilution and spread onto LB agar plates.
6. Incubate at 37 °C until CFUs can be observed (*see* **Note 21**).
7. Count CFUs in each plate and compare with control sample.

3.5 Metabolite Extraction

1. After completing incubation in **step 4** (Subheading 3.3) for a specified time, centrifuge the solution at 900 × *g*, at 4 °C for 5 min, in falcon tubes (*see* **Note 22**).
2. Discard the supernatant.
3. Add ~35 mL of ISS and hand mix for 10 s (*see* **Note 23**).
4. Repeat **steps 1–3** and discard the supernatant ISS.
5. Add 0.5 mL of cold methanol (−80 °C) to the resulting pellet.
6. Vortex for 30 s.
7. Place the falcon tubes in liquid nitrogen for 2 min.
8. Remove the falcon tubes from liquid nitrogen and wait for complete thawing (*see* **Note 24**).
9. Repeat **steps** 7 and **8** twice more.
10. After the last freeze–thaw cycle, centrifuge at 900 × *g* for 5 min, at −4 °C.
11. Transfer the supernatant into an amber glass vial (*see* **Note 25**).
12. Repeat **steps 5–11** twice more (*see* **Note 26**).
13. Thaw and mix well pooled supernatants by vortexing for 30 s.
14. Transfer half quantity of the solution to an NMR glass tube (*see* **Notes 27–29**).
15. Evaporate methanol to dryness with a gentle nitrogen stream (*see* **Note 30**).
16. Add 0.5 mL deuterated methanol in the NMR tube (*see* **Note 31**), ultrasonicate for 10 s and record the ^{1}H-NMR spectrum (*see* **Notes 32–34**).
17. Evaporate the remaining half quantity of the pooling supernatants to dryness (*see* **Note 35**) with a gentle nitrogen stream (**Notes 27**, **28**, and **30** must also apply in this step).
18. Resuspend in 200 μL of organic solvent (*see* **Note 36**) (**Notes 31–33** must also apply in this step).
19. Filter the solution through a 0.22 syringe filter and inject into UHPLC-HRMS (*see* **Note 37**).

3.6 Data Deconvolution

1. Record the ^{1}H-NMR peaks from the obtained spectrum and input to a metabolomics NMR database (*see* **Notes 38** and **39**).
2. Write down the results and record the exact mass of each metabolite (with four decimal figures).
3. Scan the UHPLC-HRMS chromatograms for the exact mass of each metabolite resulting from the above step (*see* **Note 40**).
4. Metabolite assignment should be done by matching accurate mass, isotopic distribution and fragmentation patterns with bibliographic data/database (*see* **Note 41**) and/or retention times compared with pure standards.

5. Subject metabolites to pathway analysis (*see* **Note 42**) and note down the pathways in which the metabolites are involved.

4 Notes

1. Do not add directly 1 L of water since the volume of the solution increases when the components are dissolved in water. Magnetic stirring is highly recommended for hastening the dissolution and dissolving lumps easier. Heating can be used to assist the dissolution process, but avoid unnecessary heating of the solution after dissolution is completed. After complete dissolving, the solution will have a translucent yellowish color.
2. LB broth can be stored at room temperature for a few days; storing at 4 °C is most preferred.
3. After sterilization, let cool slightly, so that the flask can be touched, but do not cool too much, since agar solidifies. It is recommended that a water bath at ~50 °C be used to keep broth at a proper temperature for handling. LB plates must be stored inverted, in plastic bags, to avoid drying out.
4. All materials are considered infectious after coming in contact with the bacteria, so they must be disinfected/sterilized before disposal/reuse.
5. Avoid using LB directly from 4 °C, since the bacteria are stressed at low temperature. Before transferring the bacteria to the LB, ensure that the growth medium has reached a temperature of 37 °C.
6. The protocol developed herein can also apply to other bacteria species. To do so, physical (i.e., temperature, pH, osmotic pressure, oxygen levels) and chemical (i.e., energy sources, growth factors) bacterial growth requirements must be met for optimum bacterial growth. Thus, LB can be substituted for another growth medium, suitable for each bacteria species.
7. Control strictly the time of incubation in order to obtain reproducible results. The two bacteria species reported herein, double in number in approximately 20 min, under optimum conditions. Thus, small variations in incubation time can result in a great deal of variation in their metabolic profiles.
8. The time needed for incubation derives from the bacterial growth curve. Incubation must stop at the end of the exponential phase, before entering stationary phase. If the growth curve for the tested bacteria species is unknown it is suggested that a curve should be drawn before conducting further experiments [7].

9. After incubation, cell preinocula must be used immediately, instead of being stored at 4 °C for later use, in order to achieve better reproducibility in the resulting metabolic fingerprint. During storage of the preinoculum, metabolic alterations progress, at a reduced rate, resulting in uncontrolled errors in the metabolic fingerprints.
10. Cell culture must be dispensed into different falcon tubes and all cells must be centrifuged simultaneously for reproducibility reasons. Avoid collecting all cells in two falcon tubes by sequential centrifugations, supernatant removal, cell culture addition etc. In this case, cell metabolic processes proceed freely and the last batch of cell culture contains cells, whose metabolome may significantly vary from the first batch of bacteria.
11. The ISS must be thermostatted at 37 °C to minimize variations in cell pellet temperature.
12. Cell pellets must be used immediately after preparation. Although they can be stored at ~20 °C after preparation, it is preferable to avoid it. This way, variations in their metabolism are minimized and higher reproducibility is ensured.
13. Before conducting the experiment, prepare a graph/table of the amount of ISS vs. the weight of the bacterial cell pellet, so that a cell suspension with $OD_{540} = 0.2$ A.U. can be prepared. Separate species-specific graphs/tables must be prepared for each microbial species.
14. Variations in the optical density among the cell suspensions must be as low as possible to ensure that samples are comparable and achieve high between-day reproducibility. Since the optical density is nearly the same for samples, almost the same number of bacterial cells is present in all samples.
15. Before adding the nanomaterial-containing ISS, make certain that nanoparticles have been well dispersed using ultrasonication, since after mixing of the two solutions no ultrasonication can be applied, because cell death definitely occurs.
16. Before mixing with the cell suspension, the solution containing the nanomaterials must be at 37 °C.
17. Since serial dilutions follow this step flush well the pipette tips to remove bacteria by pipetting 3–4 times, in order to minimize dilution errors regarding the number of bacteria.
18. At this step, a dilution of 1:10 is suggested. Other dilutions are applicable, such as 1:100 or even 1:1000. However, a scaling up of the volume of ISS and sample should be considered, in order to obtain reproducible and comparable results and minimize dilution errors. The suggested 1:10 dilution was found to be more workable in terms of reproducibility and lower consumption of ISS.

19. The plate counting method employed to assess cell viability requires 50–250 colony forming units (CFUs) in each plate. More than 250 CFUs are difficult to count, whereas lower than 50 CFUs yield statistically unreliable results. It is rather tricky to determine which of the serial dilutions finally results in the desired number of CFUs in the plate. Therefore, plating from different eppendorf/dilutions is suggested when the experiment is conducted for the first time in order to determine the most suitable dilution factor.
20. Often 3–5 serial dilutions (1:10) are needed.
21. Incubate the plates by turning them upside down. Usually, 24 h are adequate for CFUs to grow to a sufficient size; in certain situations, up to 48 h may be needed depending on the bacteria species.
22. Centrifuge the solution simultaneously, in different falcon tubes.
23. The ISS used in this step must have a temperature of 4 °C.
24. Immediately after complete thawing, snap-freeze again in liquid nitrogen.
25. Use amber glass vials to protect metabolites from light. Before repeating **steps 5–11** of Subheading 3.5, store the vial in liquid nitrogen to avoid metabolite interactions/degradation and thus metabolome alterations.
26. The supernatants from each freeze–thaw cycle are pooled together in the same amber glass vial.
27. The tube should be covered with aluminum foil to avoid exposure of the solution to light.
28. The tube is placed beforehand in a cooling bath of ice-sodium chloride (3:1 w/w).
29. The remaining quantity of the pooled supernatants either is placed in liquid nitrogen until completion of the evaporation of methanol in the NMR glass tube or is processed following **step 17** simultaneously with **step 15** of Subheading 3.5.
30. During evaporation, the tube should remain in a cooling bath.
31. Add deuterated methanol in the tube maintained in a cooling bath. Deuterated methanol must be cold (−20 °C). Then, purge the glass tube with an inert gas (e.g., nitrogen or preferably argon) and seal before proceeding to the next steps so as to protect the metabolome from oxygen.
32. The tube must be wrapped with aluminum foil until recording the NMR spectrum.
33. Deuterated methanol must be added before recording the ^{1}H-NMR data. If the spectrum is not going to be recorded immediately after evaporation of methanol, seal the NMR tube

(filled with inert gas) tightly and store in liquid nitrogen. If deuterated methanol is to be added, instruction of **Note 30** must also be followed. Our experience showed that storing in liquid nitrogen does not affect the metabolome.

34. The use of cryogenically cooled NMR probe heads is suggested to alleviate the relatively low sensitivity of the technique [8].
35. Either evaporate methanol directly in the amber glass vial or transfer it into an appropriate vial for UHPLC auto sampler.
36. The organic solvent should be the same with that used in the UHPLC mobile phase.
37. Use both positive and negative ionization modes to unveil suppressed signals [2].
38. Using the 1D-NMR search engine of ECMDB (*E. coli* metabolome database, found online at www.ecmdb.ca) is highly recommended [6]. Additionally, the 1D-NMR search engine of Human Metabolome Database [9] and/or Madison Metabolomics Consortium Database [10] can be used.
39. At this point, do not neglect any of the recorded results. All metabolites are putative and their presence cannot be ruled out until further examination of the metabolome extracts with MS is carried out.
40. Acceptable mass accuracy should be lower than 5 ppm.
41. ECMDB [6], HMDB [9], Madison Metabolomics Consortium Database [10], METLIN [11], MassBank [12], and NIST are highly suitable, since they provide adequate spectral information for each metabolite.
42. MetaboAnalyst [5] (found online at www.metaboanalyst.ca) is suggested for conducting pathway analysis.

References

1. Wang L, Hu C, Shao L (2017) The antimicrobial activity of nanoparticles: present situation and prospects for the future. Int J Nanomedicine 12:1227–1249. https://doi.org/10.2147/IJN.S121956
2. Chatzimitakos TG, Stalikas CD (2016) Qualitative alterations of bacterial metabolome after exposure to metal nanoparticles with bactericidal properties: a comprehensive workflow based on ^{1}H NMR, UHPLC-HRMS, and metabolic databases. J Proteome Res 15 (9):3322–3330. https://doi.org/10.1021/acs.jproteome.6b00489
3. Liebeke M, Lalk M (2014) Staphylococcus aureus metabolic response to changing environmental conditions – a metabolomics perspective. Int J Med Microbiol 304 (3):222–229. https://doi.org/10.1016/j.ijmm.2013.11.017
4. Kosmides AK, Kamisoglu K, Calvano SE et al (2013) Metabolomic fingerprinting: challenges and opportunities. Crit Rev Biomed Eng 41(3):205–221. https://doi.org/10.1615/CritRevBiomedEng.2013007736
5. Xia J, Wishart DS (2002) Using MetaboAnalyst 3.0 for comprehensive metabolomics data analysis. In: Current protocols in bioinformatics. John Wiley & Sons, Inc, New York, NY. https://doi.org/10.1002/cpbi.11
6. Sajed T, Marcu A, Ramirez M et al (2016) ECMDB 2.0: a richer resource for understanding the biochemistry of E. coli. Nucleic Acids Res 44(Database issue):D495–D501. https://doi.org/10.1093/nar/gkv1060

7. Chatzimitakos T, Kallimanis A, Avgeropoulos A, Stalikas CD (2016) Antibacterial, anti-biofouling, and antioxidant prospects of metal-based nanomaterials. Clean (Weinh) 44(7):794–802. https://doi.org/10.1002/clen.201500366
8. Chatzimitakos T, Exarchou V, Ordoudi SA, Fiamegos Y, Stalikas C (2016) Ion-pair assisted extraction followed by ^{1}H NMR determination of biogenic amines in food and biological matrices. Food Chem 202:445–450. https://doi.org/10.1016/j.foodchem.2016.02.013
9. Wishart DS, Jewison T, Guo AC, Wilson M et al (2013) HMDB 3.0—the human metabolome database in 2013. Nucleic Acids Res 41 (Database issue):D801–D807. https://doi.org/10.1093/nar/gks1065
10. Cui Q, Lewis IA, Hegeman AD et al (2008) Metabolite identification via the Madison Metabolomics Consortium Database. Nat Biotechnol 26:162. https://doi.org/10.1038/nbt0208-162
11. Tautenhahn R, Cho K, Uritboonthai W, Zhu Z, Patti GJ, Siuzdak G (2012) An accelerated workflow for untargeted metabolomics using the METLIN database. Nat Biotechnol 30(9):826–828. https://doi.org/10.1038/nbt.2348
12. Horai H, Arita M, Kanaya S et al (2010) MassBank: a public repository for sharing mass spectral data for life sciences. J Mass Spectrom 45 (7):703–714. https://doi.org/10.1002/jms.1777

Chapter 16

Methods to Quantify Nanomaterial Association with, and Distribution Across, the Blood–Brain Barrier In Vivo

Robert A. Yokel

Abstract

The role and functional anatomy of the blood–brain barrier (BBB) is summarized to enable the investigator to appropriately address evaluation of nanomaterial interaction with, and distribution across, it into brain tissue (parenchyma). Transport mechanisms across the BBB are presented, in relation to nanomaterial physicochemical properties. Measures and test substances to assess BBB integrity/disruption/permeation are introduced, along with how they are used to interpret the results obtained with the presented methods. Experimental pitfalls and misinterpretation of results of studies of brain nanomaterial uptake are briefly summarized, that can be avoided with the methods presented in this chapter. Two methods are presented. The in situ brain perfusion technique is used to determine rate and extent of nanomaterial distribution into the brain. The capillary depletion method separates brain parenchymal tissue from the endothelial cells that contribute to the BBB. It is used to verify nanomaterial brain tissue entry. These methods are best used together, the latter refining the results obtained with the former. Details of the materials and equipment needed to conduct these methods, and description of the procedures and data interpretation, are provided.

Key words Blood–brain barrier, Brain parenchyma enrichment, Capillary depletion, In situ brain perfusion, In vivo, Rat

1 Introduction

To appropriately address nanomaterial interaction with, and distribution across, the blood–brain barrier (BBB) requires an understanding of the BBB's roles and the functional anatomy, physiology, and biochemistry supporting its roles. The BBB has multiple roles. (1) It protects the brain from rapid changes in the level of some substances in the blood that are able to penetrate the BBB and disrupt the brain, such as amino acids. (2) It enables the distribution of some substances from blood to the brain that are needed for brain metabolism, such as glucose and iron. (3) It greatly inhibits the distribution of most pathogens and toxic substances, protecting the brain from their effects while presenting a significant challenge to the intended delivery of therapeutic agents to the brain.

Qunwei Zhang (ed.), *Nanotoxicity: Methods and Protocols*, Methods in Molecular Biology, vol. 1894, https://doi.org/10.1007/978-1-4939-8916-4_16,

The anatomical components of the BBB include the brain microvascular endothelial cells (BMECs) which line the microvessels forming the luminal side of the BBB. They have a near total absence of fenestrations through which substances might diffuse. BMECs differ from endothelial cells that line the vasculature outside of the brain by their inclusion of tight junctions which are formed between adjacent BMECs. When intact the tight junctions prevent passage of ionic substances as small as lanthanum (hydrated ionic diameter ~0.8 nm) through this paracellular barrier [1]. Proteins maintain the tight junctions, providing indicators for functional BBB alteration, including claudins, occludin, zonula occludens-1, junctional adhesion molecules (e.g., ICAM-1), cingulin, annexin A1, VE-cadherin, PECAM-1, and laminins. Microvessels totally perfuse the brain from within this organ [2]. They are comprised of 100 billion capillaries, ~400 miles (600 km) long, with a surface area of 20 m^2 in the human, providing a blood vessel within ~10 μm of every brain cell [3]. They occupy ~2% of the brain volume in the cortex and a greater space in some other brain regions [4, 5]. A basement membrane surrounds the abluminal side of the BMECs. Within the basement membrane are pericytes that cover ~30% of the BMEC surface. Astrocyte foot processes extend to cover >90% of the abluminal BMEC surface. Neurons interact with this complex of cells to form the neurovascular unit.

The ability of some substances to cross the BBB, whereas others are less or unable to do so, is a function of the physicochemical properties of the substance and the transporters and metabolic processes of the neurovascular unit, primarily in the BMECs. Diffusion of small molecules through the BBB is a product of lipophilicity and the reciprocal of their size [6, 7], limiting lipid-mediated diffusion to small molecules that are <~400 Da and that form <8 hydrogen bonds [8]. This rules out nanomaterial distribution across the intact BBB by diffusion; for example, a 1 nm^3 gold particle containing 31 atoms would be ~6100 Da. Therefore, diffusion-mediated nanomaterial brain entry requires opening the BBB tight junctions (paracellular transport) or distribution across the BMECs (transcellular transport). The BBB can be intentionally opened by osmotic insult, e.g., 25% mannitol infusion into a carotid artery which provides direct delivery of blood to the ipsilateral hemisphere. Focused ultrasound in conjunction with systemically circulating microbubbles has also been used to open the BBB, as the ultrasound causes the microbubbles to expand and contract, putting shear stress on the BBB. Both methods have been used to deliver chemotherapy drugs to treat brain tumors. Conversely, BBB opening can be an adverse effect of nanomaterials that are not intended to be delivered to the brain.

Although nanomaterials are unable to distribute across the intact BBB by diffusion they have the potential to enter the brain via transcellular, carrier-mediated, transporters. These include nutrient transporters (e.g., GLUT-1 that provides the brain with glucose that the brain cannot generate), metal transporters (e.g., that influx iron), and receptor-mediated transporters, such as for transferrin and low-density lipoprotein [9]. The mechanism of nanomaterial uptake into BMECs is via clathrin-coated pit endocytosis [10].

ATP-binding cassette transporters such as P-glycoprotein and multidrug resistance protein inhibit brain entry by effluxing many structurally diverse organics, including many drugs. Metabolic processes, including peptidases, CYP 450-linked monooxygenases, and conjugation mechanisms, also inhibit flux across the BBB.

BBB permeability in animals and/or in vitro models can be measured using substances that do not cross the intact barrier. Historically, and currently, this has been done with Evan's blue. Many substances have been used, as shown in Table 1. Small markers might indicate less extensive opening than larger ones. Some, such as sucrose, are paracellular markers; others, such as albumin, are transcellular markers. An additional use of these markers is as vascular volume/extracellular space markers in the in situ brain perfusion technique (below). These markers indicate the vascular and extracellular spaces (volume) of the perfusion fluid containing test substance (nanomaterial), compared to the brain cellular space (test substance uptake into brain parenchyma).

In vitro BBB models have been extensively studied for decades [11]. Their complexity can range from cultured BMECs to cocultures that include astrocytes, to triple cocultures that include pericytes. As complexity increases the in vivo BBB is more closely modeled. An indicator of BBB integrity, in addition to the use of chemical permeation markers (above), is the transepithelial electrical resistance (TEER) across the cells. The TEER of immortalized BMEC monoculture is usually <50 mΩ cm^2 [12] to 200 mΩ cm^2 [13]. Monocultures of primary BMECS seldom exceed 500 mΩ cm^2 [12]. A coculture of BMECs with TEER >600 mΩ cm^2 has been described [13]. The TEER of arterial and venous vessels in 21 day and older anesthetized rats averaged 1490 mΩ cm^2 and 918 mΩ cm^2, respectively, and as great as 5900 mΩ cm^2 [14]. A monoculture of human-induced pluripotent stem cells differentiated into BMECs had some TEER values exceeding 2000 mΩ cm^2, but allowed permeation of IgG to a greater extent than seen in mammalian brain [12], suggesting even this in vitro BBB model was not as impermeable as the mammalian BBB.

In addition to the above chemical and electrical indicators of BBB permeability, which indicate the pharmacokinetic integrity of the BBB as a measure of nanotoxicity, many methods have been used to indicate toxicity to BBB anatomy and function. These assays most commonly focus on junction proteins mentioned

Table 1
Substances to quantify BBB permeability (or its reciprocal, integrity) and to determine the volume of the vascular and extracellular spaces of the perfusion fluid-containing test substance (nanomaterial) in harvested brain tissue. The table lists substances in ascending order of their size and some commonly used quantification methods

Substance	Size (Da)	Concentration in intra-carotid perfusion fluid[a] Intravenous concentration or dose[b]	Quantification method(s)
^{3}H- or ^{14}C-α-amino isobutyric acid	103	^{3}H 1 or ^{14}C 0.5 μCi/mL[a] ^{14}C 10–80 μCi[b] [48, 49]	Radiation counting
^{3}H- or D-[$1\text{-}^{14}C$] mannitol	182	^{3}H 1 or ^{14}C 0.5 μCi/mL, 10 μCi[a] [50, 51] ^{3}H 15 μCi[b] [52]	Radiation counting
Fluorescein	334	0.1%[a] [53] 0.1%[b] [54]	Fluorescence (excitation λ_{max} 493 nm, emission λ_{max} 514 nm)
^{3}H- or U-^{14}C-sucrose	342	^{3}H 1 or ^{14}C 0.5 μCi/mL[a] ^{14}C 10–80 μCi[b] [48, 55]	Radiation counting
Lucifer yellow	457	5 mM[a] [56] 25 mg[b] [57]	Fluorescence (excitation λ_{max} 380 nm, emission λ_{max} 542 nm)
Gadolinium-diethylenetriamine pentaacetic acid (DTPA) complex	938	0.6 mmol/kg[a] [58] 0.4 mmol/kg[b] [50]	MRI or Gd ICP-MS elemental analysis
^{3}H- or U-^{14}C-inulin	~5000–5500	^{3}H 1 or ^{14}C 0.5 μCi/mL[a] [38] ^{3}H 30 to 50 μCi[b] [55, 59] ^{14}C 4 μCi[b] [52]	Radiation counting
Carboxyl-[^{14}C]-inulin	~6200	0.5 μCi/mL[1]	Radiation counting
Horseradish peroxidase	44,000	2.5 mg/min[a] [60] 34 mg/kg[b] [61]	Forms a brown reaction product with diaminobenzidine (λ_{max} 465) or a blue product with *o*-dianisidine (λ_{max} 460 nm)
Evan's blue + albumin complex	~66,000	0.1% Evan's blue[a] [53] 2% Evan's blue solution[b] [62, 63]	VIS spectroscopy (λ_{max} 620 nm; Evan's blue) immunocytochemistry (albumin)
FITC-albumin		10 mg/min[a] [64] 28–56 mg/kg[b] [65]	Fluorescence (excitation λ_{max} 495 nm, emission λ_{max} 525 nm) Immunohistochemistry
FITC-dextran	Variable, 70,000 typically used	5–750 mg/kg[b] [62, 66, 67]	Fluorescence (excitation λ_{max} 492 nm, emission λ_{max} 518 nm)

(continued)

Table 1
(continued)

Substance	Size (Da)	Concentration in intra-carotid perfusion fluid[a] Intravenous concentration or dose[b]	Quantification method(s)
^{3}H- or ^{14}C-dextran		^{3}H 1 or ^{14}C 0.5 μCi/mL[a] ^{3}H 30 μCi[b] [55] ^{14}C 4 μCi[b] [52]	Radiation counting
Alexa 488-labeled IgG	155,000	10 mg/kg[b] [68]	Fluorescence (excitation λ_{max} 490 nm, emission λ_{max} 525 nm)
Biotinylated IgG		28 mg/kg[b] [65]	Immunohistochemistry
IgG		Endogenous in blood	Immunohistochemistry

above; claudins, occludin, and zonula occludens-1 [15, 16], or use electron microscopy [17].

In vitro BBB models are incomplete in their cell composition, cell interactions, cell spatial relationships, and degree of impermeability compared to the in vivo neurovascular unit. Therefore, the methods described in this chapter enable the in vivo determination of nanomaterial association with, and distribution across, the BBB with verification of brain (parenchymal, neuropil) entry.

There have been studies addressing brain entry of many nanomaterials with the conclusion that they get into the brain, which is different than crossing the BBB and entering brain tissue. For most studies the methods employed were not able to confirm nanomaterial distribution into brain parenchyma because they do not account for nanomaterial in the blood within the brain's vasculature or associated with BBB components. Rats perfused to remove blood 4 h after intravenous injection of gold glyconanoparticles had only ~4% as much nanomaterial in their brain as rats that had not been perfused [18]. Similarly, vascular perfusion reduced gold in three brain regions to 7–18% of that seen in nonperfused rats after intra-abdominal nanogold injection [19]. Some studies accounted for the contribution of nanomaterial in blood to brain nanomaterial levels [5, 20, 21], however this does not address nanomaterial in nonbrain tissue sites such as adsorption to the luminal wall of brain vasculature or in cellular and membrane BBB components. After intravenous injection to rodents, nanomaterials were observed adhered to brain blood vessel walls with little to no evidence of brain tissue entry [22–24]. These observations are in agreement with a kinetic study that reported a negatively charged nanoparticle associated with the cell surface, within seconds, by Langmuir adsorption through electrostatic interaction

[25]. In several studies, nanomaterial associated with brain at short-term time points did not persist to later times. The rapid decline of nanomaterial within a few hours in the whole brain or brain regions, for example [19, 26–33], can be interpreted as not reflecting brain tissue nanomaterial entry. This is because it would not be anticipated that nanomaterials, once taken up by brain cells, would be released and distribute from brain back into blood within this time. These results suggest that not all of the nanomaterial interpreted as entering the brain distributed into brain tissue. The nanomaterial may have adhered to the luminal wall of brain vasculature or localized in cellular or membrane components of the BBB, and subsequently distributed away from these sites into circulating blood and washed out of the brain. A few reports did verify nanomaterial brain tissue entry [34, 35]. After whole body perfusion to remove blood, the capillary depletion method (described below) was used to separate brain parenchyma from brain capillaries. The percentage of the injected dose of [^{111}In]DTPA-multiwalled carbon nanotubes decreased in brain capillaries, but not brain parenchyma over 24 h, providing strong evidence of brain tissue entry of this nanomaterial [36].

The methods presented here assess whether a nanomaterial introduced into the vasculature perfusing the brain is associated with BBB components and/or crosses the BBB to enter brain tissue. Two methods are presented, the in situ brain perfusion technique and the capillary depletion method. They are best used together as the former provides a sample containing brain tissue as well as the vasculature within the brain. The latter separates BMECs from brain parenchymal tissue. The latter method is most often conducted with brain tissue obtained using the in situ brain perfusion technique, but can be used with brain tissue obtained by other methods.

The in situ brain perfusion technique can be used to determine nanomaterial entry rate and extent of distribution into the brain, or multiple brain regions and/or the choroid plexus, ipsilateral to the carotid artery perfused after a short-term (few minutes or less) intracarotid infusion of test material. It is particularly useful for materials that rapidly enter the brain, when the BBB has been opened intentionally, or in the presence of a disease that alters BBB integrity such as brain cancer. The intracarotid perfusion rate is sufficient to prevent introduction of blood into the perfused carotid artery, therefore preventing blood from entering the brain hemisphere perfused by that artery. This enables control of the chemical environment of the material tested (therefore its chemical form [speciation]), based on the perfusion fluid composition and avoidance of exposure to blood. Avoiding blood exposure avoids potential nanomaterial biotransformation (e.g., corona coating by plasma proteins, dissolution, or particle breakdown) that might change its surface properties and brain uptake. Alternatively, the influence of coating the nanomaterial with plasma proteins or any other material could be investigated by their inclusion in the perfusion fluid.

The in situ brain perfusion technique includes the evaluation of BBB integrity based on determination of vascular volume and extracellular space. This is accomplished by inclusion in the perfusion fluid, by intravenous administration, or for IgG reliance on its presence in blood, of a BBB integrity marker (Table 1) that does not significantly distribute from blood to brain across the intact BBB during the time course of brain perfusion.

The in situ brain perfusion technique can inform about the distribution of a nanomaterial out of the vascular compartment. It does not differentiate association with and distribution into BBB components from association with and uptake by brain cells.

The capillary depletion method was designed to remove the BMECs of the BBB from a brain homogenate to identify nanomaterial that transcytosed the BBB (capillary-depleted brain parenchyma). The goal is to determine nanomaterial distribution between the endothelial cells that contribute to brain capillaries vs. brain parenchyma to determine whether the nanomaterial entered brain parenchyma or if its distribution was limited to the BMECs. It is often utilized in conjunction with the in situ brain perfusion technique, but could be used after intravenous nanomaterial administration. The capillary depletion method was originally described by [37]. It is a gradient centrifugation method using dextran (~ density 1.07). As a result the BMECs are in the pellet (along with brain nuclei and erythrocytes if blood was not perfused from the brain) and the brain cells and brain extracellular fluid are in the supernatant. Given the observed association of nanomaterials with the luminal wall of BMECs [22–24] this method can help to avoid the mistaken interpretation of results as nanomaterial brain entry, when the nanomaterial is associated with the BMECs, not having crossed the BBB.

In the original description of the in situ brain perfusion technique the occipital and superior thyroid arteries were coagulated or ligated and cut and the pterygopalatine artery was ligated and cut, because these arteries do not provide blood to the brain so perfusion fluid into the carotid artery that went into these arteries was "wasted" [38, 39]. Perfusion fluid was delivered at 4–5 mL/min into the external carotid artery. This rate was chosen to minimize systemic blood flow to the contralateral hemisphere, maintain a carotid arterial perfusion pressure above the mean systolic pressure (126 mm Hg), prevent blood from entering the internal carotid artery from the circle of Willis, and provide a pressure below 160–190 mm Hg, which was shown to damage the BBB. When perfusion was to exceed 1 min a femoral artery was cannulated to enable blood withdrawal at the same rate as the carotid artery perfusion. There are many modifications of this method. We used a modification developed by the senior author of the original method [22, 37–40] that has the advantage of being less demanding of surgical skills and can be more rapidly accomplished [39]. In this modification, the common carotid artery is cannulated followed by ligation of the external carotid artery. Ligation of the occipital, superior thyroid, and pterygopalatine arteries is optional. The heart is exposed and cardiac ventricles cut within 3 s before initiation of carotid artery perfusion. This is to terminate systemic circulation and the potential for blood to enter the perfused hemisphere and provide an outlet for the perfusion fluid delivered into the carotid artery. Due to perfusion fluid flow into these common carotid artery branches that do not perfuse the brain, the rate of perfusion fluid flow should be greater than 5 mL/min. It can be varied because there is no systemic circulation providing an alternative blood source to the brain. Using this modification with ligation of only the pterygopalatine artery a perfusion rate of 10 mL/min, and without ligation of the occipital, superior thyroid, and pterygopalatine arteries, 20 mL/min was suggested [39]. We used 15 and 20 mL/min flow rates that produced comparable vascular spaces [23].

2 Materials

2.1 Both Methods

1. Ultrasonic bath/cleaner: Branson, Millipore Sigma, GT Sonic, others.
2. Ability to sterilize by autoclaving, ethylene oxide, or in a glass bead dry sterilizer: Fine Science Tools, Germinator 500, Micro Bead Sterilizer, Steri 250, others.

2.2 The In Situ Brain Perfusion Technique

2.2.1 Anesthetic

1. Injectable general anesthetic:
   (a) Ketamine: Henry Schein animal health
   (b) Xylazine: Henry Schein animal health, or dexmedetomidine: Henry Schein animal health
   (c) (*see* **Note 1**)
   (d) Plastic disposable luer-slip syringe (1 mL) and 25 g × 5/8″ needle: (VWR, others).
2. Inhalation general anesthetic: Isoflurane: Isoflurane vaporizer, supply gas, and associated equipment.

2.2.2 Equipment and Supplies

1. Citranox®: Fisher Scientific, VWR.
2. Absorbent pad: (VWR, others).
3. Sterile disposable drape/towel: (VWR, others).
4. Povidone–iodine (Betadine®: Fisher Scientific, VWR).
5. Surgery board (optional) (*see* **Note 2**).

6. Electric razor: Oster® Finisher® Narrow Blade Trimmer, Wahl from Braintree Scientific and Kent Scientific Corp.
7. Homeothermic heating blanket with rectal probe: 2biological Instruments, E-Z anesthesia, Harvard Apparatus, Kent Scientific Corp., Stoelting.
8. Scalpel handle and blade, scissors, microdissecting forceps, clamps: Fine Science Tools, George Tiemann & Co., Roboz Surgical Instrument Co.
9. Bone rongeur, curved, ~2 mm cup: Fine Science Tools, George Tiemann & Co., Roboz Surgical Instrument Co.
10. Flat stainless steel microspatula with rounded ends: Fisher Scientific.
11. Stereo boom microscope with light source: AmScope, Fisher Scientific, Microscope.com, MicroscopeNet.com.
12. 4-0 silk thread: Fine Science Tools.
13. PE 50 or PE 60 tubing: Fisher Scientific, Scientific Commodities Inc., Thomas Scientific.
14. Heparin: Cardinal Health, Henry Schein animal health, Merritt, Pfizer.
15. Plastic disposable luer-slip syringes, 1 and 5 mL, syringe needle, 20 gauge for PE-60, 23 gauge for PE-50 tubing (*see* **Note 3**).
16. Syringe pump capable of delivering 5–20 mL/min from a 20–60 mL syringe: Cole-Parmer, Harvard Apparatus Pump 11 Elite Series or earlier (11, 22, 33, 44, PHD2000), kdScientific, New Era Pump Systems, Smiths Medical.
17. Guillotine: Braintree Scientific, Nemi guillotine, or alternative method to rapidly remove the head from the body.
18. Styrofoam block with well to hold dry or liquid ice.
19. Glass plate that is laid over Styrofoam block.
20. Perfusion fluid: The perfusion fluid composition may depend on the experimental goals and nanomaterial, but should be iso-osmotic, ~ pH 7.4, and 37 °C. We used a perfusion fluid of nanomaterial containing: 153 mM Na^+, 4.2 mM K^+, 1.5 mM Ca^{2+}, 0.9 mM Mg^{2+}, 162 mM Cl^-, and 9 mM glucose. Perfusion for more than a few minutes requires addition of oxygen-carrying capacity to the perfusion fluid (*see* **Note 4**). This can be accomplished by addition of washed erythrocytes [39]. However, this may change the nature of the nanomaterial by association with the erythrocytes [40–43]. To determine BBB integrity, one of the BBB integrity markers in Table 1 can be added to the in situ brain perfusion fluid or given intravenously. Gadolinium can be quantified by elemental analysis, for example by ICP-MS concurrently with the metal(s) of the nanomaterial if present (*see* **Note 5**).

2.3 The Capillary Depletion Method

2.3.1 Equipment and Supplies

1. Buffer: 141 mM NaCl, 4 mM KCl, 2.8 mM $CaCl_2$, 1 mM NaH_2PO_4, 1 mM $MgSO_4$, 10 mM glucose, and 10 mM HEPES at pH 7.4.
2. Tenbroeck tissue grinder: Fisher Scientific, Wheaton Scientific.
3. Dextran 70,000 g/mol: Millipore Sigma.
4. Swinging bucket refrigerated centrifuge with rotor capable of $5400 \times g$.

3 Methods

3.1 Both Methods

1. Clean instruments in an ultrasonic bath/cleaner after every use.
2. Sterilize instruments.
3. Personnel should wear sterile gloves, wear proper clothing for laboratory work, and use personal protective equipment (if needed or required).

3.2 In Situ Brain Perfusion

3.2.1 Rat Preparation

1. Deeply anesthetize the rat following, if required, a governmentally and/or institutionally approved protocol using any of the following methods.
   (a) With ketamine–xylazine (75 and 5 mg/kg) or ketamine--dexmedetomidine (50–75 and 0.25 mg/kg) given ip using a 25 g 5/8″ needle, supplemented if necessary with ketamine 5 mg ip, or other suitable injectable general anesthetic (*see* **Note 1**).
   (b) With isoflurane (1–4% induction, 2–3% maintenance as needed), or other suitable inhalation general anesthetic.
2. Verify sufficient depth of anesthesia by lack of response to strong tail or foot pinch.
3. Maintain body temperature, typically by a homeothermic heating blanket with rectal probe. Alternatively maintain body temperature with a heating pad or lamp, monitored with a rectal thermometer.

3.2.2 Prepare the Surgical Work Site

1. Sterilize by spraying with Citranox® followed by 70% ethanol.
2. Lay down an absorbent pad.
3. Place a sterile disposable drape/towel containing the sterilized instruments on the absorbent pad.
4. Drape nonprocedure areas.
5. Place the anesthetized rat in dorsal recumbency (on its back) (*see* **Note 2**).

3.2.3 Cannulate the Carotid Artery

1. Shave incision areas with clippers.
2. Swab incision areas with povidone–iodine.
3. Swab incision areas with 70% alcohol.
4. Expose one carotid artery (experimenter's choice), encircle it twice with surgical thread (4-0), one below the bifurcation, the other above, and tighten the thread on the one below the bifurcation (cardiac side) to prevent blood flow (*see* **Note 6**).
5. Insert sterile (*see* **Note 7**) PE 50 or PE 60 tubing containing heparin (100 U/mL) in 0.9% NaCl into the common carotid, 4–5 mm above the bifurcation of the common carotid artery and secure it in the artery by a thread knot around the artery and indwelling tubing.
6. To contain blood released from the ligated heart, place the rat in a perfusion tray or on a grid over a sink.
7. Expose the heart by cutting through the skin and underlying tissue with a scissors in a caudal to rostral direction from the abdomen just below the xyphoid process (opening the peritoneal cavity), in a midline incision, up through the ventral thoracic cavity (opening it), avoiding lung, heart and mammary arteries. Cut the right atrial chamber or vena cava with scissors.
8. Deliver the perfusion fluid (*see* **Note 8**) using a pump and preferably a glass syringe (*see* **Notes 9–16**).
9. Decapitate the rat to end the perfusion.
10. Harvest the brain by cutting the scalp midline with a scalpel blade down to the cranium and pulling the skin to the sides. Using a bone rongeur, starting at the base of the skull, remove the skull from over the brain to expose the brain, being careful to not remove brain tissue. Cut the dura mater with the scalpel blade and pull it away from the brain. Use a flat stainless steel microspatula with rounded ends to get under the brain, cut the cranial nerves, and lift the brain from the cranial vault.
11. Place the brain sample on the cooled, moist, glass plate over the Styrofoam block containing ice.
12. Remove the meninges and surface vessels from the brain's surface with microforceps.
13. Dissect the desired brain region (typically forebrain) or regions from perfused hemisphere away from the rest of the brain and, if relevant to the brain region isolated, remove the lateral ventricle choroid plexus from the sample (*see* **Note 17**).
14. Retain a sample of the perfusion fluid for nanomaterial concentration analysis and quantitation of the BBB integrity/vascular volume/extracellular space marker.

15. Quantify the nanomaterial and BBB integrity/vascular volume/extracellular space marker in the brain sample or brain regions and perfusion fluid sample.

3.3 The Capillary Depletion Method

1. After nanomaterial dosing by carotid arterial perfusion of the in situ brain perfusion technique or any other route, blood should be perfused out of the brain before the brain is harvested. This is accomplished by systemic perfusion of the animal to remove blood from within the brain that contains nanomaterial.
2. Homogenize the tissue in 3.5 mL ice-cold buffer with 8–10 strokes in a Tenbroeck tissue grinder. Add dextran (70,000 g/mol) to 18% (w/v) and further homogenize the sample with five additional strokes.
3. Remove an aliquot of the homogenate for determination of nanomaterial content.
4. Centrifuge the sample at 5400 × *g* for 15 min in a swinging bucket centrifuge at 4 °C.
5. Carefully separate the supernatant (brain rich fraction) and pellet (capillary rich fraction) for nanomaterial measurement in each fraction (*see* **Note 18**).

3.4 Data Analysis and Interpretation of Results

3.4.1 In Situ Brain Perfusion

Flow-rate-dependent uptake is a property of some carrier-mediated transporters, but not diffusion. To identify the process of nanomaterial brain uptake, the effect of perfusion flow rate on influx rate can be determined. Diffusion-mediated nanomaterial brain uptake should be concentration independent, whereas the capacity of a carrier-mediated transporter may be exceeded. The uptake process can be further investigated by varying the nanomaterial concentration, to determine if the uptake space (see below) becomes saturated. This would not be expected for diffusion-mediated uptake during the short perfusion duration of the typical in situ perfusion experiment. Perfusion fluid flow rate- and nanomaterial concentration-dependent brain uptake would suggest non-diffusion-mediated uptake.

The influx rate (K_{in}) is the rate of nanomaterial influx in a given time into a given amount (space) of brain. It is the quotient of uptake space (Q) over time. K_{in} reflects the volume of perfusion fluid cleared of nanomaterial which is transferred into a specific mass (typically expressed per gram) of brain over a given time period. It can be determined by using multiple perfusion times, and generation of a graph of the linear least squares regression of the corrected uptake space ($Q_{nanomaterial}$) vs. perfusion time, assuming the ANOVA of corrected uptake space vs. time shows linearity. The slope of the regression line is an estimate of K_{in}. The uptake space ($Q_{nanomaterial}$), or distribution volume, derived from the in situ brain perfusion results ($Q_{nanomaterial\ total}$), is the brain tissue mass into which the nanomaterial distributes during a given perfusion duration (*see* **Note 19**). $Q_{\text{nanomaterial total}}$ is expressed as mL/g brain, and calculated as in Eq. 1 [38]:

$$\begin{aligned}&\text{mass of nanomaterial per weight brain tissue (g/g)/}\\&\text{the mass of nanomaterial per volume of perfusate (g/ml)}\end{aligned} \tag{1}$$

The uptake space is corrected for the sample's vascular/extracellular space by subtracting the uptake space of the vascular volume/extracellular space marker calculated as in Eq. 2 (obtained with a substance in Table 1), to give the corrected uptake space, calculated as in Eq. 3, and used to calculate K_{in}.

$$\begin{aligned}&\text{vascular} - \text{extracellular space marker (g/g)/vascular}-\\&\text{extracellular space marker per volume of perfusate (g/ml)}\end{aligned} \tag{2}$$

$$Q_{\text{nanomaterial}} = Q_{\text{nanomaterial total}} - Q_{\text{vascular/extracellular space marker}} \tag{3}$$

3.4.2 The Capillary Depletion Method

The percentage of nanomaterial in the capillary-enriched fraction is determined as:

(nanomaterial mass in the capillary-enriched fraction normalized to the whole brain/nanomaterial mass in the homogenized brain aliquot normalized to the whole brain) × 100%.

Mass balance can be calculated by comparing the sum of the nanomaterial in the capillary-enriched fraction normalized to the whole brain (or brain sample) plus nanomaterial in the capillary-depleted-fraction normalized to the whole brain (or brain sample), compared to the nanomaterial in the aliquot of the homogenized brain normalized to the whole brain (or brain sample).

4 Notes

1. There are now, and will be in the future, many suitable alternatives to this combination.
2. The operator may want to restrain the rat on a surgery board: Harvard Apparatus, Plas-Labs, Inc.
3. Dull the tip of needles to be inserted into PE tubing to reduce sticking oneself with the needle and puncturing the tubing while inserting the needle in the tubing. This can be done with a file, being careful to not occlude the needle lumen. Inserting stainless steel wire in the needle lumen helps avoid occlusion. The inner diameter of a 20 gauge needle is 0.34 mm and of a 23 gauge needle is 0.6 mm.
4. Introducing oxygen-carrying capacity to the perfusion fluid can be accomplished by addition of washed erythrocytes [39] or blood substitute. However, erythrocyte association may change the nature of the nanomaterial [40–43].

5. Sucrose, and perhaps some of the other markers, is a source for microorganism metabolism. If not maintained sterile it can be catabolized and the results of its use to determine the vascular space would not be valid.
6. Some videos showing carotid artery isolation are available: https://www.bing.com/videos/search?q=youtube+of+rat+carotid+artery+cannulation&view=detail&mid=5C689127E36E8933C4AA5C689127E36E8933C4AA&FORM=VIRE; https://www.youtube.com/watch?v=a_cdEJHRiVs; https://www.youtube.com/watch?v=QoGmUSOJSoM; https://www.jove.com/video/51881/catheterization-carotid-artery-jugular-vein-to-perform-hemodynamic
7. PE tubing can be sterilized by ethylene oxide or 70% ethanol immersion. Autoclaving should not be used as it melts the tubing. Tubing insertion into the carotid artery was facilitated when the artery was partially cut at an angle and the tubing end was beveled.
8. Following at least 1 h incubation at 37 °C, the perfusion fluid is bubbled for 2 min with 95/5 air/CO_2 and adjusted to pH 7.4. The perfusion fluid should be used as soon as possible, at 37 °C. Maintained at 37 °C perfusion fluid pH was shown to be stable for 4 h [44].
9. Delivery of perfusion fluid in the in situ brain perfusion technique is best accomplished using glass, rather than plastic syringes, due to lower friction of the former. Sources of glass syringes and plungers include Becton Dickinson, Hamilton 1000 series gastight syringe, Harvard Apparatus Yale Glass Syringe with Robb Tip, Leur-Loc.
10. Nanomaterials rapidly associate with proteins in blood. Protein coating, the corona, can greatly influence the nanomaterial surface properties, and "what the cell sees" [45]. The use of a blood/plasma/serum-free perfusion fluid delivering the nanomaterial to the brain in the in situ brain perfusion procedure reduces the potential for significant change to its surface chemistry, compared to its delivery to the brain in blood or blood components. Uncoated nanomaterials tend to rapidly agglomerate in the presence of ions in the surrounding solution. Nanomaterials are typically surface coated to reduce agglomeration. When the in situ brain perfusion procedure is used it would be wise to determine if the nanomaterial agglomerates in the perfusion fluid during its exposure time.
11. If there is concern that nanomaterial properties would be significantly affected by contact with blood at the beginning of the perfusion, nanomaterial-free perfusion fluid could be delivered before initiation of nanomaterial-containing perfusion fluid.

12. The duration of in situ perfusion is generally no more than 2 min to avoid anoxic injury to the BBB and brain, unless an oxygen-providing source is added to the perfusion fluid (*see* **Note 4**).
13. The "dead" volume of the carotid infusion cannula that is not filled with nanomaterial-containing perfusion fluid that will be delivered to the brain before the nanomaterial-containing perfusion fluid must be considered when determining the infusion time and amount of nanomaterial delivered to the brain. One approach is to add sufficient time to the perfusion to displace the non-nanomaterial-containing perfusion fluid and to deliver the entire intended volume of test substance-containing perfusion fluid. A better approach is to deliver the entire volume of test substance in perfusion fluid to the brain then follow its infusion with nanomaterial-free perfusion fluid, as discussed in the next note.
14. After perfusion fluid administration, cerebrovascular washout of the perfusion fluid should be conducted to remove the contribution of nanomaterial in the vascular space to apparent brain uptake. This can be conducted by perfusion of nanomaterial-free perfusion fluid for 5–20 s at the same rate as used to deliver the perfusion fluid, immediately following perfusion of the nanomaterial-containing perfusion fluid [46].
15. The rapid change from nanomaterial-containing to nanomaterial-free perfusion fluid can be accomplished with a four-way stopcock (e.g., BD M4018, BD 394910, B. Braun 455991, B. Braun 456003, B. Braun 457501).
16. For small molecules that might back diffuse from brain to blood, or substances that might be transported in that direction after entering the brain, efflux will reduce apparent brain uptake. The longer the time before decapitation including perfusion duration, the greater the potential for efflux. For nanomaterials, that are not expected to be released from cells after their uptake by phagosomes and incorporation into phagolysosomes, this should not be a concern.
17. Specific brain regions can be harvested by sectioning the brain in an acrylic matrix (Braintree Scientific, Inc.) to 1 mm thick sections with a razor blade and placing the sections on the glass plate over ice in the well of a Styrofoam block. Ice keeps the glass cold and moist, avoiding brain sticking to the glass. Specific brain regions can be dissected from the slices with guidance from a rat brain atlas (e.g., [47], http://labs.gaidi.ca/rat-brain-atlas/). When regional variation is to be studied, brain tissue is often collected from the frontal cortex, parietal cortex, occipital cortex, thalamus/hypothalamus, midbrain/colliculus, striatum, cerebellum, hippocampus, and choroid plexus. The weight of each sample is obtained in a preweighed vessel.

18. The separation should produce much higher activity of alkaline phosphatase and gamma-glutamyltransferase activity, capillary-specific enzymes, in the capillary-enriched fraction. They can be determined using enzyme activity kits (Millipore Sigma). Microscopic examination should also confirm the presence of capillary fragments in the capillary-enriched fraction, but not the capillary-poor fraction.
19. An increase of $Q_{\text{nanomaterial}}$ with increased duration of perfusion indicates nanomaterial association with BMECs and/or brain entry. It does not unequivocally demonstrate brain parenchyma entry. To determine this, the capillary depletion method can be used. One alternative to the capillary depletion method to confirm brain parenchyma nanomaterial uptake for electron dense nanomaterials is electron microscopy (and for metal-containing nanomaterials elemental analysis, such as energy-dispersive X-ray spectroscopy), to qualitatively demonstrate brain parenchyma uptake.

References

1. Sanovich E, Bartus RT, Friden PM, Dean RL, Le HQ, Brightman MW (1995) Pathway across blood-brain barrier opened by the bradykinin agonist, RMP-7. Brain Res 705:125–135
2. Zlokovic BV, Apuzzo ML (1998) Strategies to circumvent vascular barriers of the central nervous system. Neurosurgery 43:877–878
3. Boström M, Hellstroem Erkenstam N, Kaluza D, Jakobsson L, Kalm M, Blomgren K (2014) The hippocampal neurovascular niche during normal development and after irradiation to the juvenile mouse brain. Int J Radiat Biol 90:778–789
4. Ohno K, Pettigrew KD, Rapoport SI (1978) Lower limits of cerebrovascular permeability to nonelectrolytes in the conscious rat. Am J Physiol 235:H299–H307
5. Calvo P, Gouritin B, Chacun H, Desmaele D, D'Angelo J, Noel JP, Georgin D, Fattal E, Andreux JP, Couvreur P (2001) Long-circulating PEGylated polycyanoacrylate nanoparticles as new drug carrier for brain delivery. Pharm Res 18:1157–1166
6. Levin VA (1980) Relationship of octanol/water partition coefficient and molecular weight to rat brain capillary permeability. J Med Chem 23:682–684
7. Laterra J, Keep R, Betz AL, Goldstein GW (1999) Blood-brain-cerebrospinal fluid barriers. In: Siegel GJ, Agranoff BW (eds) Basic neurochemistry: molecular, cellular and medical aspects. Lippincott-Raven Publishers, Philadelphia, PA, pp 671–689
8. Pardridge WM (2012) Drug transport across the blood-brain barrier. J Cereb Blood Flow Metab 32:1959–1972
9. Yokel RA (2006) Blood-brain barrier flux of aluminum, manganese, iron and other metals suspected to contribute to metal-induced neurodegeneration. J Alzheimers Dis 10:223–253
10. Yokel RA, Grulke EA, MacPhail RC (2013) Metal-based nanoparticle interactions with the nervous system: the challenge of brain entry and the risk of retention in the organism. Wiley Interdiscip Rev Nanomed Nanobiotechnol 5:346–373
11. Madhusoodanan J (2016) Designing in vitro models of the blood-brain barrier. The Scientist (September 1)
12. Mantle JL, Min L, Lee KH (2016) Minimum transendothelial electrical resistance thresholds for the study of small and large molecule drug transport in a human *in vitro* blood-brain barrier model. Mol Pharm 13:4191–4198
13. Abbott NJ, Dolman DEM, Drndarski S, Fredriksson SM (2012) An improved in vitro blood-brain barrier model: rat brain endothelial cells co-cultured with astrocytes. Methods Mol Biol 814:415–430
14. Butt AM, Jones HC, Abbott NJ (1990) Electrical resistance across the blood-brain barrier in anaesthetized rats: a developmental study. J Physiol 429:47–62

15. Disdier C, Devoy J, Cosnefroy A, Chalansonnet M, Herlin-Boime N, Brun E, Lund A, Mabondzo A (2015) Tissue biodistribution of intravenously administrated titanium dioxide nanoparticles revealed blood-brain barrier clearance and brain inflammation in rat. Part Fibre Toxicol 12:27
16. Mendonca MCP, Soares ES, de Jesus MB, Ceragioli HJ, Batista AG, Nyul-Toth A, Molnar J, Wilhelm I, Marostica MR, Krizbai I, da Cruz-Hofling MA (2016) PEGylation of reduced graphene oxide induces toxicity in cells of the blood-brain barrier: an *in vitro* and *in vivo* study. Mol Pharm 13:3913–3924
17. Yokel RA, Florence RL, Unrine JM, Tseng MT, Graham UM, Wu P, Grulke EA, Sultana R, Hardas SS, Butterfield DA (2009) Biodistribution and oxidative stress effects of a systemically-introduced commercial ceria engineered nanomaterial. Nanotoxicology 3:234–248
18. Frigell J, Garcia I, Gomez-Vallejo V, Llop J, Penades S (2014) ^{68}Ga-labeled gold glyconanoparticles for exploring blood-brain barrier permeability: preparation, biodistribution studies, and improved brain uptake via neuropeptide conjugation. J Am Chem Soc 136:449–457
19. Sela H, Elia P, Zach R, Zeiri Y, Sela H, Karpas Z, Zeiri Y, Cohen H (2015) Spontaneous penetration of gold nanoparticles through the blood brain barrier (BBB). J Nanobiotechnol 13:71
20. Schleh C, Semmler-Behnke M, Lipka J, Wenk A, Hirn S, Schaeffler M, Schmid G, Simon U, Kreyling WG (2012) Size and surface charge of gold nanoparticles determine absorption across intestinal barriers and accumulation in secondary target organs after oral administration. Nanotoxicology 6:36–46
21. Buzulukov YP, Arianova EA, Demin VF, Safenkova IV, Gmoshinski IV, Tutelyan VA (2014) Bioaccumulation of silver and gold nanoparticles in organs and tissues of rats studied by neutron activation analysis. Biol Bull 41:255–263
22. Gessner A, Olbrich C, Schroder W, Kayser O, Muller RH (2001) The role of plasma proteins in brain targeting: species dependent protein adsorption patterns on brain-specific lipid drug conjugate (LDC) nanoparticles. Int J Pharm 214:87–91
23. Dan M, Tseng MT, Wu P, Unrine JM, Grulke EA, Yokel RA (2012) Brain microvascular endothelial cell association and distribution of a 5 nm ceria engineered nanomaterial. Int J Nanomedicine 7:4023–4036
24. Baghirov H, Karaman D, Viitala T, Duchanoy A, Lou Y-R, Mamaeva V, Pryazhnikov E, Khiroug L, de lange C, Sahlgren C, Rosenholm JM (2016) Feasibility study of the permeability and uptake of mesoporous silica nanoparticles across the blood-brain barrier. PLoS One 11:e0160705
25. Wilhelm C, Gazeau F, Roger J, Pons JN, Bacri JC (2002) Interaction of anionic superparamagnetic nanoparticles with cells: kinetic analyses of membrane adsorption and subsequent internalization. Langmuir 18:8148–8155
26. Gao K, Jiang X (2006) Influence of particle size on transport of methotrexate across blood brain barrier by polysorbate 80-coated polybutylcyanoacrylate nanoparticles. Int J Pharm 310:213–219
27. Al Zaki A, Hui JZ, Higbee E, Tsourkas A (2015) Biodistribution, clearance, and toxicology of polymeric micelles loaded with 0.9 or 5 nm gold nanoparticles. J Biomed Nanotechnol 11:1836–1846
28. Tsai Y-M, Chien C-F, Lin L-C, Tsai T-H (2011) Curcumin and its nano-formulation: the kinetics of tissue distribution and blood-brain barrier penetration. Int J Pharm 416:331–338
29. Tröster SD, Müller U, Kreuter J (1990) Modification of the body distribution of poly(methyl methacrylate) nanoparticles in rats by coating with surfactants. Int J Pharm 61:85–100
30. Fundarò A, Cavalli R, Bargoni A, Vighetto D, Zara GP, Gasco MR (2000) Non-stealth and stealth solid lipid nanoparticles (SLN) carrying doxorubicin: pharmacokinetics and tissue distribution after i.v. administration to rats. Pharmacol Res 42:337–343
31. Guerrero S, Araya E, Fiedler JL, Arias JI, Adura C, Albericio F, Giralt E, Arias JL, Fernandez MS, Kogan MJ (2010) Improving the brain delivery of gold nanoparticles by conjugation with an amphipathic peptide. Nanomedicine 5:897–913
32. Wen Z, Yan Z, He R, Pang Z, Guo L, Qian Y, Jiang X, Fang L (2011) Brain targeting and toxicity study of odorranalectin-conjugated nanoparticles following intranasal administration. Drug Deliv 18:555–561
33. Martins SM, Sarmento B, Nunes C, Lucio M, Reis S, Ferreira DC (2013) Brain targeting effect of camptothecin-loaded solid lipid nanoparticles in rat after intravenous administration. Eur J Pharm Biopharm 85:488–502
34. Chen Y-S, Hung Y-C, Lin L-W, Liau I, Hong M-Y, Huang GS (2010) Size-dependent impairment of cognition in mice caused by

the injection of gold nanoparticles. Nanotechnology 21:485102

35. Dziendzikowska K, Gromadzka-Ostrowska J, Lankoff A, Oczkowski M, Krawczynska A, Chwastowska J, Sadowska-Bratek M, Chajduk E, Wojewodzka M, Dusinska M, Kruszewski M (2012) Time-dependent biodistribution and excretion of silver nanoparticles in male Wistar rats. J Appl Toxicol 32:920–928
36. Kafa H, Wang JT-W, Rubio N, Venner K, Anderson G, Pach E, Ballesteros B, Preston JE, Abbott NJ, Al-Jamal KT (2015) The interaction of carbon nanotubes with an *in vitro* blood-brain barrier model and mouse brain *in vivo*. Biomaterials 53:437–452
37. Triguero D, Buciak J, Pardridge WM (1990) Capillary depletion method for quantification of blood-brain barrier transport of circulating peptides and plasma proteins. J Neurochem 54:1882–1888
38. Takasato Y, Rapoport SI, Smith QR (1984) An in situ brain perfusion technique to study cerebrovascular transport in the rat. Am J Physiol 247:H484–H493
39. Smith QR (1996) Brain perfusion systems for studies of drug uptake and metabolism in the central nervous system. Pharm Biotechnol 8:285–307
40. Geiser M, Rothen-Rutishauser B, Kapp N, Schurch S, Kreyling W, Schulz H, Semmler M, Im Hof V, Heyder J, Gehr P (2005) Ultrafine particles cross cellular membranes by nonphagocytic mechanisms in lungs and in cultured cells. Environ Health Perspect 113:1555–1560
41. Wang J, Zhou G, Chen C, Yu H, Wang T, Ma Y, Jia G, Gao Y, Li B, Sun J, Li Y, Jiao F, Zhao Y, Chai Z (2007) Acute toxicity and biodistribution of different sized titanium dioxide particles in mice after oral administration. Toxicol Lett 168:176–185
42. Nemmar A, Beegam S, Yuvaraju P, Yasin J, Shahin A, Ali BH (2014) Interaction of amorphous silica nanoparticles with erythrocytes *in vitro*: role of oxidative stress. Cell Physiol Biochem 34:255–265
43. Antonelli A, Sfara C, Manuali E, Bruce IJ, Magnani M (2011) Encapsulation of superparamagnetic nanoparticles into red blood cells as new carriers of MRI contrast agents. Nanomedicine 6:211–223
44. Crossgrove JS, Allen DD, Bukaveckas BL, Rhineheimer SS, Yokel RA (2003) Manganese distribution across the blood-brain barrier. I. Evidence for carrier-mediated influx of managanese citrate as well as manganese and manganese transferrin. Neurotoxicology 24:3–13
45. Walczyk D, Bombelli FB, Monopoli MP, Lynch I, Dawson KA (2010) What the cell "sees" in bionanoscience. J Am Chem Soc 132:5761–5768
46. Crossgrove JS, Yokel RA (2004) Manganese distribution across the blood-brain barrier III. The divalent metal transporter-1 is not the major mechanism mediating brain manganese uptake. Neurotoxicology 25:451–460
47. Paxinos G, Charles W (2013) The rat brain in stereotaxic coordinates, 7th edn. Academic Press, Cambridge, MA
48. Weyerbrock A, Walbridge S, Saavedra JE, Keefer LK, Oldfield EH (2011) Differential effects of nitric oxide on blood-brain barrier integrity and cerebral blood flow in intracerebral C6 gliomas. Neuro Oncol 13:203–211
49. Blasberg RG, Fenstermacher JD, Patlak CS (1983) Transport of α-aminoisobutyric acid across brain capillary and cellular membranes. J Cereb Blood Flow Metab 3:8–32
50. Alaofi A, On N, Kiptoo P, Williams TD, Miller DW, Siahaan TJ (2016) Comparison of linear and cyclic his-ala-val peptides in modulating the blood-brain barrier permeability: impact on delivery of molecules to the brain. J Pharm Sci 105:797–807
51. Laksitorini MD, Kiptoo PK, On NH, Thliveris JA, Miller DW, Siahaan TJ (2015) Modulation of intercellular junctions by cyclic-ADT peptides as a method to reversibly increase blood-brain barrier permeability. J Pharm Sci 104:1065–1075
52. Sisson WB, Oldendorf WH (1971) Brain distribution spaces of mannitol-^{3}H, inulin-^{14}C, and dextran-^{14}C in the rat. Am J Physiol 221:214–217
53. Hawkins BT, Egleton RD (2006) Fluorescence imaging of blood-brain barrier disruption. J Neurosci Methods 151:262–267
54. Euser AG, Bullinger L, Cipolla MJ (2008) Magnesium sulphate treatment decreases blood-brain barrier permeability during acute hypertension in pregnant rats. Exp Physiol 93:254–261
55. Smith QR, Ziylan YZ, Robinson PJ, Rapoport SI (1988) Kinetics and distribution volumes for tracers of different sizes in the brain plasma space. Brain Res 462:1–9
56. Wolff CB, Sarker MH, Fraser PA (1995) Cerebral microvascular permeability and CSF pH in anaesthetized rats. Exp Physiol 80:1053–1055
57. Miller RD, Monsul NT, Vender JR, Lehmann JC (1996) NMDA- and endothelin-1-induced increases in blood-brain barrier permeability quantitated with Lucifer yellow. J Neurol Sci 136:37–40

58. Tabanor K, Lee P, Kiptoo P, Choi I-Y, Sherry EB, Eagle CS, Williams TD, Siahaan TJ (2016) Brain delivery of drug and MRI contrast agent: detection and quantitative determination of brain deposition of CPT-glu using LC-MS/MS and Gd-DTPA using magnetic resonance imaging. Mol Pharm 13:379–390
59. Alyaudtin RN, Reichel A, Lobenberg R, Ramge P, Kreuter J, Begley DJ (2001) Interaction of poly(butyl cyanoacrylate) nanoparticles with the blood-brain barrier *in vivo* and *in vitro*. J Drug Target 9:209–221
60. Carvey PM, Zhao CH, Hendey B, Lum H, Trachtenberg J, Desai BS, Snyder J, Zhu YG, Ling ZD (2005) 6-Hydroxydopamine-induced alterations in blood-brain barrier permeability. Eur J Neurosci 22:1158–1168
61. Bertram KJ, Shipley MT, Ennis M, Sanberg PR, Norman AB (1994) Permeability of the blood-brain barrier within rat intrastriatal transplants assessed by simultaneous systemic injection of horseradish peroxidase and Evans blue dye. Exp Neurol 127:245–252
62. Hoffmann A, Bredno J, Wendland M, Derugin N, Ohara P, Wintermark M (2011) High and low molecular weight fluorescein isothiocyanate (FITC)-dextrans to assess blood-brain barrier disruption: technical considerations. Transl Stroke Res 2:106–111
63. Shim KH, Jeong K-H, Bae SO, Kang MO, Maeng EH, Choi CS, Kim Y-R, Hulme J, Lee EK, Kim M-K, An SSA (2014) Assessment of ZnO and SiO_2 nanoparticle permeability through and toxicity to the blood-brain barrier using Evans blue and TEM. Int J Nanomedicine 9:225–233
64. Zhang J, Ke K-F, Liu Z, Qiu Y-H, Peng Y-P (2013) Th17 cell-mediated neuroinflammation is involved in neurodegeneration of Aβ1-42-induced Alzheimer's disease model rats. PLoS One 8:e75786
65. Michalski D, Grosche J, Pelz J, Schneider D, Weise C, Bauer U, Kacza J, Gaertner U, Hobohm C, Haertig W (2010) A novel quantification of blood-brain barrier damage and histochemical typing after embolic stroke in rats. Brain Res 1359:186–200
66. Pinard E, Engrand N, Seylaz J (2000) Dynamic cerebral microcirculatory changes in transient forebrain ischemia in rats: involvement of type I nitric oxide synthase. J Cereb Blood Flow Metab 20:1648–1658
67. Li Y, Xu L, Zeng K, Xu Z, Suo D, Peng L, Ren T, Sun Z, Yang W, Jin X, Yang L (2017) Propane-2-sulfonic acid octadec-9-enyl-amide, a novel PPARα/γ dual agonist, protects against ischemia-induced brain damage in mice by inhibiting inflammatory responses. Brain Behav Immun 66:289–301
68. Jacob A, Hack B, Chiang E, Garcia JGN, Quigg RJ, Alexander JJ (2010) C5a alters blood-brain barrier integrity in experimental lupus. FASEB J 24:1682–1688

Chapter 17

Evaluation of Genotoxicity of Nanoparticles in Mouse Models

Sameera Nallanthighal and Ramune Reliene

Abstract

Owing to new and unique properties, engineered nanoparticles (NPs) likely pose different risks than their constituent chemicals and these risks need to be understood. In particular, it is important to assess genotoxicity, since genotoxicity is a precursor to carcinogenicity. Here we describe a battery of tests for the assessment of genotoxicity of NPs in vivo in mice. Mice can be exposed to NPs for various exposure durations and by any route of exposure, provided NPs are absorbed into the systemic blood circulation. The testing battery measures three well-established markers of DNA damage: oxidative DNA damage, double strand breaks (DSBs) and chromosomal damage. These markers are measured in peripheral blood cells by microscopic techniques. 8-oxo-7,8-dihydro-2-deoxyguanine (8-oxoG), indicative of oxidative DNA damage, and phosphorylated histone 2AX (γ-H2AX) foci, indicative of DSBs, are determined in white blood cells by immunofluorescence. Micronuclei, indicative of chromosomal damage, are examined in erythrocytes on Giemsa-stained peripheral blood smears. This testing battery can be easily integrated in general toxicology studies or studies examining carcinogenic potential of NPs.

Key words Nanoparticles, Genotoxicity, Oxidative damage, Double strand breaks, Micronuclei, Cancer

1 Introduction

Owing to unique physicochemical properties, biological effects of engineered nanoparticles (NPs) are distinct from their constituent chemicals. Unique properties of NPs, while form the basis for new and improved products, can also result in unwanted health effects and, therefore, warrant safety evaluations in controlled experiments. In particular, it is important to assess genotoxicity, since genotoxicity is a precursor to carcinogenicity.

Genotoxic effects of NPs have been reported in the scientific literature, especially, for metal and metal oxide NPs [1–8]. These data suggest that it is necessary to incorporate genotoxicity tests in safety evaluations of new NPs. In this article, we describe a battery of tests for the assessment of genotoxicity of NPs in vivo in mice.

Qunwei Zhang (ed.), *Nanotoxicity: Methods and Protocols*, Methods in Molecular Biology, vol. 1894, https://doi.org/10.1007/978-1-4939-8916-4_17,

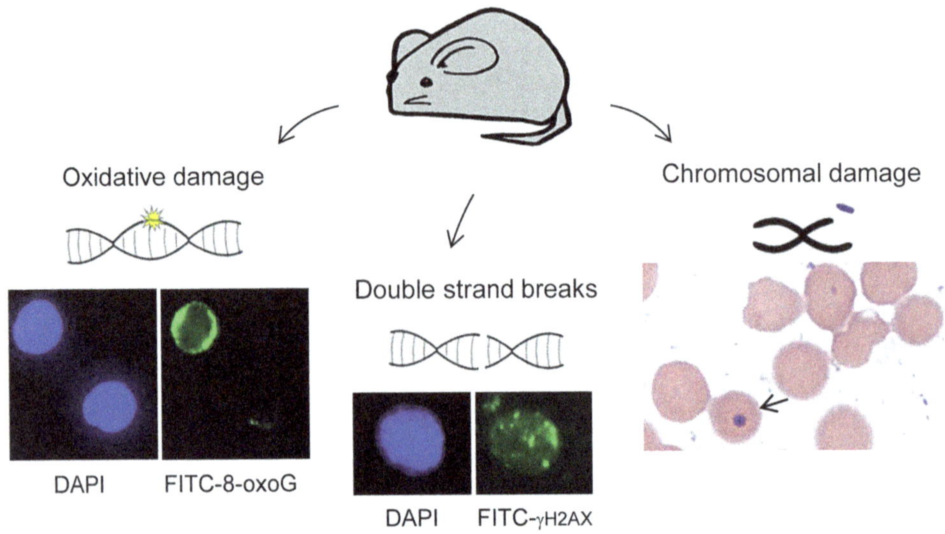

Fig. 1 Genotoxicity assays in vivo in mice. Oxidative DNA damage is measured by immunofluorescence of 8-oxoG. DAPI staining visualizes cellular nuclei and FITC staining visualizes 8-oxoG in the nuclear DNA. One of two nuclei shown in the figure emits bright fluorescence. Thus, this cells is considered positive for 8-oxoG. DSBs are measured by immunofluorescence of γ-H2AX. DAPI staining visualizes cellular nucleus and FITC staining visualizes γ-H2AX foci in the same nucleus. The nucleus shown in the figure contains more than four discrete foci. Thus, this cell is considered positive for γ-H2AX foci. Chromosomal damage is measured by micronucleus assay. A micronucleated erythrocyte highlighted by an arrow is shown on a Giemsa-stained peripheral blood smear

The battery consists of three test assays that are performed on peripheral blood samples using microscopic techniques. About 100 μL of blood is sufficient for all assays. This volume of blood can be harvested by nonterminal bleeding techniques and, thus, allows for follow-up observation in the same animals. Genotoxic effects of NPs can be examined after oral ingestion, inhalation, intravenous injection, or other routes of exposure, provided NPs are absorbed into the systemic blood circulation.

The testing battery measures three well-established markers of DNA damage: oxidative DNA damage, double strand breaks (DSBs) and chromosomal damage (Fig. 1). Oxidative DNA damage is assessed by examining 8-oxo-7,8-dihydro-2-deoxyguanine (8-oxoG) on nuclear DNA by immunofluorescence. 8-oxoG is an oxidative modification of guanine (G) and is a promutagenic lesion. For example, 8-oxoG often mispairs with adenine (A) leading to C:G to A:T transversion mutations, which are the most frequently found mutations in human cancers [9, 10]. DSBs are assessed by measuring phosphorylated histone 2AX (γ-H2AX) foci by immunofluorescence. γ-H2AX foci rapidly form on DNA, where DSBs are induced, and are therefore used as a sensitive marker of DSBs [11]. The possible outcomes of DSBs are cell death and/or genome rearrangements (chromosomal translocations, inversions or deletions) [12]. Genome rearrangements can affect many genes simultaneously. In particular, deleterious are genome rearrangements that inactivate tumor suppressers and/or activate proto-oncogenes, which drive carcinogenesis. Both oxidative DNA damage and DSBs are measured in nucleated blood cells, that is, white blood cells, most of which are lymphocytes. Chromosomal damage is assessed by measuring micronucleus formation. Micronuclei are the result of chromosome fragmentation and/or loss occurring in dividing erythroblasts. In mice, micronuclei can be scored in peripheral blood since damaged erythroblasts complete cell division and maturation in the bone marrow and subsequently enter the systemic circulation [13, 14]. While erythrocytes lose their nuclei during cell maturation, micronuclei remain and can be easily detected in otherwise enucleated cytoplasm of erythrocytes.

A good concordance between the 8-oxoG, γ-H2AX, and micronucleus assay results is possible, but should not be anticipated because different NPs can have different effects on DNA damage and these effects may be cell type- and tissue-specific. Of note, immunofluorescent 8-oxoG and γ-H2AX assays detect the damage occurring in circulating white blood cells, while micronuclei occur in the precursors of erythrocytes that reside in the bone marrow.

Experimental design includes the utilization of young (2--3 months) sexually mature male and female mice (wild type or genetically engineered mice) to assure their bone marrow cells are actively proliferating and to account for possible sex differences, respectively. Mice can be treated with NPs for various durations and followed-up after exposure cessation for a desired period of time. In our studies, we exposed mice orally to silver nanoparticles (AgNPs) for up to 7 days and examined genotoxicity at different time points: at 1, 7, and/or 14 days post-exposure [1–3]. Any nonterminal bleeding technique can be used for blood harvest, but the sub-mandibular bleeding using a lancet is a preferred method. This technique is a humane, efficient and economical method for bleeding of laboratory mice, allows for multiple blood draws and does not require anesthesia [15]. Each experiment should contain a treatment group and a negative control (mice exposed to vehicle only) and data in the treatment group should be compared with a concurrent negative control. Inclusion of a concurrent negative control is critical because background levels can vary from experiment to experiment, especially, in immunofluorescent assays. Positive controls can be included, especially, at early stages of investigations, when techniques need to be established in the laboratory. Since 8-oxoG, DSBs and micronuclei are induced by ionizing radiation, mice exposed to ionizing radiation can serve as a positive control in all three assays [16, 17].

In summary, this testing battery measures well-established markers of genotoxicity ranging from oxidative DNA damage to chromosomal damage. The testing battery can be easily integrated in general toxicology studies or studies focused on the assessment of carcinogenic potential of NPs.

2 Materials

2.1 Buffers and Stains

1. Cell attachment solution: 0.1 mg/mL of poly-D-lysine in water (*see* **Note 1**). Prepare a 1 mg/mL stock solution by dissolving 100 mg of poly-D-lysine in 100 mL water. Store in 5 mL aliquots at −20 °C. When ready to use, dilute 1 part of stock solution with 9 parts of water to prepare 0.1 mg/mL working solution.
2. Erythrocyte lysis buffer: 155 nM (8.3 g/L) ammonium chloride (NH_4Cl) in 0.01 M Tris–HCl, pH 7.4. To make 500 mL of erythrocyte lysis buffer, add 4.15 g NH_4Cl to 50 mL of 0.1 M Tris–HCl, add deionized water to get a final volume of 500 mL, adjust pH to 7.4 with HCl and store at RT.
3. Fixative: 4% paraformaldehyde in 0.1 M Phosphate buffer, pH.7.4 (*see* **Note 2**). Solution may be stored at RT or 4 °C.
4. Phosphate Buffer Saline (PBS): 8 g/L NaCl, 0.2 g/L KCl, 1.44 g/L $Na_2HPO_4 \cdot 2H_2O$, 0.24 g/L KH_2PO4, pH. 7.4. Store at RT.
5. Permeabilization buffer: 0.5% Triton X-100 in PBS. Store at RT.
6. Blocking buffer: 10% fetal bovine serum (FBS) in PBS. To make 100 mL of blocking buffer, add 10 mL of FBS to 10 mL of 10× PBS and add deionized water to get a final volume of 100 mL. Store in 10 mL aliquots at −20 °C. When ready to use, take one aliquot and thaw at RT or 37 °C.
7. Washing buffer: 0.1% Triton X-100 in PBS. Store at RT.
8. Giemsa stain: 0.4% w/w modified Giemsa stain in a buffered methanol solution, pH 6.9 (Sigma-Aldrich). Store at RT.
9. Mounting medium: VECTASHIELD Hardset Antifade Mounting Medium with DAPI (Vector laboratories). Store at 4 °C.
10. Microscope immersion oil. Store at RT.

2.2 Disposables

1. 5 mm Goldenrod animal lancet for blood collection (BrainTree Scientific).
2. 1.3 mL EDTA-coated blood collection tubes (Sarstedt, catalog #SAR-411395105).

3. Microscope slides (25 × 75 × 1 mm).
4. Glass coverslips for microscope slides (22 × 22 mm).
5. Micropipette tips (20, 200, 1000 μL).
6. 6-well flat bottom culture plates.
7. Paper towel.
8. Parafilm.
9. Aluminum foil.

2.3 Antibodies

1. Primary γ-H2AX antibody: Anti-phospho-Histone H2A.X (Ser 139) antibody, clone JBW301 (EMD Millipore, catalog #05-636).
2. Primary 8-oxoG antibody: Anti-8-oxoguanine antibody, clone 483.15 (EMD Millipore, catalog #MAB3560).
3. Secondary antibody: Fluorescein (FITC) AffiniPure Goat Anti-Mouse IgG, Fcγ fragment specific (Jackson ImmunoResearch Laboratories, catalog #115-095-008).

2.4 Equipment

1. Fluorescent microscope with DAPI and FITC filters and a 100× oil immersion objective.
2. Bright field microscope with a 100× oil immersion objective.
3. "Humidifying chamber": an empty micropipette tip box half-filled with warm water. Coverslips are placed on a micropipette tip rack for incubation with primary and secondary antibodies (Fig. 2). The holes in the rack allow for water to evaporate and create a humid environment, which prevents drying of antibodies and coverslips.
4. Dumont Forceps: Inox, 110 mm length (BrainTree Scientific).
5. Wheaton Coplin staining jars: five slide glass jars with plastic screw cap (Sigma-Aldrich).
6. Rotary shaker.
7. A manual cell counter: a Unico L-BC3 two key differential counter.

3 Methods

3.1 Blood Collection

Draw peripheral blood (~120 μL) from the facial (sub-mandibular) vein using a 5 mm goldenrod animal lancet into EDTA-coated blood collection tubes [15] (*see* **Note 3**). Code blood samples in order not to reveal the treatment groups to investigators who will perform microscopic analyses. From harvested blood, 100 μL of blood will be used for immunofluorescent assays examining 8-oxoG and γ-H2AX foci and the rest of blood will be used for

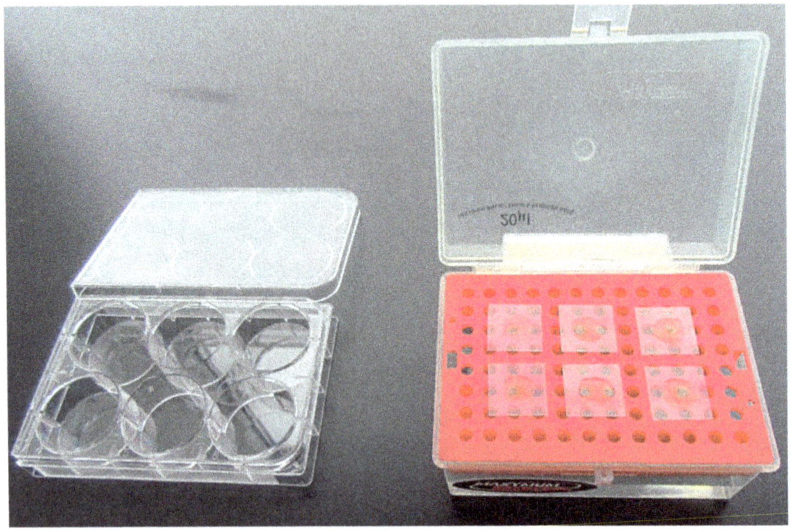

Fig. 2 Transfer of coverslips from a culture plate to a "humidifying chamber". After incubation in blocking solution that is performed in 6-well tissue culture plates coverslips are placed on a "humidifying chamber" with cells facing up for incubation with antibodies. A 6-well plate and a "humidifying chamber" with six coverslips containing adhered cells are shown

micronucleus assay. A flowchart below depicts experimental procedures described in detail in subsequent sections (Fig. 3).

3.2 Immuno-fluorescent Detection of 8-oxoG and γ-H2AX Foci

3.2.1 Preparation of Coverslips for Cell Adherence

1. Clean coverslips by acid wash (*see* **Note 4**). Submerge coverslips in 1 M HCl in a glass container and incubate for 2 h. Then place a large volume of deionized water and leave overnight. Be sure to wash out the acid between the stuck coverslips. Store cleaned coverslips in 100% ethanol.
2. Take coverslips using Dumont forceps and place on a sheet of paper towel or clean bench. Leave coverslips to air-dry for 5–10 min or flame-dry to remove ethanol.
3. Place coverslips in 6-well plates using Dumont forceps, one coverslip per well. Add 2 mL of cell attachment solution (0.1 mg/mL poly-D-lysine), make sure coverslips are submerged, and incubate for 5 min at RT. Remove coverslips using forceps, put on a sheet of paper towel and allow the surface to dry.

3.2.2 Erythrocyte Lysis and Cell Adherence on Coverslips

1. Transfer 100 μL of freshly collected blood to 15 mL Falcon centrifuge tube, add 1 mL (i.e., 10 volumes) of Erythrocyte lysis buffer and mix the blood by gently inverting tubes 2–4 times. Observe turbidity to evaluate erythrocyte lysis. Once the solution becomes clear, lysis is complete. Typically, the solution becomes clear after 1–2 min incubation in lysis buffer.

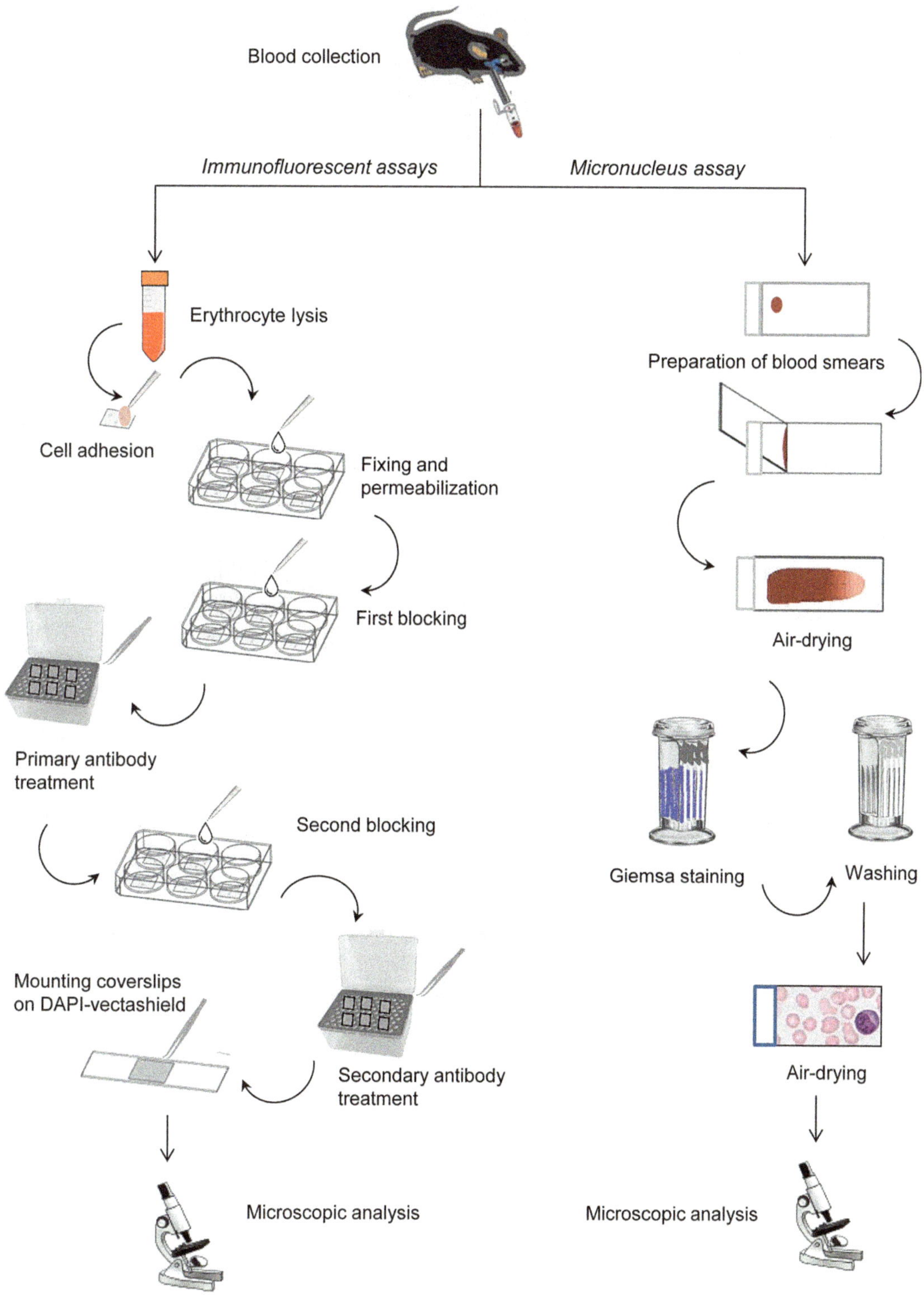

Fig. 3 A flowchart of experimental procedures

2. Add 10 mL (i.e., 10 volumes) of PBS to stop the lysis reaction and centrifuge at 500 × *g* for 5 min at RT. Gently decant the supernatant (*see* **Note 5**).
3. Suspend pelleted cells in the residual volume (~100–120 μL) of PBS, measure the final volume and divide into two aliquots. One aliquot will be used for determination of 8-oxoG and another aliquot will be used for determination of γ-H2AX foci.
4. Drop cells onto two poly-D-lysine coated coverslips, one coverslip for determination of 8-oxoG and another coverslip for determination of γ-H2AX foci. Spread cells evenly over the surface of the coverslip by dispersing the cell suspension in a circular motion with a clean pipette tip. Incubate for 5 min at RT to allow cells to adhere.
5. Place coverslips in 6-well plates and add 2 mL of PBS to prevent drying.

3.2.3 Cell Fixation and Permeabilization

1. Remove PBS by aspiration, add 2 mL of fixative and incubate for 10 min at RT.
2. Aspirate fixative and wash cells with PBS, that is, add 2 mL of PBS, incubate for 3 min at RT, and aspirate the solution.
3. Add 2 mL of permeabilization buffer and incubate for 10 min at RT.
4. Aspirate permeabilization buffer and wash five times with PBS, that is, add 2 mL of PBS, aspirate the solution, and add fresh PBS, repeat five times.

3.2.4 First Blocking

1. Add 2 mL of blocking buffer and incubate for 1 h at RT. Alternatively, incubation can be carried out at +4 °C overnight.

3.2.5 Incubation with Primary Antibodies

1. Prepare working dilutions of primary antibodies in blocking buffer (*see* **Note 6**). To calculate the required volume of diluted antibody solutions, consider that each cover slip will require 50 μL.
2. Transfer coverslips from 6-well plates using Dumont forceps and place them on a "humidifying chamber" (i.e., an empty micropipette tip box that is half-filled with water) with cells facing up (Fig. 2). Use separate "humidifying chambers" for incubation with 8-oxoG and γ-H2AX antibodies (*see* **Note 7**).
3. Pipette 50 μL of primary antibody solution onto each coverslip.
4. Cut a piece of Parafilm (~75 mm × ~75 mm) and place over the coverslips to spread antibodies uniformly over the surface of the coverslips and prevent drying. Close "humidifying chambers" by putting on a micropipette tip box cover.
5. Incubate for 1.5 h at RT.

3.2.6 Second Blocking

1. Transfer coverslips to 6-well plates and wash three times with 2 mL of washing buffer for 5 min each time, that is, add 2 mL of washing buffer, incubate for 5 min at RT, aspirate the solution, and add fresh washing buffer, repeat three times.
2. Aspirate washing buffer, add 2 mL of blocking buffer and incubate for 1 h at RT (or overnight at +4 °C).

3.2.7 Incubation with Secondary Antibodies

1. Prepare working dilution of secondary antibodies in blocking buffer at a dilution of 1:200. To calculate the required volume of antibodies, consider that each cover slip will require 50 μL.
2. Transfer coverslips from 6-well plates using forceps and place them back on "humidifying chambers".
3. Pipet 50 μL of secondary antibody solution onto each coverslip, place a piece of Parafilm over coverslips to ensure even distribution of antibodies and prevent drying. Close "humidifying chambers" by putting on a micropipette tip box cover. Put a piece of aluminum foil over the chambers to minimize light exposure to fluorescent (FITC-conjugated) secondary antibodies.
4. Incubate for 1 h at RT.
5. Transfer coverslips to 6-well plates and wash three times with 2 mL of washing buffer for 5 min each time, that is, add 2 mL of washing buffer per well, incubate for 5 min at RT, aspirate the solution, and add fresh washing buffer, repeat three times.

3.2.8 Mounting Coverslips on Microscope Slides

1. Apply a drop of mounting medium to the surface of a prelabeled microscope slide.
2. Take a coverslip from a 6-well plate using Dumont forceps. Remove excess liquid by dabbing edges of a coverslip on a paper towel.
3. Slowly tip the coverslip with cells facing down onto the mounting medium. Avoid creating bubbles as you lower it into place. Let the slides stand for 15 min at RT to allow mounting medium to harden, which will immobilize the coverslip.
4. Place microscopic slides in a slide holder and keep in the dark to minimize light exposure. Analyze γ-H2AX foci and 8-oxoG within a few days due to gradual decay of fluorophore.

3.2.9 Microscopic Analysis of Immunofluorescence

1. Place a slide under a fluorescent microscope.
2. Analyze 8-oxoG and γ-H2AX foci under a 100× oil immersion objective.
3. Visualize cellular nuclei under a DAPI filter and then switch to the FITC filter to observe immunofluorescence in the nuclei (*see* **Note 8**).

4. To analyze 8-oxoG, score 100 nuclei and record brightly fluorescent nuclei. To analyze γ-H2AX foci formation, count the number of fluorescent foci in each nucleus in a total of 100 nuclei. Tabulate data into an XLS worksheet.
5. Present data as the percentage of cells positive for 8-oxoG and the percentage of cells positive for γ-H2AX foci (*see* **Note 9**).
6. Decode slides, calculate mean ± SD per group, and perform statistical data analysis.

3.3 Micronucleus Assay

3.3.1 Preparation of Blood Smears

1. Place a clean microscope slide on a flat surface and pipette 3 μL of blood on one end of the slide.
2. Take another clean slide, and holding at an angle of about 45°, touch the blood with one end of the slide so the blood runs along the edge of the slide by capillary action. Maintaining firm contact with the bottom slide push carefully along the length of the bottom slide to produce a thin smear of blood. Prepare at least two blood smears per animal. Label slides clearly and let them air-dry.

3.3.2 Staining of Blood Smears

1. Place air-dried blood smears in undiluted Giemsa stain in a Coplin staining jar for 2 min. Giemsa stain in methanol solution combines cell fixation and staining.
2. Remove slides from a Coplin jar, dab excess liquid on a paper towel and rinse them twice in water, that is, immerse slides in water in Coplin jars, place jars on a rotary shaker, and incubate for 3 min each time.
3. Let slides air-dry and place them in a slide holder.

3.3.3 Microscopic Analysis of Micronuclei

1. Place a slide under a bright field microscope.
2. Analyze micronuclei under a 100× oil immersion objective.
3. Score 2000 erythrocytes using a manual cell counter (*see* **Note 10**). Record the number of micronucleated erythrocytes per 2000 erythrocytes. Tabulate data into an XLS worksheet.
4. Decode slides, calculate mean ± SD per group, and perform statistical data analysis.

4 Notes

1. Poly-D-Lysine is available at Sigma-Aldrich as lyophilized powder of poly-D-Lysine hydrobromide in several molecular weight ranges (30,000–70,000, 70,000–150,000, >300,000, and others). We use 30,000–70,000 molecular weight Poly-D-Lysine, but all molecular weights promote cell adhesion to solid substrates.

2. Fixative (phosphate buffered 4% paraformaldehyde) can be purchased from Sigma-Aldrich and other providers as ready-to-use solution. Alternatively, fixative can be made in a laboratory. To make 500 mL of fixative, heat 200 mL of deionized water to ~80 °C. In a chemical fume hood, place hot water on a stir plate, add 20 g paraformaldehyde crystals while stirring, add drops (~20) of 1.0 N NaOH slowly until paraformaldehyde is well dissolved. Add 250 mL 0.2 M sodium phosphate buffer (210 mL dibasic and 40 mL monobasic). Transfer to graduated cylinder and add deionized water to get a final volume of 500 mL. Adjust pH to 7.4 and store at RT or 4 °C.
3. Do not freeze blood, use immediately, that is, on the same day.
4. Although coverslips may look clean, they may have a thin film of grease on them and, therefore, should routinely be washed with acid or base solutions to remove this film. A clean coverslip will help cell adhesion and enhance poly-amino acid coating.
5. A pink-red cell pellet is anticipated after cell centrifugation following erythrocyte lysis, because immature erythrocytes (reticulocytes) are very difficult to lyse. Erythrocyte lysis step can be repeated, but is not necessary because a small number of residual erythrocytes does not interfere with the subsequent use of cells.
6. We use anti-8-oxoguanine antibody at a dilution of 1:500 and anti-γ-H2AX antibody at a dilution of 1:400. It is recommended however that investigators perform dilution series in their own laboratories to establish optical working dilutions that give the best staining with minimum background.
7. We recommend using separate "humidifying chambers" for incubations with γ-H2AX and 8-oxoG antibodies to avoid possible antibody cross-contamination.
8. γ-H2AX foci and 8-oxoG are analyzed in mononuclear white blood cells (mainly lymphocytes). These cells represent majority of nucleated blood cells and have large round nuclei as opposed to multilobed nuclei of granulocytes.
9. We use the following criteria to identify cells positive for 8-oxoG and/or γ-H2AX foci formation. A cell that displays strong fluorescence in the nucleus is considered positive for the 8-oxoG formation, while a cell that is negative for 8-oxoG (i.e., majority of normal undamaged cells) emits very low, if any, fluorescence (Fig. 1). A cell that exhibits more than four discrete foci in the nucleus is considered positive for γ-H2AX foci formation (Fig. 1).
10. Micronuclei appear as dark-blue smooth round remnants of nuclear chromatin in otherwise enucleated cytoplasm of erythrocytes (Fig. 1). Usually 2000 erythrocytes per animal are

scored. The revised OECD (Organization for Economic Co-operation and Development) test guideline TG-474 recommends scoring 4000 erythrocytes [14].

Acknowledgment

This work was supported by NIEHS grant ESO24123 and the Dominic Ferraioli Foundation, both received by RR.

References

1. Kovvuru P, Mancilla PE, Shirode AB, Murray TM, Begley TJ, Reliene R (2015) Oral ingestion of silver nanoparticles induces genomic instability and DNA damage in multiple tissues. Nanotoxicology 9:162–171
2. Nallanthighal S, Chan C, Bharali DJ, Mousa SA, Vasquez E, Reliene R (2017) Particle coatings but not silver ions mediate genotoxicity of ingested silver nanoparticles in a mouse model. NanoImpact 5:92–100
3. Nallanthighal S, Chan C, Murray TM, Mosier AP, Cady NC, Reliene R (2017) Differential effects of silver nanoparticles on DNA damage and DNA repair gene expression in Ogg1-deficient and wild type mice. Nanotoxicology 11:996–1011
4. Patlolla AK, Hackett D, Tchounwou PB (2015) Genotoxicity study of silver nanoparticles in bone marrow cells of Sprague-Dawley rats. Food Chem Toxicol 85:52–60
5. Dobrzynska MM, Gajowik A, Radzikowska J, Lankoff A, Dusinska M, Kruszewski M (2014) Genotoxicity of silver and titanium dioxide nanoparticles in bone marrow cells of rats in vivo. Toxicology 315:86–91
6. Ghosh M, Sinha S, Jothiramajayam M, Jana A, Nag A, Mukherjee A (2016) Cyto-genotoxicity and oxidative stress induced by zinc oxide nanoparticle in human lymphocyte cells in vitro and Swiss albino male mice in vivo. Food Chem Toxicol 97:286–296
7. Magdolenova Z, Collins A, Kumar A, Dhawan A, Stone V, Dusinska M (2014) Mechanisms of genotoxicity. A review of in vitro and in vivo studies with engineered nanoparticles. Nanotoxicology 8:233–278
8. Pati R, Das I, Mehta RK, Sahu R, Sonawane A (2016) Zinc-oxide nanoparticles exhibit genotoxic, clastogenic, cytotoxic and actin depolymerization effects by inducing oxidative stress responses in macrophages and adult mice. Toxicol Sci 150:454–472
9. Hirano T (2008) Repair system of 7, 8-dihydro-8-oxoguanine as a defense line against carcinogenesis. J Radiat Res 49:329–340
10. Greenman C, Stephens P, Smith R et al (2007) Patterns of somatic mutation in human cancer genomes. Nature 446:153–158
11. Rogakou EP, Boon C, Redon C, Bonner WM (1999) Megabase chromatin domains involved in DNA double-strand breaks in vivo. J Cell Biol 146:905–916
12. van Gent DC, Hoeijmakers JH, Kanaar R (2001) Chromosomal stability and the DNA double-stranded break connection. Nat Rev Genet 2:196–206
13. Hayashi M, MacGregor JT, Gatehouse DG et al (2000) In vivo rodent erythrocyte micronucleus assay. II. Some aspects of protocol design including repeated treatments, integration with toxicity testing, and automated scoring. Environ Mol Mutagen 35:234–252
14. Hayashi M (2016) The micronucleus test-most widely used in vivo genotoxicity test. Genes Environ 38:18
15. Golde WT, Gollobin P, Rodriguez LL (2005) A rapid, simple, and humane method for submandibular bleeding of mice using a lancet. Lab Anim (NY) 34:39–43
16. Soultanakis RP, Melamede RJ, Bespalov IA et al (2000) Fluorescence detection of 8-oxoguanine in nuclear and mitochondrial DNA of cultured cells using a recombinant Fab and confocal scanning laser microscopy. Free Radic Biol Med 28:987–998
17. Nallanthighal S, Shirode AB, Judd JA, Reliene R (2016) Pomegranate Intake Protects Against Genomic Instability Induced by Medical X-rays In Vivo in Mice. Nutr Cancer 68:1349–1356

Chapter 18

Evaluation of Pulmonary Toxicity of Nanoparticles by Bronchoalveolar Lavage

Yiqun Mo, Yue Zhang, and Qunwei Zhang

Abstract

Nanoparticles can enter the body via the lungs, the digestive tract, and the skin. The pulmonary effects of nanoparticles and the underlying mechanisms may be investigated by histopathological examination, immunostaining, bronchoalveolar lavage (BAL), and so on. BAL is a simple, fast, and inexpensive method that is commonly used to investigate the immune cells and acellular components in the lungs, which reflect the health state of the lungs. In this chapter, we describe the detailed procedures of performing BAL on mouse lungs. In a typical procedure, a catheter is inserted in the exposed trachea of a mouse, through which a phosphate-buffered saline (PBS) solution containing ethylenediaminetetraacetic acid (EDTA) is instilled into the lungs by a syringe. BAL fluid (BALF) is collected by gently retracting the instilled solution and massaging the thoracic cavity to maximize BALF retrieval and to minimize shearing forces. The type and number of differentiated immune cells in the BALF are analyzed, and the soluble factors such as total proteins, chemokines, and cytokines in the BALF are determined by protein assay, ELISA, etc.

Key words Nanoparticles, Bronchoalveolar lavage, BALF, Mouse lungs, Immune cells

1 Introduction

Bronchoalveolar lavage (BAL) is a simple, fast, and inexpensive technique that is commonly used to determine the health state of the lungs by counting the type and number of immune cells and by analyzing the soluble factors such as cytokines and chemokines in the BAL fluid (BALF). It is widely used to examine immune cells, pathogens, proteins, and the expression levels of inflammation-related and other genes in the cells. Nanoparticles can enter the body via the lungs, the digestive tract, and the skin, resulting in inflammation locally and systemically. After entering the lungs, nanoparticles may cause immune cells such as neutrophils, macrophages, and eosinophils to infiltrate the lumen of lungs and cause acellular contents, such as cytokines and chemokines, to be secreted. Therefore, BAL is an efficient way to determine the effects of nanoparticles on the lungs and to elucidate the underlying

Qunwei Zhang (ed.), *Nanotoxicity: Methods and Protocols*, Methods in Molecular Biology, vol. 1894, https://doi.org/10.1007/978-1-4939-8916-4_18,

mechanisms of nanoparticle-induced lung effects. In addition, performing BAL is simple and does not need special tools or equipment. Here, we will describe the detailed procedures for performing BAL on mouse lungs, for identifying and enumerating different types of inflammatory cells using Giemsa and May Grünwald stains, and for determining the total protein concentration by Bio-Rad Protein Assay. However, evaluating the cellular composition in the BALF by flow cytometry [1], immunostaining [2], or PCR [3], and determining the acellular composition by enzyme-linked immunosorbent assay (ELISA) [4], immunoblot [5], or the simultaneous analysis of multiple cytokines by a cytokine bead array [6], are not within the scope of this chapter.

2 Materials

All animal use in this chapter was reviewed and approved by the University of Louisville Institutional Animal Care and Use Committee. A clean lab coat and disposable gloves should always be worn.

1. 0.5 M ethylenediaminetetraacetic acid (EDTA, pH 8.0): Add 18.6 g of disodium EDTA·$2H_2O$ to 80 mL of ultrapure water. Stir vigorously on a magnetic stirrer. Adjust the pH to 8.0 with NaOH (~2 g of NaOH pellets). Add water to 100 mL by using a graduated cylinder. Autoclave and store at room temperature (*see* **Note 1**).
2. Phosphate-buffered saline (1× PBS): Weigh 8 g NaCl, 0.2 g KCl, 1.44 g Na_2HPO_4, and 0.24 g KH_2PO_4, and dissolve in 800 mL water. Adjust pH to 7.4 with HCl. Add water to 1000 mL by using a graduated cylinder. Autoclave and store at room temperature.
3. Lavage fluid (1× PBS with 0.4 mM EDTA): Add 400 μL of 0.5 M EDTA to 500 mL of 1× PBS. Store at 4 °C (*see* **Note 2**).
4. Catheter: SURFLO® PTFE I.V. catheter, 20G × 1–1/4″, Terumo (Philippines) Corporation (Fig. 1).
5. 70% ethanol: Mix 350 mL of 100% ethanol and 150 mL of ddH_2O to make a 500 mL of 70% ethanol.
6. Anesthetics (*see* **Note 3**): 300 mg/kg body weight of 2, 2, 2-tribromoethanol (*see* **Note 4** for detailed preparation procedure) in the abdominal cavity using a hypodermic needle. An additional dose (175 mg/kg of 2, 2, 2-tribromoethanol) will be used if needed.
7. Trypan Blue Solution: 0.4% (w/v), in normal saline. Store at room temperature.

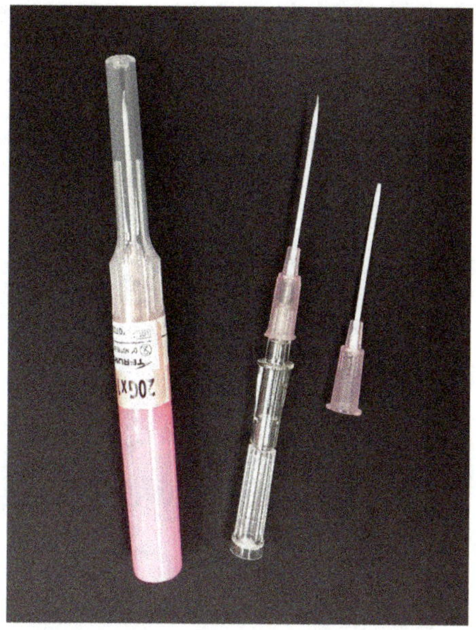

Fig. 1 Catheter for BAL. SURFLO® PTFE I.V. catheter, 20G × 1–1/4″, Terumo (Philippines) Corporation

8. May-Grünwald Stain: 0.25% (w/v), in methanol. Store at room temperature.
9. Giemsa Stain, modified: 0.4% (w/v), in a buffered methanol solution, pH 6.9, with stabilizers. Store at room temperature.
10. Bio-Rad Protein Assay Dye Reagent Concentrate: Bio-Rad, Hercules, CA, USA.
11. Protein standards: bovine gamma globulin (BGG, lyophilized, Bio-Rad) or bovine serum albumin (BSA, lyophilized, Bio-Rad). When reconstituted, it provides 20 mL of 1.4 ± 0.2 mg/mL of BGG or BSA.

3 Methods

3.1 Animal Preparation

1. Weigh the mice prior to bronchoalveolar lavage (BAL).
2. Anesthetize the mouse by administration of 300 mg/kg body weight of 2, 2, 2-tribromoethanol in the abdominal cavity using a hypodermic needle. With this dosage the mice are usually anesthetized within 5–10 min (*see* **Note 5**). An additional dose (175 mg/kg of 2, 2, 2-tribromoethanol) will be used if needed.
3. Place the mouse in supine position on a surgical plate and fix the limbs of the mouse by rubber bands, tape, pins, needles, etc. (Fig. 2a).

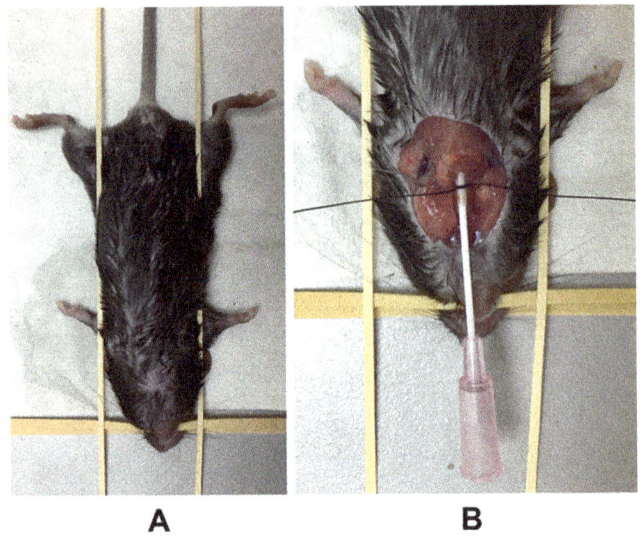

Fig. 2 Mouse bronchoalveolar lavage

4. Dampen the mouse from neck to abdomen with 70% ethanol (Fig. 2a).
5. Open the abdominal cavity using scissors by making an incision in the abdominal skin.
6. Sacrifice the mouse by severing major blood vessels in the abdominal cavity such as abdominal aorta, inferior vena cava, and renal artery and vein.
7. Soak up blood with Kimwipes.

3.2 Catheter Placement

1. Make an incision on the neck skin near the trachea using a scalpel or scissors.
2. Separate the salivary glands in the mouse neck by using forceps to expose the sternohyoid muscle.
3. Gently incise the muscle around the trachea using forceps to expose the trachea.
4. Use forceps to insert a ~10 cm-long cotton or silk string under the trachea.
5. Insert the catheter about 0.5 cm into the exposed trachea between two cartilage rings (*see* **Note 6**). Take care not to damage the trachea.
6. Carefully withdraw the needle and discard it in a sharps container. Only leave the catheter hub in the trachea.
7. Tie the trachea around the catheter hub using the preplaced string to stabilize the catheter hub (*see* **Note 7**) (Fig. 2b).

3.3 Collecting the BALF

1. Load a 1 mL syringe with 0.8 mL of ice-cold lavage fluid.
2. Connect the syringe to the catheter hub and gently inject the lavage fluid into the lungs.
3. Aspirate the solution gently while massaging the thorax of the mouse. If no fluid is aspirated, carefully insert the catheter a little further down or up the trachea.
4. Remove the syringe from the catheter hub. Transfer the recovered lavage fluid into a 1.5 mL Eppendorf tube on ice (*see* **Note 8**).
5. Repeat **steps 1–4** four more times and save the lavage fluid in a 15 mL tube (*see* **Note 9**).
6. Estimate and record the volume of BALF collected according to the marks on the 1.5 mL and 15 mL tubes.

3.4 Obtaining the Noncellular and Cellular Components of the BALF

1. Centrifuge the first lavage fluid in the 1.5 mL Eppendorf tube for 5 min at 200 × *g* and 4 °C.
2. Collect the supernatant in two 0.5 mL Eppendorf tubes (210 μL per tube) and keep the remaining supernatant in a 1.5 mL Eppendorf tube for further analysis such as ELISA, determination of protein concentration, etc. Store the supernatant at −80 °C if not used immediately.
3. Add 0.5 mL of ice-cold lavage fluid into the first 1.5 mL Eppendorf tube with the cell pellet.
4. Mix and transfer the cell suspension into the 15 mL tube containing lavage fluid samples 2–5 on ice (Subheading 3.3, **step 5**).
5. Centrifuge the cell suspension in the 15 mL tube for 10 min at 200 × *g* and 4 °C.
6. Remove and discard the supernatant by aspiration.
7. Resuspend cell pellet in 0.5 mL of ice-cold lavage fluid. This is the cellular part of the BALF.

3.5 Determining the Total Number of Cells in BALF

1. From the cell suspension tube in Subheading 3.4, **step 7**, mix 10 μL of cell suspension with 10 μL of 0.4% (w/v) of Trypan Blue Solution, and immediately load 10 μL of mixture into a hemocytometer.
2. Count the cells in the two of nine 1 × 1 mm (1 mm^2) squares (*see* **Note 10**).
3. The concentration of cells in BAL is calculated as the following (cells/mL): the average cell count from each of the corner 1 × 1 mm square × 10^4 × 2.
4. The total number of cells in BAL is calculated as the following: the concentration of cells in BAL (cells/mL) × the total volume of the cell suspension (0.5 mL).

3.6 Preparation of Cytospin Slides

1. Mix cell suspension and ice-cold lavage fluid to give 25,000–50,000 cells in 200 μL in a 1.5 mL Eppendorf tube.
2. Load all 200 μL of cell suspension sample into cytospin bucket/filter/glass slide assembly and spin at 600 rpm for 3 min at room temperature by using a Thermo Scientific® Cytospin® 4 Cytocentrifuge.
3. Disassemble and let slides dry completely (*see* **Note 11**).
4. Centrifuge the remaining cell suspension in the 1.5 mL Eppendorf tube for 5 min at 200 × g and 4 °C.
5. Remove the supernatant. The cell pellets can be lysed for RNA or protein extraction. Store the cells at −80 °C if not used immediately.

3.7 Analysis of the Different Cell Types in the BALF

To analyze the different cell types in the BAL fluid, both cell counting on a stained cytospin slide or flow cytometry may be used. Flow cytometry is a specialized technique that uses a specific fluorophore-conjugated antibody to recognize a specific surface antigen on each particular cell type. It is relatively expensive and requires access to a machine and trained personnel to perform. Since this chapter focuses on the technique of bronchoalveolar lavage, we will not discuss flow cytometry here. Instead, we will introduce a common, simple, inexpensive, and relatively fast method to analyze the different cell types in the BAL by counting cells on a stained cytospin slide. There are several ways to stain the cytospin slides, such as by using DIFF-QUIK stain kit, Wright-Giemsa stain, etc. Here we will introduce a method using Giemsa and May Grünwald stains to stain the cytospin slides.

1. Dilute Giemsa Stain 1:20 with ddH_2O (*see* **Note 12**).
2. Place slides in May-Grünwald stain for 5 min (*see* **Note 13**).
3. Briefly rinse slides in 1× PBS.
4. Place slides in diluted Giemsa solution from **step 1** for 15–20 min.
5. Rinse slides briefly in ddH_2O (*see* **Note 14**).
6. Air-dry completely and evaluate. A minimum of 400 cells will be examined under a light microscope (*see* **Note 15**) (Fig. 3).

3.8 Determination of the Total Protein Concentration in the BALF

The concentration of total protein in the BALF can be determined by the Bradford method using Bio-Rad Protein Assay (Bio-Rad, Hercules, CA). It is a simple and relatively accurate procedure for determining the relative concentration of solubilized protein by comparison to a standard curve.

1. Reconstitute the protein standards (lyophilized bovine gamma globulin, BGG, or bovine serum albumin, BSA) by adding

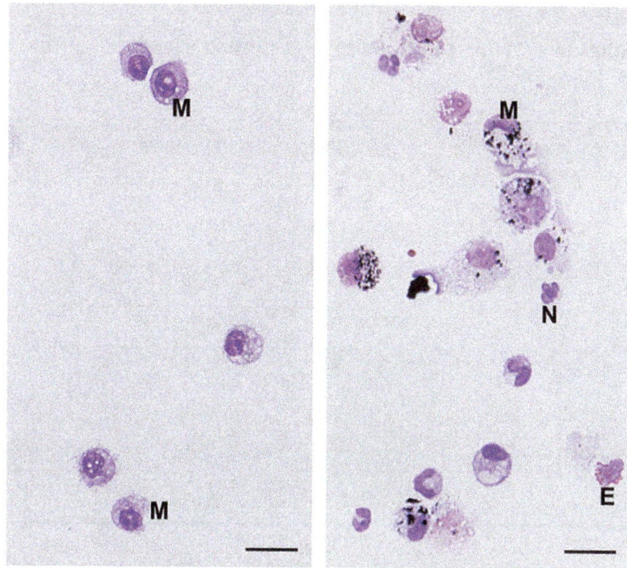

Fig. 3 Cells in lung lavage fluid (BALF). C57BL/6J mice were intratracheally instilled with 50 μg per mouse of nickel nanoparticles (Nano-Ni) . Control mice were instilled with normal saline. Cells in BALF were collected from mice at day 3 after exposure, and stained with May-Grünwald/Giemsa stains (Sigma-Aldrich, St. Louis, MO). *M* macrophage, *N* neutrophil, *E* eosinophil. Scale bar: 20 μm

20 mL of ddH_2O and mix until dissolved. The solution is 1.4 mg/mL and should be aliquoted and frozen at −20 °C.

2. Dilute the protein standard solution to 0.1 mg/mL with ddH_2O.
3. Prepare 1× dye reagent by diluting 1 part Dye Reagent Concentrate with 4 parts ddH_2O. Filter through Whatman #1 filter (or equivalent) to remove particulates (*see* **Note 16**).
4. Prepare a series of dilutions of a protein standard. The total volume of the solution is 100 μL (*see* **Note 17**) (Table 1).
5. Pipet 5–20 μL of BALF samples into a clean and dry 1.5 mL Eppendorf tube (*see* **Note 18**). Protein solutions are normally assayed in duplicate or triplicate.
6. Add ddH_2O to dilute the BALF sample to 100 μL.
7. Add 900 μL of 1× dye reagent to each tube of standards and samples and vortex.
8. Incubate at room temperature for at least 5 min, but less than 1 h (*see* **Note 19**).
9. Measure absorbance at 595 nm (*see* **Note 20**).
10. Calculate the protein concentration in the BALF according to the standard curve.

Table 1
Preparation of a series of dilutions of a protein standard, bovine serum albumin (BSA, lyophilized, Bio-Rad, Hercules, CA, USA)

Tube No.	BSA (0.1 mg/mL) (μL)	ddH_2O (μL)	1xdye reagent (μL)	Total (μL)	Final BSA concentration (μg/mL)
1	0	100	900	1000	0
2	10	90	900	1000	1
3	20	80	900	1000	2
4	40	60	900	1000	4
5	60	40	900	1000	6
6	80	20	900	1000	8
7	100	0	900	1000	10

4 Notes

1. The disodium salt of EDTA will not dissolve until the pH of the solution is adjusted to ~8.0 by the addition of NaOH pellets.
2. To measure the protein level in the BAL fluid (BALF), it is recommended to add protease inhibitors to prevent protease activity in the BALF.
3. Since inhaled anesthesia may have an influence on the BAL fluid content, we suggest using injected anesthesia. For example, CO_2 can influence the pH of the blood and consequently cause the redistribution of certain compounds.
4. 2, 2, 2-Tribromoethanol (TBE, >96.5%) will be dissolved in tertiary-amyl alcohol in a 1 g/1 mL ratio, labeled with an expiration date of 6 months from the time of preparation, and kept in a dark bottle away from light and tightly sealed. Stirring on magnetic stirrer and heating to approximately 40–50 °C may help dissolve the TBE. To make a working solution, the stock solution will be diluted 1:80 in warm normal saline, resulting in a final concentration of 12.5 mg/mL. The solution will be sterilized by 0.2 μm filtration in a Class II biological safety cabinet and stored in sterile vials with rubber septum to maintain sterility. The solution will be labeled with an expiration date of 2 weeks from the time of preparation and stored protected from light at 4 °C. Do not use any stock or working solution that is discolored, and/or has any evidence of a precipitate.

5. Anesthetic depth will be assessed by an inability to remain upright, loss of voluntary movement, loss of blink reflex, muscle relaxation, and loss of response to reflex stimulation (toe pinch with firm pressure).
6. Ensure that the catheter is not inserted too far down into the trachea, as this can damage the lung structure or result in incomplete lavage.
7. If the catheter hub is not tied sufficiently, it will result in lavage fluid leakage. The lavage fluid may also flow toward the upper part of the respiratory tract instead of down into the lungs.
8. Normally, 500–700 μL of BAL is recovered from 0.8 mL of injected solution.
9. After performing BAL with 4× 0.8 mL of ice-cold lavage fluid, a volume between 2.8 and 3.2 mL should be recovered.
10. We usually count the cells in the two of four corner 1 × 1 mm (1 mm^2) squares.
11. It requires a wait of at least 10 min after removing bucket and filter paper.
12. For bluer coloration, water buffered at pH 7.2 may be used in place of ddH_2O.
13. If slides will not be stained immediately, cells on the slides can be fixed in 100% methanol or −20 °C acetone for 5–7 min. Let slides air-dry for later staining.
14. We usually dip slides once in a large container of water (about 2 s).
15. If slides need to be stored for longer periods of time, they can be immersed in 100% xylene twice, 5 min each time and mounted using a coverslip and a small drop of Permount.
16. This diluted reagent may be used for approximately 2 weeks when kept at room temperature.
17. The linear range of the assay for BSA is about 1.2–10.0 μg/mL, whereas with BGG the linear range is about 1.2 to 25 μg/mL.
18. We usually use 20 μL of BALF samples obtained from the control mice to determine their protein concentration. However, for BALF samples obtained from nanoparticle-treated mice, the volume of BALF used varies and pretest is needed to find the appropriate volume of BALF. For example, we usually use 5 μL of BALF obtained from mice intratracheally instilled with nickel or cobalt nanoparticles.
19. Absorbance will increase over time; samples should incubate at room temperature for no more than 1 h.

20. The Bio-Rad Protein Assay can also be used with a microplate reader. We suggest reading the manufacturer's instruction carefully before conducting this experiment.

Acknowledgment

This work was partly supported by the NIESH/NIH (ES023693 and ES028911), KSEF-148-502-16-381, Kentucky Lung Cancer Research Program, and an Intramural Research Incentive Grants (50992) from UofL to Dr. Qunwei Zhang.

References

1. Van Hoecke L, Job ER, Saelens X, Roose K (2017) Bronchoalveolar lavage of murine lungs to analyze inflammatory cell infiltration. J Vis Exp 123:e55398. https://doi.org/10.3791/55398
2. Mo Y, Chen J, Schlueter CF, Hoyle GW (2013) Differential susceptibility of inbred mouse strains to chlorine-induced airway fibrosis. Am J Physiol Lung Cell Mol Physiol 304(2): L92–L102. https://doi.org/10.1152/ajplung.00272.2012
3. Mo Y, Wan R, Zhang Q (2012) Application of reverse transcription-PCR and real-time PCR in nanotoxicity research. Nanotoxicity: Method and Protocols. In the series: Methods in Molecular Biology, edited by John Walker, Springer Protocol. (www.SpringerProtocols.com). Humana Press. DOI: https://doi.org/10.1007/978-1-62703-002-1; Methods Mol. Biol; 926: 99–112
4. Wan R, Mo Y, Zhang Z, Jiang M, Tang S, Zhang Q (2017) Cobalt nanoparticles induce lung injury, DNA damage and mutations in mice. Part Fibre Toxicol 14:38. https://doi.org/10.1186/s12989-017-0219-z
5. Gallagher S, Chakavarti D (2008) Immunoblot analysis. J Vis Exp 16:759. https://doi.org/10.3791/759
6. Mo Y, Chen J, Humphrey DM Jr, Fodah RA, Warawa JM, Hoyle GW (2015) Abnormal epithelial structure and chronic lung inflammation after repair of chlorine-induced airway injury. Am J Physiol Lung Cell Mol Physiol 308(2): L168–L178. https://doi.org/10.1152/ajplung.00226.2014

Chapter 19

Pulmonary Function Testing in Animals

Gary W. Hoyle, Connie F. Schlueter, and Sadiatu Musah

Abstract

Nanoparticles possess a number of useful properties that make them useful for a variety of industrial and commercial applications. The small size of nanoparticles means that they are respirable and can penetrate deep into the lung when inhaled. Because of this, there is interest in assessing possible toxic effects of nanoparticles on the respiratory system. Measurement of respiratory mechanics and pulmonary function represents a sensitive way of detecting pathological effects of inhaled substances on the lungs. Here we describe a procedure for conducting pulmonary function measurements in mice using the forced oscillation technique. Measurements of baseline lung mechanics are conducted in anesthetized, mechanically ventilated mice, followed by repeated measurements subsequent to inhalation challenge with aerosolized methacholine. General guidelines for data analysis are provided, and sample results are presented.

Key words Pulmonary function testing, Forced oscillation technique, Lung resistance, Lung compliance

1 Introduction

Nanoparticles have unique chemical and physical properties that have made them useful in a variety of industrial, medical, and consumer applications [1]. However, the rapid expansion in the use of nanoparticles has been coupled with concerns regarding the toxicity of nanomaterials resulting from their unusual characteristics [2]. The respiratory system is a major portal of entry for exogenous substances into the body. Because of their small size, nanoparticles are readily inhaled and penetrate deep into the lung, where they have the potential to cause adverse health effects [3]. Nanoparticles have been reported to produce a variety of toxic effects on the lung, including inflammation [4, 5], oxidative stress [3], DNA damage [5], and inhibition of surfactant function [6]. Pulmonary toxicities such as these have the potential to cause lung disease de novo as well as to exacerbate preexisting pulmonary conditions.

Pulmonary function testing provides a sensitive measure of lung health and is capable of detecting even subtle manifestations

Qunwei Zhang (ed.), *Nanotoxicity: Methods and Protocols*, Methods in Molecular Biology, vol. 1894, https://doi.org/10.1007/978-1-4939-8916-4_19, © Springer Science+Business Media, LLC, part of Springer Nature 2019

of acute or chronic lung injury. Such manifestations of injury include airway and parenchymal remodeling, airway hyperreactivity, and changes in airway tone and lung compliance. In humans, lung function is most commonly assessed by spirometry, which allows for measurement of air flow through the respiratory tract as well as certain lung volumes, including forced vital capacity. Other types of lung function procedures include whole body plethysmography for measuring lung volumes and diffusing capacity for measuring the ability of gases to pass between the air spaces and bloodstream. An alternative to spirometry for measuring lung function is impulse oscillometry, which involves measurement of pressure and volume changes in the respiratory tract in response to the application of defined oscillatory signals [7]. The impulse oscillometry technique has the advantage of requiring only the passive cooperation of the subject, as opposed to spirometry, which requires the subject to perform active, forced exhalation maneuvers that may be difficult in children, the elderly, or patients with lung disease. Likewise, for measurement of lung function in animals, a technique not requiring cooperation of the subject is needed, and a related method, forced oscillation technique (FOT), has been used [8]. FOT allows for the measurement of lung resistance and compliance, and, with the use of appropriate mathematical modeling, can dissociate lung functional impairment between the central airway tree and the distal lung [9, 10]. FOT has been used to assess lung function in mice and rats exposed to nanoparticles [11–14]. A method for measuring lung mechanics via FOT in mice with lung injury caused by exposure to nanoparticles or other toxic agents is the subject of the present chapter.

For measurement of lung function in mice by FOT, the subject is anesthetized, mechanically ventilated, and treated with a neuromuscular blocking agent to inhibit endogenous breathing effort. Baseline measurements are collected by applying pressure/volume perturbations to the respiratory system and measuring the corresponding changes in airway opening pressure. The derived signals are used to calculate lung mechanics parameters. A single frequency perturbation at 2.5 Hz is used to derive resistance and compliance, and a broadband perturbation from 1 to 20.5 Hz is analyzed to derive parameters via the constant phase model, which can be used to attribute functional changes to the central airways or distal lung [9, 10]. Once baseline measurements are made, the response of the lung to challenge with increasing doses of the bronchoconstricting drug methacholine is assessed. Methacholine inhalation is the basis of a bronchoprovocation test that is sometimes used clinically in the diagnosis of asthma. Diseased lungs often exhibit an exaggerated response to methacholine challenge, which is a phenomenon known as airway hyperreactivity. Thus, measuring the response to methacholine is a potential way to detect subtle pulmonary abnormalities that may not be apparent from the baseline measurements.

2 Materials

2.1 Equipment

1. SCIREQ flexiVent system including base unit, controller, ventilator module 1 for mice, flexiWare software, and AeroNeb nebulizer unit.

2.2 Solutions

1. Dulbecco's phosphate buffered saline, calcium and magnesium-free (D-PBS): 2.67 mM potassium chloride, 1.47 mM potassium phosphate monobasic, 138 mM sodium chloride, 8.1 mM sodium phosphate dibasic.
2. Normal saline: 0.9% sodium chloride.
3. 15 mg/ml tribromoethanol (*see* **Note 1**).
4. 0.08 mg/ml pancuronium bromide in D-PBS.
5. 50 mg/ml methacholine chloride in D-PBS; twofold serial dilutions of this stock are performed to produce solutions for the methacholine dose–response curve.

3 Methods

3.1 Data Collection

1. Turn on computer and flexiVent system. Enter mouse subject data, including weight, into system.
2. Calibrate pressure transducers and tracheal cannula according to SCIREQ instructions.
3. Anesthetize mouse with 375 mg/kg tribromoethanol by intraperitoneal injection and check for absence of toe-pinch reflex before starting procedure. Additional doses of 50–100 mg/kg tribromoethanol may be given if needed until the animal is unresponsive.
4. Place mouse on 35 °C warming pad, and attach EKG leads to paws for monitoring of heart rate during procedure.
5. Place tracheal cannula and start mechanical ventilation. This is done by making a 1 cm longitudinal incision in the skin over the ventral midline of the neck. The salivary glands over the tracheal muscle are reflected, and a small longitudinal incision is made in the muscle overlying the trachea. A small incision is made in the trachea to allow insertion of the tracheal cannula (a blunt-end 19 g × ½" needle). After insertion of the cannula, the mouse is connected to the ventilator equipped with transducers to measure the cylinder and airway opening pressures. Mice are mechanically ventilated with a tidal volume of 10 ml/kg at 150 breaths/min and a positive end-expiratory pressure of 3 cm of water.
6. Inject additional doses of 50–100 mg/kg tribromoethanol as needed to stabilize mouse on ventilator with a heart rate of

250–300 beats per minute. Inject additional tribromoethanol as needed throughout the procedure to maintain the heart rate in this range.

7. Inject mouse intraperitoneally with 0.8 mg/kg pancuronium bromide to inhibit endogenous breathing effort. Wait 3 min after injection before starting perturbations and data collection.
8. Start perturbations and collect data for baseline lung function (*see* **Note 2**).
9. Add 50 μl D-PBS (i.e., 0 mg/ml methacholine dose) to the AeroNeb chamber. Start the methacholine dose-response by nebulizing the solution for 10 s followed by performing perturbations and collecting data (*see* **Note 3**). Remove residual liquid from AeroNeb chamber, load the next methacholine dose, and start perturbations and data collection. Repeat for the remaining methacholine doses (*see* **Note 4**).
10. Euthanize mouse while still anesthetized by making an abdominal incision and cutting the abdominal aorta and diaphragm.
11. Export data from the flexiWare system into Excel.

3.2 Data Analysis

1. Analysis of baseline data. For baseline data, the repeated measurements for each parameter are averaged to produce a single value per mouse for each parameter. The values are then averaged over all mice in a treatment group (e.g., exposed to nanoparticles vs. unexposed). Figure 1 shows an example of baseline data for healthy mice vs. those with lung injury.
2. Analysis of methacholine challenge data. For methacholine dose-response data, the 15 values collected for each parameter following each methacholine dose are averaged (eliminating any with coefficients of determination <90%) to produce a single value for each parameter for each dose for each mouse (*see* **Note 5**). Values are then averaged over the animal treatment groups. Figure 2 shows an example of the effect of methacholine challenge on respiratory system resistance in healthy mice and those with lung injury.
3. Analysis of input impedance data. In addition to analysis using the constant phase model, the input impedance data collected in response to the Quick Prime-3 perturbation can be analyzed directly. This approach can be advantageous because it does not require parameter fitting based on a model of normal lung, and hence can be used even in situations where there is severe lung injury or exaggerated bronchoconstriction. In addition, this type of data analysis is analogous to that used for impulse oscillometry studies in humans [7], thus affording better linking of phenotypes among species. Impedance is a complex value, having both real and imaginary components at each

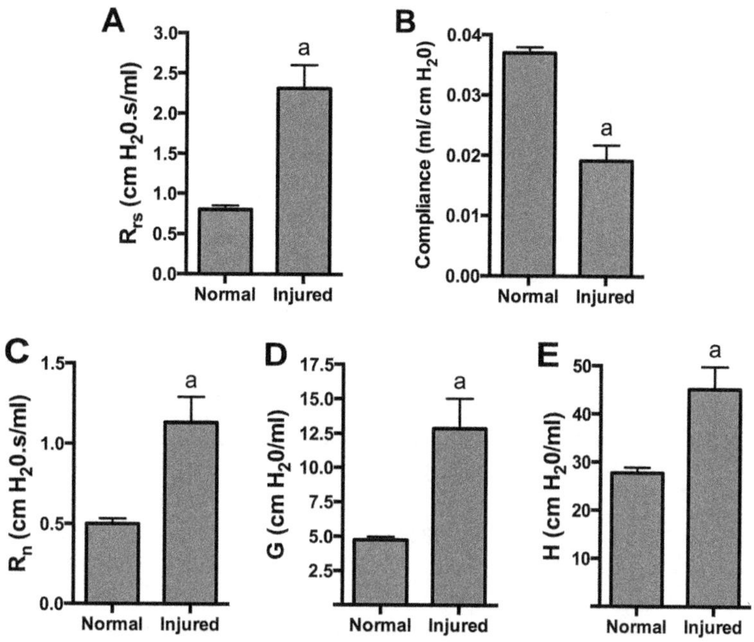

Fig. 1 Baseline lung mechanics. Baseline measurement of parameters derived from the SnapShot-150 (**a** and **b**) or Quick Prime-3 (**c**–**e**) perturbations. (**a**) Respiratory system resistance (R_{rs}). (**b**) Compliance. (**c**) Newtonian resistance (Rn, a measurement of central airways resistance). (**d**) Tissue damping (G, related to tissue resistance). (**e**) Tissue elastance (H). a $p < 0.01$ vs. normal

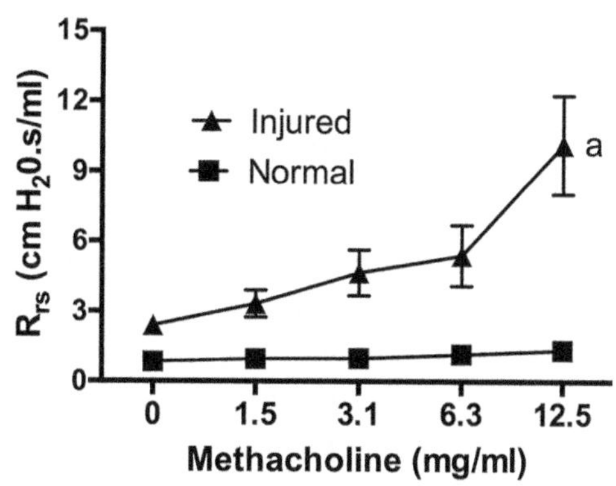

Fig. 2 Methacholine challenge dose-response. Dose–response curves for the effect of methacholine challenge on respiratory system resistance in mice with normal or injured lungs. Error bars on the normal curve are smaller than the symbols. a, dose–response curve different from normal at $p < 0.0001$ by repeated measures ANOVA

frequency. The real part of impedance can be plotted as resistance vs. frequency and the imaginary part can be plotted as reactance vs. frequency. This type of data analysis can be used to dissociate the responses of the central and peripheral

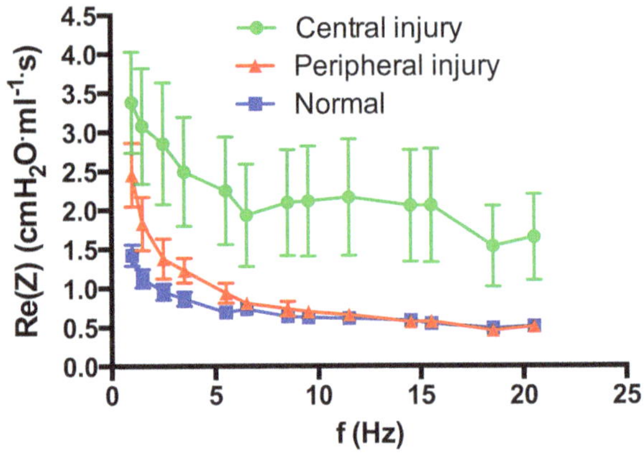

Fig. 3 Impedance data. Resistance is plotted as the real part of input impedance as a function of frequency. The curves show the effects of injury to different parts of the lung. Injury to the central portion of the respiratory tract produces increased resistance at both high and low frequencies (circles). Injury to the distal lung causes increased resistance specifically at low frequencies (triangles)

portions of the respiratory system, with effects at low frequencies indicative of responses in the peripheral lung. Figure 3 shows a comparison of frequency-dependent resistance derived from impedance data from mice with central or peripheral lung disease.

4 Notes

1. Tribromoethanol stock solution is made by adding 1 g of tribromoethanol to 1 ml of tert-amyl alcohol and warming to 45 °C to dissolve. This produces a stock solution of 770 mg/ml tribromoethanol. The working solution of 15 mg/ml is obtained by diluting the stock solution 1:50 with normal saline and sterilizing by filtration. The stock and working solutions should be stored at 4 °C protected from light. Any unused working solution should be discarded 2 weeks after preparation.
2. A variety of perturbations is available through the flexiWare software to assess lung mechanics. For baseline lung function, we typically use SnapShot-150 to measure resistance and compliance using the single compartment model, Quick Prime-3 to measure frequency-dependent impedance and parameters derived from the constant phase model, and PVs-P to perform a quasi-static pressure–volume curve. The perturbations can be run manually or can be executed automatically using scripts. We typically perform the SnapShot-150, Quick Prime-3, and PVs-P perturbations in series and then repeat the series twice more to collect a total of three baseline measurements for each

parameter. If any measurements have coefficients of determination <90%, the perturbations are repeated to collect a minimum of three acceptable measurements per parameter.

3. We typically perform 15 SnapShot-150 and Quick Prime-3 perturbations following each methacholine dose. Collection of this number of data points allows the peak responses after methacholine challenge to be identified.
4. Considerations for choosing the concentrations of methacholine for the dose–response curve include the type of mouse and extent of lung injury. An upper limit of 50 mg/ml produces a moderate increase in respiratory system resistance in wild-type mice without lung disease, but this dose may produce a severe response in genetically altered mice with abnormal lung structure or in wild-type mice with lung injury or disease. In some cases, an exaggerated bronchoconstrictive response may produce data that do not fit well to the underlying analysis models, resulting in low coefficients of determination. In this case, a lower dose for the upper end of the curve (e.g., 12.5 or 25 mg/ml) is recommended. Once the appropriate highest dose is determined, other doses can be generated by twofold serial dilutions of the highest dose. Typically, 4–5 doses (plus D-PBS alone as 0 mg/ml dose) are performed, which represents a balance between a full range dose–response curve and the time it takes to perform the measurements. Therefore, an example of a methacholine dose–response curve for a healthy wild-type mouse would involve challenge with doses of 0, 3.13, 6.25, 12.5, 25, and 50 mg/ml methacholine. The time to prepare the subject and perform the baseline measurements and methacholine dose-response will be approximately 40–60 min for each mouse. An abbreviated challenge involving fewer or even a single methacholine dose can be done if time is a particularly important consideration.
5. An alternative data analysis strategy is to use the peak (or trough) value for each parameter after each methacholine dose. This approach will highlight the maximum effects of methacholine, but may produce curves with increased variance caused by sporadic high (or low) values.

References

1. Chan-Remillard S, Kapustka L, Goudey S (2009) Nanotechnology. In: Linkov I, Steevens J (eds) Nanomaterials: risks and benefits. Nato science for peace and security series C: environmental security. Springer, Dordrecht
2. Wu T, Tang M (2018) Review of the effects of manufactured nanoparticles on mammalian target organs. J Appl Toxicol 38(1):25–40
3. Madl AK, Plummer LE, Carosino C, Pinkerton KE (2014) Nanoparticles, lung injury, and the role of oxidant stress. Annu Rev Physiol 76:447–465
4. Shoeb M, Kodali V, Farris B, Bishop LM, Meighan T, Salmen R, Eye T, Roberts JR, Zeidler-Erdely P, Erdely A, Antonini JM (2017) Evaluation of the molecular

mechanisms associated with cytotoxicity and inflammation after pulmonary exposure to different metal-rich welding particles. Nanotoxicology 11(6):725–736

5. Wan R, Mo Y, Zhang Z, Jiang M, Tang S, Zhang Q (2017) Cobalt nanoparticles induce lung injury, DNA damage and mutations in mice. Part Fibre Toxicol 14(1):38
6. Beck-Broichsitter M, Ruppert C, Schmehl T, Gunther A, Seeger W (2014) Biophysical inhibition of synthetic vs. naturally-derived pulmonary surfactant preparations by polymeric nanoparticles. Biochim Biophys Acta 1838 (1 Pt B):474–481
7. Smith HJ, Reinhold P, Goldman MD (2005) Forced oscillation technique and impluse oscillometry. Eur Respir Mon 31:72–105
8. Bates JH, Irvin CG, Farre R, Hantos Z (2011) Oscillation mechanics of the respiratory system. Compr Physiol 1(3):1233–1272
9. Hantos Z, Daroczy B, Suki B, Nagy S, Fredberg JJ (1992) Input impedance and peripheral inhomogeneity of dog lungs. J Appl Physiol 72 (1):168–178
10. Irvin CG, Bates JH (2003) Measuring the lung function in the mouse: the challenge of size. Respir Res 4, 4
11. Ambalavanan N, Stanishevsky A, Bulger A, Halloran B, Steele C, Vohra Y, Matalon S (2013) Titanium oxide nanoparticle instillation induces inflammation and inhibits lung development in mice. Am J Physiol Lung Cell Mol Physiol 304(3):L152–L161
12. Botelho DJ, Leo BF, Massa CB, Sarkar S, Tetley TD, Chung KF, Chen S, Ryan MP, Porter AE, Zhang J, Schwander SK, Gow AJ (2016) Low-dose AgNPs reduce lung mechanical function and innate immune defense in the absence of cellular toxicity. Nanotoxicology 10(1):118–127
13. Jonasson S, Gustafsson A, Koch B, Bucht A (2013) Inhalation exposure of nano-scaled titanium dioxide (TiO2) particles alters the inflammatory responses in asthmatic mice. Inhal Toxicol 25(4):179–191
14. Seiffert J, Buckley A, Leo B, Martin NG, Zhu J, Dai R, Hussain F, Guo C, Warren J, Hodgson A, Gong J, Ryan MP, Zhang JJ, Porter A, Tetley TD, Gow A, Smith R, Chung KF (2016) Pulmonary effects of inhalation of spark-generated silver nanoparticles in Brown-Norway and Sprague-Dawley rats. Respir Res 17(1):85

Chapter 20

Nanotoxicity Assessment Using Embryonic Zebrafish

Eduard Dumitrescu, Kenneth Wallace, and Silvana Andreescu

Abstract

The emergence of nanomaterials in industrial processing and consumer products has generated an increased presence of nano-enabled products in the environment and now pose an increased risk of exposure to living organisms. However, assessing the risks of nanomaterials is a challenging task because of a large variety and great variability in their properties. Here, we describe a methodology for assessing toxicity and evaluate potential risks posed by nanomaterials using zebrafish embryos as a model organism. Zebrafish are a well-established organism that has a number of advantages over other biological models. These include optical transparency, similar structure and arrangement of organs, and conserved genetic pathways compared to other vertebrates. Their rapid development and high numbers of embryos enables high throughput screening to study toxicity of a large number of nanomaterials. The method described in this chapter can be used as a universal screening approach to assess toxicity of any type of nanomaterials, determine both lethal and sublethal effects, measure LD50 doses, evaluate morphological and organ defects, cell apoptosis, and production of reactive species.

Key words Nanomaterials, Nanoparticles, Nanotoxicity, Zebrafish embryos, Viability assay, Histology, Apoptosis, Oxidative stress

1 Introduction

The rapid growth of nanotechnology in the last few decades has led to the development and implementation of a large number of nanomaterials in many industrial processes and consumer products [1, 2]. As exposure to nanomaterials continues to increase [3], questions have been raised regarding their interaction with live organisms and potential environmental health and safety (EHS) risks [4]. The main challenge in assessing these risks comes from the great variability in type and properties of nanomaterials such as size, surface coating, surface charge and aggregation tendency, solubility and reactivity, mobility in environmental conditions, and interaction with other species in the surrounding environment [5].

The zebrafish is an established in vivo model for toxicity studies [6, 7] with demonstrated advantages when applied to the study of

Qunwei Zhang (ed.), *Nanotoxicity: Methods and Protocols*, Methods in Molecular Biology, vol. 1894, https://doi.org/10.1007/978-1-4939-8916-4_20,

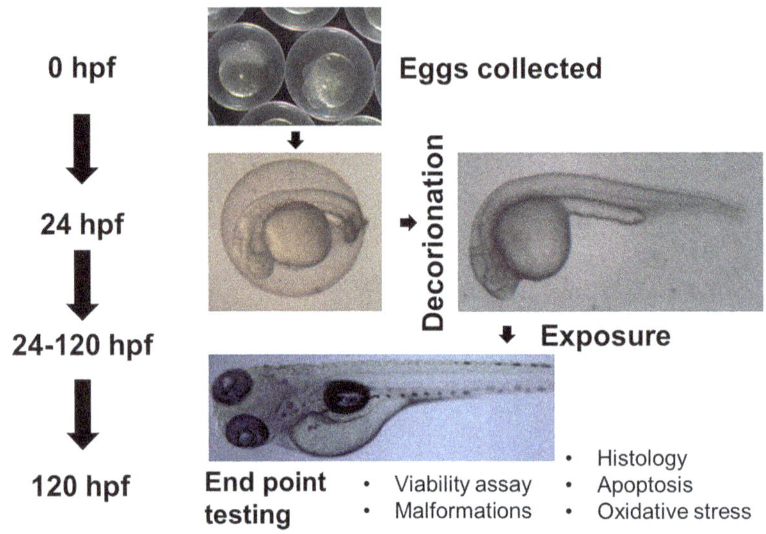

Fig. 1 Schematic representation of the main procedure steps during zebrafish embryos nanotoxicity assessment, including initial preparation, exposure period, and end point analysis

nanomaterial toxicity [8–10]. General approaches to study development and genetics of zebrafish embryos have been previously described [11, 12]. The fecundity, short embryogenesis period, and ease of manipulation make zebrafish embryos a good model for high-throughput testing and evaluation of a large number of materials in a short time. Moreover, zebrafish shares similar organ structure and function as well as genetic information with other vertebrates, which allows for translation of toxicity information to higher organisms, including humans. Zebrafish are well-characterized organisms, and a broad range of tools exist to study embryonic development, which can be applied to nanotoxicity studies.

This chapter describes some of the routine procedures used in the assessment of nanotoxicity using zebrafish embryos, which include (1) determination of mortality, lethal dose, and morphological defects, (2) internalization of nanomaterials and study of their effect on organ development using histological analysis, (3) cellular level effects using apoptosis imaging, and (4) assessment of oxidative stress and the redox imbalance in individual organs through monitoring of reactive oxygen/nitrogen species. Figure 1 shows a general experimental approach that can be used to study nanomaterial effects in zebrafish.

2 Materials

2.1 Exposure Protocol

1. Zebrafish embryos are collected and grown in petri dishes. Exposure experiments are performed in six-well plates. Fixing and storage of embryos is done in 1.5 mL microcentrifuge

tubes. Handling and visualization of embryos is done under a stereomicroscope.

2. E3 embryo medium: 5 mM NaCl, 0.17 mM KCl, 0.33 mM $CaCl_2$, and 0.33 mM $MgSO_4$ in distilled, deionized water (dH_2O). For preparation of E3 medium stock, dissolve 7.3 g NaCl, 0.325 g KCl, 1.1 g $CaCl_2$, and 2.025 $MgSO_4$ in about 300 mL dH_2O and then bring to 500 mL. Dilute the stock 50 times in dH_2O to obtain the E3 embryo medium. 0.003% PTU (1-phenyl-2-thiourea) is added in the E3 medium for pigment inhibition (*see* **Note 1**). Store at 28.5 °C when not in use (*see* **Note 2**).
3. Nanomaterial dispersion for exposure: weigh the amount of nanomaterial to be studied, add a proper volume of E3 with PTU medium, and sonicate for at least 15 min (*see* **Note 3**).
4. 0.4% tricaine (ethyl 3-aminobenzoate) solution: 400 mg tricaine in 97.9 mL dH_2O adjusted to pH 7 using 1 M Tris, pH 9 (*see* **Note 4**). Store at room temperature.
5. 4% PFA (paraformaldehyde) solution: 4 g PFA in 100 mL PBS (*see* **Note 5**).
6. 0.1 M phosphate buffer, pH 7.3: mix 80 mL 0.1 M Na_2HPO_4 with 20 mL 0.1 M NaH_2PO_4.
7. PBS solution: mix 8 g NaCl, 0.2 g KCl, and 200 mL phosphate buffer, and dilute to 1 L in dH_2O. Store at room temperature.
8. PBST solution: 1 mL 100% Tween in 1 L PBS. Store at room temperature.

2.2 Histology Protocol

1. Glycol methacrylate (JB-4 Plus embedding kit, Polysciences).
2. Embedding molds (Polyethylene Molding Cup Trays, Polysciences) and plastic block holders (Polysciences).
3. Azure II–Methylene blue solution: 0.130 g Methylene Blue and 0.020 g Azure II in 50 mL dH_2O, 30 mL PBS solution, 10 mL glycerol, and 10 mL methanol. Store at room temperature.
4. Permount mounting medium (Fisher Chemical). Store at room temperature.
5. Xylenes mixture, to be used as solvent for the mounting medium. Store in a fume hood.

2.3 Apoptosis Protocol

1. 5 μg/mL acridine orange solution in E3 medium (*see* **Note 6**).
2. Antifade mounting medium with DAPI (Vectashield, Vector Laboratories), used for counterstaining. Store at 4 °C.

2.4 Nitrosative Stress Imaging

1. 5 mM DAF-FM DA (4-Amino-5-methylamino-2′,7′-difluorofluorescein diacetate) solution: prepared in E3 medium (*see* **Note 7**).
2. 3 mM L-NAME (N$^{\omega}$-Nitro-L-arginine methyl ester hydrochloride) solution: 8.1 mg L-NAME in 10 mL E3 medium (*see* **Note 8**).
3. 100 μM Spermine NONOate (*N*-[4-[1-(3-Aminopropyl)-2-hydroxy-2-nitrosohydrazino]butyl]-1,3-propanediamine) solution: 0.3 mg Spermine NONOate in 10 mL E3 medium (*see* **Note 8**).

3 Methods

3.1 Viability Assay and Malformations Assessment

1. Collect zebrafish embryos immediately after fertilization and place in petri dishes containing E3 medium.
2. Sort out viable embryos under stereomicroscope based on developmental stage. Place approximately 50 eggs per petri dish in E3 with PTU medium.
3. Grow embryos in 28.5 °C incubator until about 22 hpf (hours post-fertilization).
4. Manually dechorionate the embryos between 22 and 24 hpf under the microscope using forceps.
5. Separate embryos in six-well plates, 20 embryos per well with a small volume of E3 medium.
6. Prepare nanomaterial dispersions fresh just before the start of exposure (at 24 hpf).
7. Replace E3 with 3 mL nanomaterial dispersion in E3 with PTU medium.
8. Grow embryos at 28.5 °C throughout the exposure until 120 hpf.
9. Inspect embryos every 24 h, until end of exposure at 120 hpf. Remove dead embryos from each well. Count remaining live embryos. Inspect embryos for malformations: head malformation (ocular edema, opaque head region), pericardial or submandibular edema, yolk malformation (opaque yolk, yolk not depleted, yolk sac edema), and bent spine or tail (Fig. 2).
10. Calculate the LD50 value (the concentration value that causes the death of 50% of embryos in the test sample) for each different sample according to Miller and Tainter method [13].
11. Use live embryos for apoptosis assessment or NO imaging (*see* Subheadings 3.3 and 3.4).

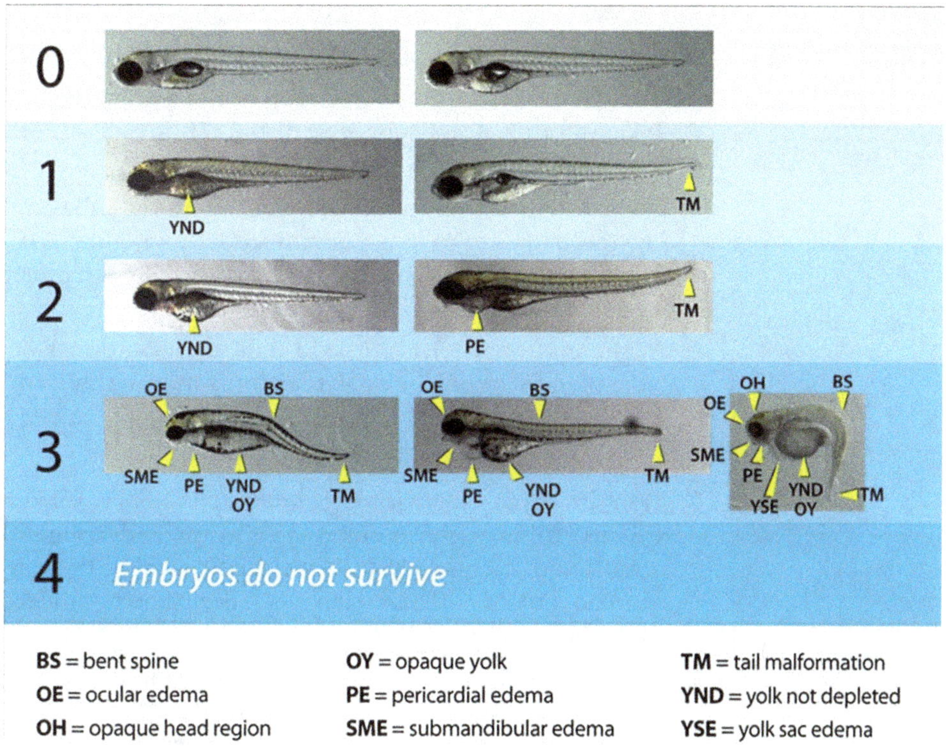

Fig. 2 Following exposure to a nanomaterial, the zebrafish embryos can be scored based on the severity of their morphological defects. Scores range from 0 through 4, with 0 indicating no visible toxic effects and 4 indicating death. Intermediate scores correspond to various degrees of morphological anomalies. For example, a score of 1 would indicate one to two minor toxic effects; 2: one moderate or 3–4 minor toxic effects; and 3: one or more severe effects or more than four minor toxic effects. Developmental abnormalities include: nondepleted or malformed yolk; malformations of spine, tail, and caudal fin; formations around the pericardial sacs or yolk; delayed hatching; stunted body or eye growth; degraded and opaque tissues; uncharacterized chorionic excretions; and edema in the body cavity, pericardial sac, or yolk sac regions. (reproduced from ref. 8 with permission from Elsevier and ref. 10 with permission from Wiley)

12. Wash the embryos three times with E3 medium in six well plates to remove nanomaterial and transfer embryos back to petri dishes.
13. Euthanize embryos with 0.4% tricaine solution by adding and mixing.
14. Transfer embryos to 1.5 mL tubes.
15. Remove E3 medium and add 1 mL of 4% PFA solution.
16. Rock the embryos for 2 h at room temperature.
17. Wash the embryos three times with PBST and three times with methanol, mixing through inversion.
18. Store embryos in methanol at −20 °C for at least 2 h before use in immunohistochemistry or histological analysis (*see* Subheading 3.2).

3.2 Organ Development Analysis

1. Prepare several blocks of glycol methacrylate.
2. Cut the preformed blocks in half and put them at the bottom of the embedding mold.
3. Take Solution A and mix it with 0.0125 g catalyst/mL in a centrifuge tube (*see* **Note 9**).
4. For infiltration, remove the methanol from the tubes containing the fixed embryos to be embedded (*see* **Note 10**), add 0.5 mL Solution A + catalyst, and keep on a rocking platform for 10 min.
5. At the end of the 10 min, add 0.04 mL Solution B/mL to remaining Solution A + catalyst and mix thoroughly by vortex.
6. Transfer Solution A + catalyst + Solution B mixture to each mold enough to overfill it.
7. Transfer glycol methacrylate infiltrated embryos from the 1.5 mL tube to the mold using forceps and arrange them parallel with each other, with the head touching the top edge of the mold. This step is performed under the stereomicroscope.
8. Wait for 5–10 min until the solution around the embryos slightly cures and then cover each mold with a plastic cover, being careful not to let bubbles form under the cover.
9. Allow the blocks to fully cure 2 h to overnight.
10. Remove the cured blocks from the embedding mold and superglue the block containing the embedded embryos onto a JB4 plastic block holder, with the heads of the embryos oriented away from the block holder.
11. Cut 5 μm sections of embryos on a microtome using a glass knife.
12. Float sections on room temperature water and transfer to a slide (usually 7–8 sections per slide).
13. Dry slides before staining.
14. Stain slides for 25–30 s in the Azure II–Methylene Blue solution and wash in dH_2O.
15. Allow the slides to dry at 65 °C for 15 min or at room temperature overnight.
16. For mounting, dip each slide in xylene (*see* **Note 11**).
17. Dispense Permount using a pipette along the middle of the slide and carefully press a coverslip over sections.
18. Remove excess Permount by dipping in xylene and cleaning slide.
19. Allow Permount to harden at room temperature and store.

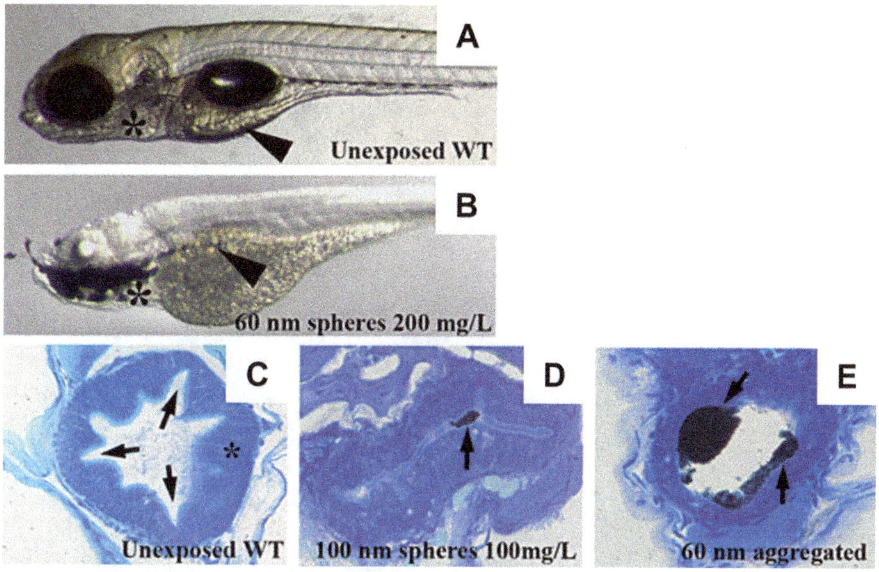

Fig. 3 Nickel nanoparticles accumulate within the lumen of the digestive system to different levels. Unexposed wild-type embryos in whole mount (**a** arrowhead) and in cross section (**c** arrows) have highly folded anterior intestines and columnar epithelial cells (**c** asterisks). Ni NPs can aggregate within the pharynx and intestine to high enough levels to be observed in whole mount (**b** pharynx asterisks and intestine arrowhead, 60 nm Ni NPs). Intestinal sections show the variation in Ni NP accumulation between exposures. Often small accumulations of Ni NP are present (arrow in **d**, 100 nm Ni NPs) while in some cases a much larger quantity will aggregate (arrows in **e**, dendritic aggregates of 60 nm). (reproduced from ref. 14 with permission from American Chemical Society)

20. Observe slides under a compound microscope. One of the main targets of nanomaterial exposure is the digestive system and the organs part of it. The digestive system opens to the exterior environment by 96 hpf, and nanomaterials can enter and become trapped by developing folds in the intestine. Typical features observed in exposed embryos are accumulation of nanomaterials between intestinal folds (Fig. 3) and defects in the structure of skeletal muscle fibers (Fig. 4).

3.3 Apoptosis Assessment

1. Wash the live embryos three times with E3 medium in the 6-well plate.
2. Add 3 mL 5 μg/mL acridine orange to each well and incubate for 30 min at 28.5 °C.
3. Wash the embryos three times with E3 medium to remove excess dye. Leave in last wash and keep in the 6-well plate.
4. For whole-mount imaging, add 5–10 drops of tricaine solution to each well, mix and wait until embryos do not move.
5. Transfer individual embryos to a depression slide with E3 medium.

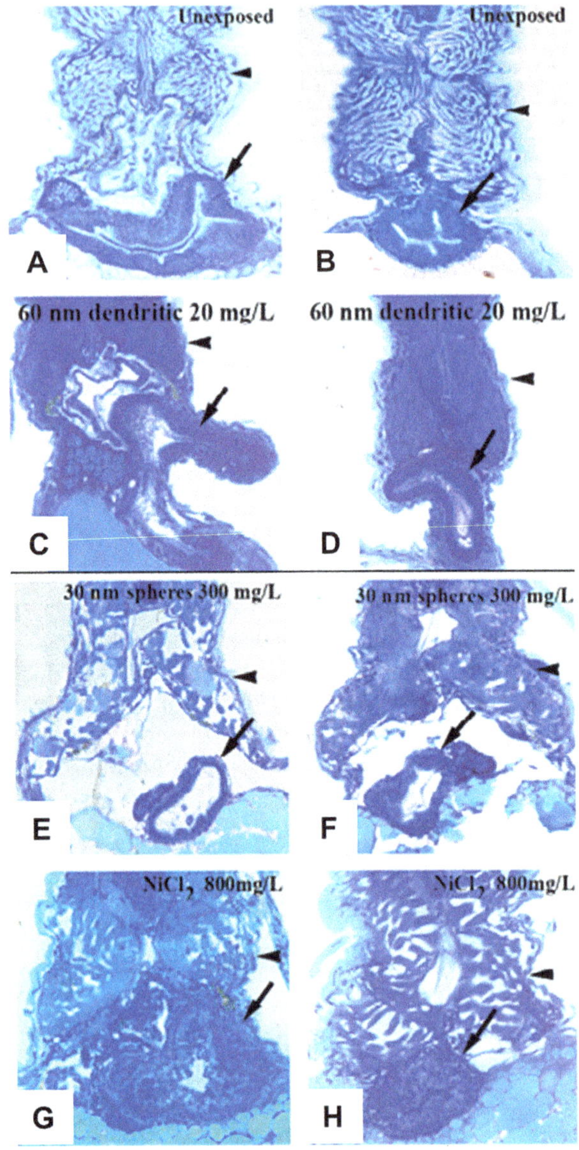

Fig. 4 Nanoparticle nickel and soluble nickel generate different defects in zebrafish embryos. Cross sections of unexposed embryo intestines have columnar epithelial cells with multiple folds (anterior, arrow in **a** and posterior, arrow in **b**). Skeletal muscle throughout the trunk is organized and continuous (arrowhead **a** and **b**). Exposure of nickel nanoparticles to concentrations around the LD10 results in thin intestine with cuboidal epithelial cells (anterior, arrow in **c** and posterior, arrow in **d**, dendritic aggregates) and unaffected skeletal muscle (anterior, arrowhead in C and posterior, arrowhead in **d**). Embryos exposed to NPs at concentrations around the LD50 still have thin walled intestines (anterior, arrow in **e** and posterior, arrow in **f**, 30 nm Ni NPs) but now skeletal muscle fibers have become separated throughout the trunk (anterior, arrowhead in **e** and posterior, arrowhead in **f**). Embryos exposed to soluble nickel have columnar epithelial cells and multiple folds (anterior, arrow in **g** and posterior, arrow in **h**)

6. Observe embryos under a fluorescence microscope (for acridine orange, the excitation wavelength is 500 nm, and the emission wavelength 526 nm).
7. For sectioning, fix the embryos in 4% PFA (*see* Subheading 3.1, **steps 12–19**).
8. Perform the embedding and sectioning according to Subheading 3.2, **steps 1–13**.
9. For mounting, add 2–3 drops of antifade mounting medium with DAPI along the middle of the slide and cover carefully with a coverslip.
10. Wipe excess antifade mounting medium (*see* **Note 12**).
11. Store slides in a microscope slide case at 4 °C for long-term preservation.
12. Observe the slides under a fluorescence microscope using the same setup as for the whole-mount imaging (*see* **step 6**). The DAPI counterstaining can be visualized using excitation wavelength at 360 nm and emission wavelength at 460 nm. Overlay of the images gives a complete picture of the nature of the cells within different organs of the embryo (Fig. 5).

3.4 NO Imaging

1. For negative control, remove the E3 medium from each well at 96 hpf and add 3 mL L-NAME solution. Keep the embryos at 28.5 °C until 120 hpf.
2. For positive control, remove the E3 medium from each well at 119 hpf and add 3 mL Spermine NONOate solution. Keep the embryos at 28.5 °C until 120 hpf.
3. Wash the live embryos (control, negative control, positive control, nanomaterial exposed) three times with E3 medium in the 6-well plate.
4. Add 3 mL 5 μM DAF-FM DA solution to each well and incubate for 2 h at 28.5 °C.
5. Wash the embryos three times with E3 medium to remove any excess dye and finally keep in about 3 mL E3 medium.
6. Before fluorescence imaging, add 5–10 drops tricaine solution to each well and mix until the embryos cease movement.
7. Transfer individual embryos to a depression slide with E3 medium.

Fig. 4 (continued) in the intestine even at concentrations well over the LD50. Separated skeletal muscles are first observed at concentrations in the 800 mg/L range (anterior, arrowhead in **g** and posterior, arrowhead in **h**). (reproduced from ref. 14 with permission from American Chemical Society)

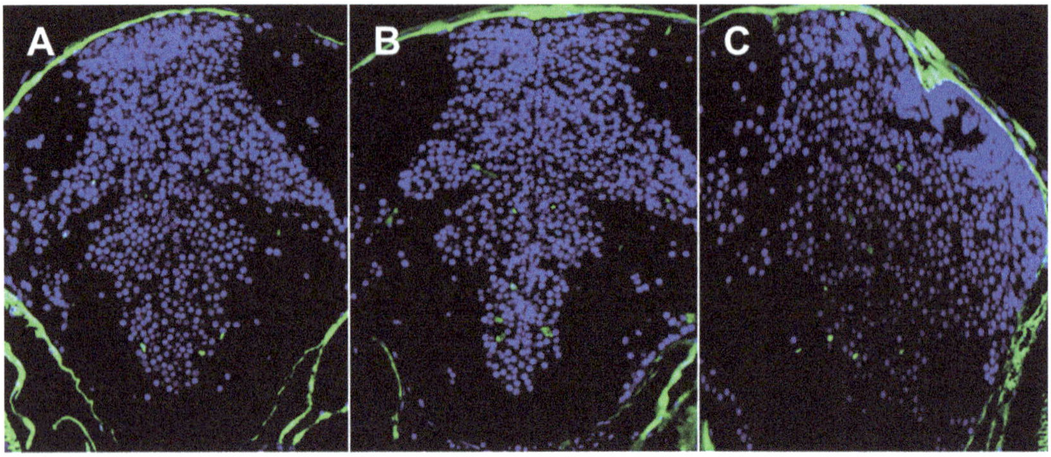

Fig. 5 Cross sections through the head of embryos at 96 hpf, control (**a**) and exposed to 1 mg/mL SNPs (**b**) and 1 mg/mL glycine-SNPs (**c**), stained with acridine orange. Nuclei of dead cells stained with acridine orange are shown in green color, while the nuclei of live cells are counterstained (shown in blue color). (reproduced from ref. 15 with permission from Elsevier)

8. Observe the embryos in whole-mount under a fluorescence microscope (for DAF-FM DA, the excitation wavelength is 495 nm, and the emission wavelength is 515 nm). Significant concentrations of NO are localized within the intestine of the embryos. Compare fluorescence intensity in the intestinal region between the exposed embryos and control embryos. Exposure to L-NAME, a potent inhibitor of NO producing enzymes, decreases the level of intestinal NO and it can be used as a negative control. On the other hand, exposure to Spermine NONOate, a NO donor, increases the level of intestinal NO and can be used as a positive control. Exposure to nanomaterials can either decrease or increase the level of intestinal NO. Some nanomaterials which are redox active (e.g., CeO_2) can scavenge NO due to their ROS scavenging properties, thus decreasing the NO level, while others can increase NO concentrations and induce a local inflammatory response (e.g., CuO) (Fig. 6).

4 Notes

1. E3 medium with and without PTU should be prepared. E3 with PTU medium needs to be used only for storing the embryos between 0 and 24 hpf and for preparation of exposure solutions. Any steps requiring washing after the exposure period can be performed using E3 medium without PTU.
2. Formation of fungus may occur sometimes in the petri dishes with eggs between 0 and 24 hpf which may affect the

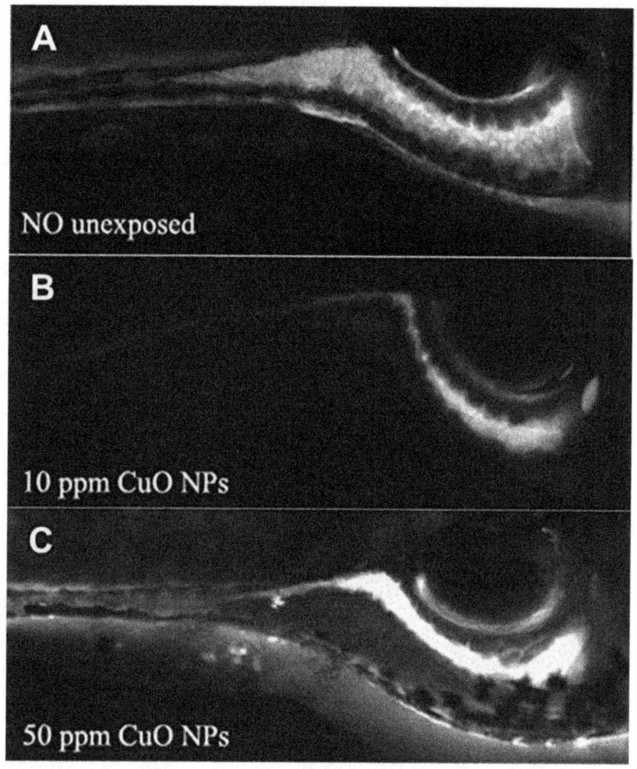

Fig. 6 Imaging of intestinal NO using DAF-FM DA after exposure to CuO NPs: fluorescence images obtained from embryos, control and exposed to 10 ppm and 50 ppm CuO NPs. Fluorescence images display similar intensities for both control embryos and embryos exposed to 10 ppm CuO NPs. Increase in the fluorescence intensity is visibly observed for embryos exposed to 50 ppm CuO NPs. (reproduced from ref. 16 with permission from Wiley)

development of the embryos and makes the dechorionation step difficult. In order to avoid this issue, methylene blue is added to the E3 medium (2 mL 0.1% methylene blue/L of E3 medium).

3. The preparation of nanomaterial dispersions should be done as close as possible to the start of the exposure period. If preparing a stock dispersion, sonicate and vortex well the stock until homogenous before preparing any further dilutions.
4. Tricaine powder can degrade rapidly. Buy tricaine powder in small quantities and store in the freezer. Prepare fresh tricaine solution as often as possible.
5. Prepare a larger volume of PFA solution at once and store it as 1 mL aliquots in plastic vials at −20 °C. Thaw the number of needed vials right before use at 37 °C.
6. Prepare a stock solution of acridine orange by diluting 1 mg in 1 mL dH_2O. Distribute in 1.5 mL vials, 5 μL per vial, and store

at −20 °C. For use, dilute the content of each vial with 995 μL E3 medium.

7. For preparation of DAF-FM DA stock, the dye is diluted first in dimethyl sulfoxide (final concentration 1 μg/μL). The stock is then diluted in E3 medium, 1 μL in 1 mL E3 medium (final concentration 5 mM). Prepare only the necessary amount of DAF-FM DA powder for each experiment.
8. Prepare a concentrated stock solution in dimethyl sulfoxide and store at −20 °C. Dilute in E3 medium to the working concentration right before exposure experiments.
9. Based on our experience, it is recommended to start with 1 mL Solution A for each new block or cover block needed, plus 0.5 mL Solution A for each sample that needs to be infiltrated.
10. We recommend inexperienced users to start with 5–8 embryos for each sample. Ideally, a maximum of 15 embryos could be embedded in the same block.
11. For this step and the following two steps, working with gloves and in the chemical fume hood is mandatory.
12. Distilled H_2O can be used to clean the excess antifade mounting medium.

References

1. Roco MC (2011) The long view of nanotechnology development: the National Nanotechnology Initiative at 10 years. J Nanopart Res 13 (2):427–445. https://doi.org/10.1007/s11051-010-0192-z
2. Vance ME, Kuiken T, Vejerano EP, McGinnis SP, Hochella MF, Rejeski D, Hull MS (2015) Nanotechnology in the real world: redeveloping the nanomaterial consumer products inventory. Beilstein J Nanotechnol 6:1769–1780. https://doi.org/10.3762/bjnano.6.181
3. Keller AA, Lazareva A (2014) Predicted releases of engineered nanomaterials: from global to regional to local. Environ Sci Technol Lett 1(1):65–70. https://doi.org/10.1021/ez400106t
4. Service RF (2004) Nanotechnology grows up. Science 304(5678):1732–1734. https://doi.org/10.1126/science.304.5678.1732
5. Andreescu S, Gheorghiu M, Özel RE, Wallace KN (2011) Methodologies for toxicity monitoring and nanotechnology risk assessment. In: Biotechnology and nanotechnology risk assessment: minding and managing the potential threats around US, vol 1079. ACS Symposium Series, vol 1079. American Chemical Society, pp. 141–180. doi:https://doi.org/10.1021/bk-2011-1079.ch007
6. Hill AJ, Teraoka H, Heideman W, Peterson RE (2005) Zebrafish as a model vertebrate for investigating chemical toxicity. Toxicol Sci 86 (1):6–19. https://doi.org/10.1093/toxsci/kfi110
7. Scholz S, Fischer S, Gündel U, Küster E, Luckenbach T, Voelker D (2008) The zebrafish embryo model in environmental risk assessment—applications beyond acute toxicity testing. Environ Sci Pollut Res 15(5):394–404. https://doi.org/10.1007/s11356-008-0018-z
8. Fako VE, Furgeson DY (2009) Zebrafish as a correlative and predictive model for assessing biomaterial nanotoxicity. Adv Drug Deliv Rev 61(6):478–486. https://doi.org/10.1016/j.addr.2009.03.008
9. George S, Xia T, Rallo R, Zhao Y, Ji Z, Lin S, Wang X, Zhang H, France B, Schoenfeld D, Damoiseaux R, Liu R, Lin S, Bradley KA, Cohen Y, Nel AE (2011) Use of a high throughput screening approach coupled with in vivo zebrafish embryo screening to develop hazard ranking for engineered nanomaterials. ACS Nano 5(3):1805–1817. https://doi.org/10.1021/nn102734s

10. Bar-Ilan O, Albrecht RM, Fako VE, Furgeson DY (2009) Toxicity assessments of multisized gold and silver nanoparticles in zebrafish embryos. Small 5(16):1897–1910. https://doi.org/10.1002/smll.200801716
11. Westerfield M (2007) The zebrafish book: a guide for the laboratory use of zebrafish (Danio rerio), 5th edn. University of Oregon Press, Eugene, OR
12. Nusslein-Volhard C, Dahm R (2002) Zebrafish. Oxford University Press, New York
13. Randhawa MA (2009) Calculation of LD50 values from the method of Miller and Tainter, 1944. J Ayub Med Coll Abbottabad 21 (3):184–185
14. Ispas C, Andreescu D, Patel A, Goia DV, Andreescu S, Wallace KN (2009) Toxicity and developmental defects of different sizes and shape nickel nanoparticles in zebrafish. Environ Sci Technol 43(16):6349–6356. https://doi.org/10.1021/es9010543
15. Dumitrescu E, Karunaratne DP, Prochaska MK, Liu X, Wallace KN, Andreescu S (2017) Developmental toxicity of glycine-coated silica nanoparticles in embryonic zebrafish. Environ Pollut 229(Supplement C):439–447. https://doi.org/10.1016/j.envpol.2017.06.016
16. Özel RE, Alkasir RSJ, Ray K, Wallace KN, Andreescu S (2013) Comparative evaluation of intestinal nitric oxide in embryonic zebrafish exposed to metal oxide nanoparticles. Small 9 (24):4250–4261. https://doi.org/10.1002/smll.201301087

Chapter 21

Application of *Daphnia magna* for Nanoecotoxicity Study

Zhizhen Xu, Yingying Liu, and Yuqian Wang

Abstract

Daphnia magna (D. magna), an aquatic invertebrate, is the most commonly used test organism in ecotoxicological studies on manufactured nanomaterials (MNs). Although standard protocols for undertaking acute and chronic toxicity tests of dissolved chemicals with *D. magna* have been endorsed by several national and international organizations, comprehensive guidance on aquatic toxicology testing of MNs with *D. magna* are in their infancy. Here we describe the acute and chronic toxicity methods with *D. magna* as test organism for nanoecotoxicity study. These methods may provide reference for the next step toward developing prescriptive aquatic toxicity standard tests for MNs with *D. magna*.

Key words Nanomaterials, *Daphnia magna*, Nanoecotoxicity, Acute toxicity, Chronic toxicity

1 Introduction

The increased production and widespread usage of manufactured nanomaterials (MNs) with unique and enhanced properties inevitably result in their release into environment. The potential ecotoxicological effects induced by MNs must, therefore, be evaluated to protect ecological safety. With regard to ecotoxicological tests on MNs, *Daphnia magna* (*D. magna*) is the most commonly used invertebrate species, which is also included in several guidelines and international standards for acute and chronic tests (e.g., Organization of Economic Cooperation and Development (OECD), International Organization for Standardization) [1]. These standard test guidelines were originally intended for dissolved chemicals. However, the exposure of test organisms to MNs involves colloids and particle-sediment mixtures besides dissolved chemicals. Due to the difference of intrinsic properties between MNs and dissolved chemicals, the applicability of these standard methods for ecotoxicity assessment of MNs with *D. magna* as test organism should be improved by additional guidance [2]. Several recent publications have discussed the key issues and specific considerations, including standard terminology (MNs suspensions, intrinsic toxicity, and

Qunwei Zhang (ed.), *Nanotoxicity: Methods and Protocols*, Methods in Molecular Biology, vol. 1894,
https://doi.org/10.1007/978-1-4939-8916-4_21,

physical effects), MN behavior in aquatic media, quantification of MNs in aqueous media, to develop additional guidance document for nanoecotoxicity tests [2–6]. However, no consensus on some test details (e.g., MN suspension preparation and MN dosimetry type) has been reached. Referring to already published articles on aquatic ecotoxicity testing of MNs, OECD test guidelines about the acute and chronic toxicity testing of chemicals using *D. magna* and our laboratory experience, we present here detailed method descriptions about nanoecotoxicity assessment with *D. magna*.

2 Materials

2.1 Equipment

Standard laboratory equipment, including but not limited to:

1. Test vessels: Prepare test vessels or other apparatus made of glass or other chemically inert material for sample preparation.
2. Artificial climate chamber: Culture daphnids and algae with the control of temperature, humidity, lighting regime, and light intensity.
3. Refrigerator: Store samples at 4 °C.
4. Ultrasonic probe: Disperse MN suspension.
5. Inductively coupled plasma mass spectrometry (ICP-MS) or inductively coupled plasma optical emission spectrometry (ICP-OES): Analyze the mass concentration of metal and metal oxide nanomaterials in medium.
6. Refrigerated centrifuge: Centrifuge samples.
7. Zetasizer Nano ZS system: Measure the hydrodynamic diameter and zeta potential of MNs.
8. X-ray photoelectron spectroscopy (XPS): Determine chemical composition of MNs.
9. Brunauer–Emmett–Teller (BET): Determine specific surface areas of MNs.
10. Transmission electron microscopy (TEM): Observe nanostructures and morphology of MNs.
11. Stereomicroscope: Measure the body length of daphnids.

2.2 MN Dispersion

1. Simplified Elendt medium (SM7): Prepare mixture solution of 293.8 mg/L $CaCl_2$, 123.3 mg/L $MgSO_4$, 0.184 mg/L K_2HPO_4, 0.274 mg/L $NaNO_3$, 64.8 mg/L $NaHCO_3$, 10 mg/L Na_2SiO_3, 0.175 mg/L H_3BO_3, 5.8 mg/L KCl, and 0.143 mg/L KH_2PO_4, with a water hardness of 250 mg $CaCO_3$ per L and pH of 7.8–8.2 according to the OECD Guideline 211 [7] and the previous report [8]. Prepare all solutions using ultrapure deionized water (18 MΩ.cm sensitivity) and analytical grade reagents.

2. MN stock suspension: Prewet known mass MN dry power in ultrapure water into wet-paste form for 24 h. Prepare MN stock suspension by dispersing the MN wet paste into known volume of SM7 medium (*see* **Note 1**). Disperse MN stock suspension with a calibrated sonication probe as follows:
   (a) Add MN stock suspension into a glass beaker which is placed in an >1 L ice bath and secure against moving.
   (b) Place the tip of the ultrasonic probe in the center of the beaker, 2.5 cm below the surface (*see* **Note 2**).
   (c) Add 40 W output power for 10 min.
   (d) Store the prepared MN dispersion in an amber glass container at 4 °C. Redisperse by probe sonication according to b and c after more than 3 h (*see* **Note 3**), referring to the OECD Guideline 318 [9]. Store MN dispersion no longer than 14 days. Dispersant with little or no toxicity can be used if necessary to reduce agglomeration and settling rates.
3. MN test suspension: Prepare suspensions with different concentrations used for acute and chronic toxicity by diluting the MN stock suspension with SM7 medium followed by probe sonication in ice bath for 30 s before exposure.

2.3 D. magna Culture

1. Culture medium: Glass-fiber filtered unpolluted natural water or moderately hard reconstituted water (SM7) (*see* **Note 4**). Renew three times a week at least.
2. Culture condition: Culture daphnids under a 16: 8 light–dark cycle within the temperature range of 18–23.5 °C (*see* **Note 5**) in climate chamber [10, 11].
3. Feeding: Feed daphnids with freshwater alga cells at a cell density of 10^4 cells per mL (for daphnia <3 days old) and 10^5 cells per mL (for daphnids >3 days old) every day [12] (*see* **Note 6**).
4. Daphnia density: 1 individual per 10 mL culture medium.

3 Methods

3.1 Characterization of MNs

1. Chemical composition: Determine for the dry MNs by XPS or elemental analyzer.
2. Specific surface area: Determine for the dry MNs by BET method.
3. Nanostructure and morphology: Observe via TEM. Drip several drops of the MN suspension onto the clean carbon grid or micrograte and dry at room temperature before TEM analysis (*see* **Note 7**).

4. Suspension stability (average hydrodynamic diameter and zeta potential): Detect by a Zetasizer Nano ZS system (*see* **Note 8**).
5. Solubility of metal ions or residue: Determine by ICP-MS or ICP-OES. Centrifuge 10 mL MN test suspension for 10 min using a refrigerated centrifuge and collect the supernatant to determine metal content (*see* **Note 9**).
6. Quantification of MNs in test media:
   (a) Mass concentration: For metal and metal oxide nanomaterials, determine by ICP-MS. MNs in test media are digested in 68% nitric acid at 110 °C until the dissolution is complete. After digestion, the samples are diluted with 2% HNO_3 for metal concentration analysis.

   For carbon nanomaterials (e.g., single-walled carbon nanotube (SWCNs), multiwalled carbon nanotube (MWCNs), graphene (GN) and fullerene (C60)), determine by UV–visible spectroscopy or sodium dodecyl sulfate-polyacrylamide gel electrophoresis (SDS-PAGE) method [13, 14].
   (b) Particle concentration: Calculate according to the formula: $N = M/\rho V$, where N is the number of particles in the suspension, M is the mass of the powder to prepare the suspension, ρ (kg/m^3) is the density of the particle material (known value), V (m^3) is the volume of particles taken from existing material information or calculated from DLS size-measurements (*see* **Note 10**).

3.2 Toxicity Tests

1. Daphnids sensitivity: Check monthly using potassium dichromate ($K_2Cr_2O_7$) to ensure EC_{50}-24 h within the range 0.6–2.1 mg/L (*see* **Note 11**) [15].
2. Control: Solution containing the solvent or dispersant used for preparing MN test suspension as control. The concentration of control solution should be same as that used in MN test suspension.
3. MN test concentration: Expose at least five young daphnids aged less than 24 h old to MN test suspension at widely spaced concentrations for 24 h. Find out the lowest and highest MN test concentrations which result in no observable effect and 100% immobilization, respectively (*see* **Note 12**). Determine at least five MN test concentrations between and including the lowest and highest test concentrations for acute toxicity test [10, 15]. Determine MN test concentrations to be sublethal for chronic toxicity test.
4. Acute toxicity: Exposure of young daphnids aged less than 24 h old to MN test suspension at a range of concentrations for 48 h. Fill appropriate volumes of MN test suspension in the test vessels and keep identical ratio of air–water in the vessels.

Provide at least 2 mL of MN test suspension for each animal (e.g., 10 mL MN test suspension for five daphnids per test vessels) [13]. Employ three replicates for each concentration. No feeding during test. Conduct the same test with controls. Record immobilization of daphnids at 24 h and 48 h.

5. Chronic toxicity: Exposure of young daphnids aged less than 24 h old to MN test suspension at a range of concentrations test for 21 days. Keep one daphnids per test vessel and one individual per 10 mL MN test suspension. Employ 15 replicates for each concentration [13]. Feed daphnids every day. Renew MN test suspension every day. Remove offspring in a timely fashion, count living offspring daily after the first brood and record dead offspring. Record survival of parents, time of first brood, number of living offspring produced per surviving parent, and body length daily during exposure (*see* **Note 13**). Conduct the same test with controls (*see* **Note 14**).

3.3 Test Results

3.3.1 Acute Toxicity

1. Mortality: Calculate based on the surviving daphnids.
2. EC_{50}: Plot the percentages immobilized at 24 h and 48 h against test concentrations. Analyze the data and calculate the EC_{50} at 48 h.
3. Body burden: After exposure, ten surviving daphnids from each treatment are rinsed three times with ultrapure water. Then, the daphnids are put in 2 mL centrifuge tubes.

For metal and metal oxide nanomaterials, all tubes are placed in a dry oven at 60 °C to constant dry weight and then digested in 68% nitric acid at 110 °C until the dissolution is complete. After digestion, the samples are diluted with 2% HNO_3 for metal concentration analysis via ICP-MS [16, 17].

For carbon nanomaterials (e.g., SWCNT, MWCNT, and GN), the daphnid tissues are quickly homogenized in a 200 μL mixture of 1% SDS, 1 mM $MgCl_2$, and 1 mM $CaCl_2$ in an ice bath using an ultrasonic wave cell pulverizer, after which the homogenate is incubated for 2 h in a 37 °C water bath. Then 20 μg of deoxyribonuclease I is used to treat samples at 37 °C for 2 h to further release the DNA and reduce the viscosity. The supernatant is removed by centrifuging at 10,000 × *g* for 10 min to obtain the substrate samples containing carbon nanomaterials. Finally, the concentration of carbon nanomaterials is determined by SDS-PAGE method [13]. For carbon nanomaterials (C60), their concentrations in the daphnids are measured by extracting the substrate samples into toluene. Subsequently, the absorbance of the toluene extract is measured at 332 nm or 337 nm by UV–visible spectroscopy [18, 19] (*see* **Note 15**).

3.3.2 Chronic Toxicity

1. Daphnid size: Analyze the effects of MNs on the body length of adult daphnids after 21 days of exposure.
2. Reproduction: Calculate the total number of living offspring per parent animal. Analyze the effects of MNs on the time of first brood and the number of neonates in the first brood.
3. Body burden: Use the same procedure as for the detection of body burden in acute toxicity above.

4 Notes

1. The recommended concentration of MN stock suspension shall not exceed the concentration of MN test suspension by a factor of more than 20 [9].
2. High aspect ratio nanomaterials could be sonicated by bath sonication to avoid destruction of nanomaterials.
3. Place the sonication probe in the bottle of the NM stock suspension when performing redispersion.
4. If glass-fiber filtered unpolluted natural water is used, the quality parameters including heavy metals (e.g., conductivity and total organic carbon or chemical oxygen demand, Cu, Pb, Zn, Hg, Cd, Ni) should be measured twice a year or whenever the characteristics may have changed greatly. If moderately hard reconstituted water is used, the water should be aerated prior to use to ensure sufficient dissolved oxygen in the water.
5. The temperature should not vary by more than 2 °C within the limit of 18–23.5 °C.
6. If *Chlamydomonas reinhardtii* is used as food of daphnids, centrifuging alga suspension at 12,000 × g for 10 min using a refrigerated centrifuge at 4 °C should be conducted followed by resuspension in Daphnids culture medium.
7. A micrograte is generally used when nanomaterials with large aspect ratio (in the form of thin sheets or plates) are characterized by TEM.
8. The average hydrodynamic diameter of MNs is usually measured using DLS method. However, the analysis of DLS results is based on spherical nanoparticles. This limitation of current DLS techniques should be noted if nanoparticles with other shapes (e.g., sheet or plate shaped nanoparticles) are monitored.
9. The rotating speed of centrifuge changes according to different MNs.
10. V (m^3) is calculated from DLS size measurement, using the formula for the volume of a sphere and the most frequent

diameter of the intensity weighted distribution of the autocorrelation function, not the intensity weighted mean hydrodynamic size measured by DLS.

11. EC_{50}: The concentration estimated to immobilize 50% of the daphnids within a stated exposure period.
12. Immobilization: No swimming of daphnids within 15 s after gentle agitation.
13. Body length of daphnids: The length of the daphnids from the top of the head to the base of the apical spine [20] measured by stereomicroscope.
14. Validity of the chronic toxicity test: In the controls, the mortality of the parent daphnids does not exceed 20% after exposure and the surviving number of offspring produced by per parent daphnids is not less than 60.
15. Other carbon nanomaterials (e.g., SWCNT, MWCNT, and GN) can also be measured by UV–visible spectroscopy.

Acknowledgment

This work was supported by the Youth Core Plan of Beijing Academy of Science and Technology (No. 201703).

References

1. Baun A, Hartmann NB, Grieger K, Kusk KO (2008) Ecotoxicity of engineered nanoparticles to aquatic invertebrates: a brief review and recommendations for future toxicity testing. Ecotoxicology 17(5):387–395
2. Petersen EJ, Diamond SA, Kennedy AJ, Goss GG, Ho K, Lead J, Hanna SK, Hartmann NB, Hund-Rinke K, Mader B, Manier N, Pandard P, Salinas ER, Sayre P (2015) Adapting OECD aquatic toxicity tests for use with manufactured nanomaterials: key issues and consensus recommendations. Environ Sci Technol 49(16):9532–9547
3. Skjolding LM, Sørensen SN, Hartmann NB, Hjorth R, Hansen SF, Baun A (2016) Aquatic ecotoxicity testing of nanoparticles—the quest to disclose nanoparticle effects. Angew Chem Int Ed Engl 55(49):15224–15239
4. Hansen SF, Sørensen SN, Skjolding LM, Hartmann NB, Baun A (2017) Revising REACH guidance on information requirements and chemical safety assessment for engineered nanomaterials for aquatic ecotoxicity endpoints: recommendations from the EnvNano project. Environ Sci Eur 29(1):1–15
5. Hartmann NB, Ågerstrand M, Lützhøft HCH, Baun A (2017) NanoCREDA transparent framework to assess' the regulatory adequacy of ecotoxicity data for nanomaterials–relevance and reliability revisited. NanoImpact 6:81–89
6. Hund-Rinke K, Baun A, Cupi D, Fernandes TF, Handy R, Kinross JH, Navas JM, Peijnenburg W, Schlich K, Shaw BJ, Scott-Fordsmand JJ (2016) Regulatory ecotoxicity testing of nanomaterials–proposed modifications of OECD test guidelines based on laboratory experience with silver and titanium dioxide nanoparticles. Nanotoxicology 10 (10):1442–1447
7. Organisation for Economic Cooperation and Development (2012) Daphnia magna Reproduction Test. OECD Guideline 211 Paris, France
8. Samel A, Ziegenfuss M, Goulden CE, Banks S, Baer KN (1999) Culturing and bioassay testing of *Daphnia magna* using Elendt M4, Elendt M7, and COMBO media. Ecotoxicol Environ Saf 43(1):103–110
9. Organisation for Economic Cooperation and Development (2017) Dispersion stability of

nanomaterials in simulated environmental media. OECD Guideline 318 Paris, France
10. Standard methods for bioassay of daphnia magna straus. GB/T 16125–2012. Ministry of health, China
11. US Environmental Protection Agency (2003) Standard operating procedure # 204 for moderately hard reconstituted water. SoBran, Dayton, OH
12. Liu Y, Fan W, Xu Z, Peng W, Luo S (2017) Transgenerational effects of reduced graphene oxide modified by au, Ag, Pd, Fe_3O_4, Co_3O_4 and SnO_2 on two generations of *Daphnia magna*. Carbon 122:669–679
13. Fan W, Liu Y, Xu Z, Wang X, Li X, Luo S (2016) The mechanism of chronic toxicity to: *Daphnia magna* induced by graphene suspended in a water column. Environ Sci Nano 3(6):1405–1415
14. Yu ZG, Wang WX (2013) Influences of ambient carbon nanotubes on toxic metals accumulation in *Daphnia magna*. Water Res 47 (12):4179–4187
15. Organisation for Economic Cooperation and Development (2004) Daphnia sp., Acute Immobilisation Test. OECD Guideline 202 Paris, France
16. Adam N, Leroux F, Knapen D, Bals S, Blust R (2015) The uptake and elimination of ZnO and CuO nanoparticles in *Daphnia magna* under chronic exposure scenarios. Water Res 68(6):249–261
17. Fan W, Wang X, Cui M, Zhang D, Zhang Y, Yu T, Guo L (2012) Differential oxidative stress of octahedral and cubic Cu_2O micro/nanocrystals to *Daphnia magna*. Environ Sci Technol 46(18):10255–10262
18. Oberdörster E, Zhu S, Blickley TM, McClellan-Green P, Haasch ML (2006) Ecotoxicology of carbon-based engineered nanoparticles: effects of fullerene (C60) on aquatic organisms. Carbon 44(6):1112–1120
19. Tervonen K, Waissi G, Petersen EJ, Akkanen J, Kukkonen JVK (2010) Analysis of fullerene-C60 and kinetic measurements for its accumulation and depuration in *Daphnia magna*. Environ Toxicol Chem 29(5):1072–1078
20. Arndt DA, Chen J, Moua M, Klaper RD (2014) Multigeneration impacts on *Daphnia magna* of carbon nanomaterials with differing core structures and functionalizations. Environ Toxicol Chem 33(3):541–547

Chapter 22

The Overview of Methods of Nanoparticle Exposure Assessment

Peng Zhao and Yuanbao Zhang

Abstract

Nanotechnology is now widely used in industry as well as consumer products, such as electrical devices, cosmetics, medicine, and household appliances. In the life cycle of the nano-products, including production, use, and disposal, nanoparticles may be released to the environment. However, there is no current consensus on the best method for evaluating and characterizing nanoparticle exposure. Therefore, this chapter focuses on the nanoparticle exposure assessment methods and sampling techniques.

Key words Nanomaterial, Nanoparticles, Exposure assessment, Sampling techniques

1 Introduction

The standards, ISO/TS 27687 [1] and ISO/TS 80004-1 [2], have listed terms and definitions related to particles and core terms in the field of nanotechnology. Though they are intended to facilitate the development of the nanotechnology, they also provide some basis of exposure assessment of nanoparticles. In the field of occupational and environmental health, the exposure assessment for nanoparticles is a new challenge. Although there are several standard methods of exposure assessment of non-nanoscale particles, these conventional methods are not suitable for nanoparticles due to their small particle size and large surface area [3], so a set of quite distinct sampling and assessment techniques and methods, no matter in workplace or environment, is urgently needed.

As for engineered nanomaterials (ENMs), there is no consensus so far on the optimal sampling methods to evaluate the exposure characteristics of nanoparticles. In most cases, we can only qualitatively identify the emission source and exposure mitigation through the comparison of nanoparticle concentrations and the difference in background particle concentrations. The National Institute for Occupational Safety and Health (NIOSH) published only three

Qunwei Zhang (ed.), *Nanotoxicity: Methods and Protocols*, Methods in Molecular Biology, vol. 1894, https://doi.org/10.1007/978-1-4939-8916-4_22,

mass concentration based recommended exposure limits (RELs) and sampling guidance for titanium dioxide (TiO_2) [4], carbon nanotubes (CNTs), and carbon nanofibers (CNFs) [5], and no other exposure assessment methods for nanoparticles have been established except mass concentration. Because of their specific properties such as small size and high surface area, nanoparticles exhibit more toxicity than non-nanoscale particles [6]; therefore, other methods for evaluating the exposure of nanoparticles are required far more than mass concentration. This chapter describes the development trend of nanoparticle exposure assessment technology.

2 Physicochemical Characterization of Nanomaterials Related to Exposure Assessment

In this chapter, we focus on the physicochemical properties related to exposure assessment. Particle size and size distribution have effects on their surface area and quantities of particle, thus such properties are very important for exposure assessment. Due to their high surface energy, nanomaterials are subject to agglomeration or aggregation, so the nanomaterials detected in the workplace are not single dispersed particles, but rather condensed or aggregated nano-objects. In two technical reports published by International Standardization Organization (ISO), ISO/TR 13014 recommended eight physicochemical parameters for the toxicity assessment of nanomaterials, and ISO/TR 13329 recommended eight physicochemical parameters mainly for workplace environment management and worker protection. Although two reports are based on different goals, the physicochemical parameters recommended are very similar.

3 Relevant Standards for Nanoparticle Exposure Assessment

At present, for the complexity, uncertainty, and the lack of scientific nature of the nanomaterial evaluation, there are no universally recognized standards for the exposure evaluation of nanoparticles. Nevertheless, guidelines or reports on the exposure evaluation of nanomaterials have been published. British Standards Institution (BSI) published "Guide to assessing airborne exposure in occupational settings relevant to nanomaterials" (BSI PD 6699-3) [7]. Organization for Economic Co-operation and Development (OECD) published "Strategies, techniques and sampling protocols for determining the concentrations of manufactured nanomaterials in air at the workplace (OECD, 2017)," "Grouping and read-across for the hazard assessment of manufactured nanomaterials

(OECD, 2016)," "Harmonized tiered approach to measure and assess the potential exposure to airborne emissions of engineered nano-objects and their agglomerates and aggregates at workplaces (OECD, 2015)," "Compilation and comparison of guidelines related to exposure to nanomaterials in laboratories" (OECD, 2010), "Identification, compilation and analysis of guidance information for exposure measurement and exposure mitigation: manufactured nanomaterials" (OECD, 2009), and "Emission assessment for identification of sources and release of airborne manufactured nanomaterials in the workplace: compilation of existing guidance" (OECD, 2009). Meanwhile, ISO also provided several guides of action about nanoparticle exposure assessment, including ISO/TR 12885 (ISO, 2008) and ISO/TS 12901-1 (ISO, 2012), which recommended general guides for assessing the exposure of nanoparticles. Later, they published a standard, ISO/TS 12901-2 (2014), which provides the control banding approach to mitigate the risks associated with occupational exposure to engineered nanomaterials. A new project to establish the occupational exposure limits of nanomaterials and their aggregates and agglomerations will also be implemented. However, despite such advances, due to the challenges of nanoparticle sampling and characterization techniques, the evaluation criteria for nanoparticle exposure have not yet been established.

4 Instruments for Exposure Assessment

In order to characterize and measure the airborne nanoparticles, different detection devices can be used based on different detection purposes. Figure 1 shows detection equipment corresponding to detection purposes. Currently, there is an international standard method for detecting aerosol mass concentration based on filter sampling technology. However, as to nanoparticles, the information obtained from the filter sampling method cannot be used to fully assess the occupational exposure characteristics of nanoparticles. Toxicity studies showed that particle toxicity increases as they become smaller. Therefore, besides the mass concentration, the parameters, such as number concentration, surface area concentration, size, and morphology, are needed to be analyzed for comprehensive characterizing nanoparticle exposure, and the instruments needed are shown in Table 1.

4.1 Tapered Element Oscillating Microbalance (TEOM)

Generally, aerosol mass concentration is detected by collecting aerosols on the filter, followed by measuring the deposited mass. At present, TEOM can automatically measure the mass concentration of aerosol in a single step, with a detection range fromμg/m^3 to g/m^3. TEOM is mainly used in environmental air quality monitoring. It can bring about the quickly detection of PM_{10}, $PM_{2.5}$,

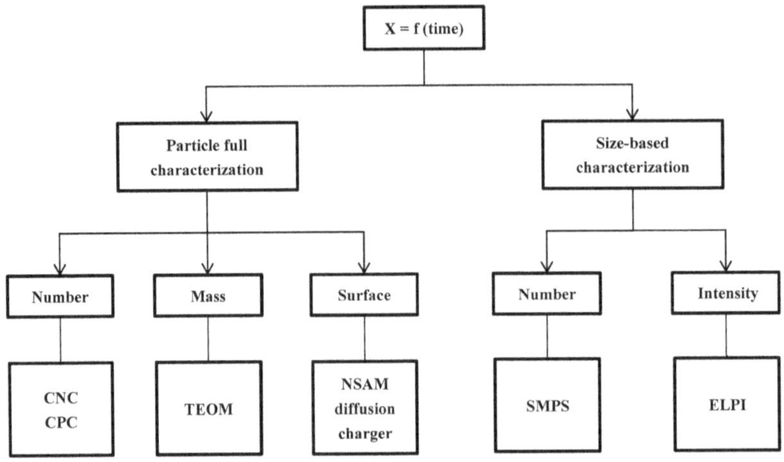

Fig. 1 Classification of instruments [18] (*CNC* Condensation nuclei counter, *CPC* Condensation particle counter, *TEOM* Tapered element oscillating microbalance, *NSAM* Nanoparticle surface aerosol monitor, *SMPS* Scanning mobility particle sizer, *ELPI* Electrical low pressure impactor)

and $PM_{1.0}$ with aerodynamic cutoff diameters, and satisfy the demand of the environmental monitoring [8]. However, it is not fully satisfactory to the requirement of the occupational hygiene standards. Occupational exposure detection needs to determine the mass concentration of the inhalable particles with the size less than 4 μm [9]. In addition, due to its own weight and volume limit, it is difficult for TEOM to meet the needs of individual sampling.

4.2 Cascade Impactor

Cascade impact sampler consists of a series of particle impaction plates in series. The more stages of the impaction plate, the smaller the particle size that can be collected. Each stage collects particles with a specific particle size, the particles with size larger than the cut size are collected on the impaction plate and the smaller particles follow the air flow into the next impaction plate, so that the larger number stages of impaction plate collect the smaller particles. The Nano-micro orifice uniform deposit impactor (Nano-Moudi) made by the MSP company has up to 13 stages that can collect the particles with the size range from 10 nm to 10 μm [10]. The deposit particles can be used for further detection and analysis, such as weighing, electron microscopy, and elemental analysis.

Electrical low pressure impactor (ELPI) is an improved cascade impactor [11]. It has a corona charger at the instrument inlet, which can make particles charged. The particles are collected on the impaction plate, which is accompanied with a sensitive electrometer, depending on their aerodynamic diameter. In addition to collecting particles in specific size, it can calculate the number of particles based on the electric current. Therefore, the particle

Table 1
Nanoparticle monitoring devices

Measured parameter	Instruments	Real-time	Remarks	Examples	Size range (μm)
Mass	TEOM (tapered element oscillating microbalance)	YES	Sensitive real-time monitor, can be used to measure the nanoaerosol mass concentration on-line, with a suitable size-selective inlet	PDM3700	1.0–10
	OPC (optical particle counter)	YES	Measures total number of particles within specific size range, calculates mass concentration by a specific model	DUSTTRAKII 8530	0.1–10
	LPCI (low pressure cascade impactor)	NO	Collects particles on the impactors according to particle size range, Provides off-line gravimetric measurement of collected samples	Nano-moudi 122R	0.01–10
	Particles sampler	NO	Collects particles on the microporous filters using a sampler with a suitable size-selective inlet, but no current device offers cut-off point of 100 nm, Provides off- line gravimetric measurement of filter sample	SKC	1.0–10
Number	CPC (condensation particle counter)	YES	CPCs provide real-time particle number measurements form per cubic centimetre of air (particles/cm^3)	NANO-5403	0.01–10
	OPC (optical particle counter)	YES	Measures total number of particles within specific size range	DUSTTRAK II 8530	0.1–10
	SMPS (scanning mobility particle sizer)	YES	Real-time size-selective (mobility diameter) detection of number concentration giving number-based size distribution	GRIMM SMPS+E	0.0025–1
	FMPS (fast mobility particle sizer)	YES	Measures particles within specific size range, offering a total of 32 channels of resolution	FMPS 3091	0.0056–0.56
	ELPI (electrical low pressure impactor)	YES	Measures particle sizes and particle concentrations in real time, particles can be collected on substrates for microscopic analysis	HR-ELPI+	0.006–10

(continued)

Table 1
(continued)

Measured parameter	Instruments	Real-time	Remarks	Examples	Size range (μm)
			or additional measurements of mass or composition		
Surface area	NS AM (nanoparticle surface aerosol monitor)	YES	Real-time measurement of aerosol active surface area, active surface-area does not scale directly with geometric surface-area above 100 nm. Note that not all commercially available diffusion chargers have a response that scales with particle active surface-area below 100 nm. Diffusion chargers are only specific to nanoparticles if used with appropriate inlet pre-separator	AEROTRAK 9000	0.01–1
	ELPI (electrical low pressure impactor)	YES	Real-time size-selective (aerodynamic diameter) detection of active surface area concentration. Active surface-area does not scale directly with geometric surface-area above 100 nm	HR-ELPI+	0.006–10
Size distribution	SMPS (scanning mobility particle sizer)	YES	Measures size distribution of particles in real time	GRIMM SMPS+E	0.0025–1
	FMPS (fast mobility particle Sizer)	YES	Measures size distribution of particles in real time	FMPS 3091	0.0056–0.56
	ELPI (electrical low pressure impactor)	YES	Measures size distribution of particles in real time	HR-ELPI+	0.006–10
Composition and shape	LIBS (laser-induced breakdown spectroscopy)	YES	Offers direct chemical analysis for virtually every element in virtually all solid materials	TSI 3766	–
	ICP-MS (inductively coupled plasma mass spectrometry)	NO	Collects airborne particles using cascade impactor or aerosol sampler, analysis chemical composition information and shape of particles	–	–
	TEM-EDX (transmission electron microscopy-energy-dispersive X-ray) or SEM-EDX	NO	Collects airborne particles on a TEM grid using mini particle sampler (MPS), TEM-EDX or SEM-EDX offers a very comprehensive tool for individual particle analysis allowing the determination of size, morphology, specific surface, and elemental composition	INERIS MPS,TSI Model 3089, Grimm Model 5.561	0.1–1

concentration and size distribution can be shown in real time. Also the mass concentration and surface area concentration of particles can be calculated by specific model, and particles collected on substrates can be used to electron microscope analysis and elemental analysis.

4.3 Particle Counter

Particle counters include optical particle counter (OPC) and condensation particle counter (CPC). OPC is mostly used to determine the number concentration of lager size particles (larger than 100 nm), and the mass concentration could be calculated by the mathematical model [12]. While the number concentration of small size particles (less than 100 nm) is under detection, the CPC is needed. CPC is the most popular counter for nanoparticles currently, with a detective range from 10 nm to 10 μm. The nanoparticles, as condensation nuclei, coagulate organic matter in saturated organic vapor (such as isopropyl alcohol), which would result in an increase in the volume of particle, and thus the number of particles could be calculated by laser detector in the CPC [11, 13].

4.4 Particle Sizer

Scanning mobility particle sizer (SMPS) is a commonly used particle size detector, which is composed of a differential mobility analyzer (DMA) and a condensation particle counter (CPC). The particles enter from the DMA inlet and are charged by corona discharge, and under the influence of an electric field, the particles are graded according to the size of the particles. The particle size distribution is calculated by measuring the number of particles in a specific particle size range by CPC [14]. For example, the SMPS+E produced by GRIMM in Germany can detect the particle size distribution in the range of 2.5 nm to 1 μm in 64 channels. Similar instrument is fast mobility particle sizer (FMPS) model 3091 by TSI company, which is capable of rapidly detecting the particle size distribution and number concentration [15].

4.5 Nanoparticle Surface Aerosol Monitor (NSAM)

Nanoparticle surface aerosol monitor (NSAM) possesses two particle surface area detection modes, bronchial deposition mode and alveolar deposition mode. The testing principle is that the particles are charged at the entrance by the corona, then collected by a filter and the resulting current is measured simultaneously. Since the amount of charge is related to the particle surface area, the surface area concentration of the particles could be calculated. But it could not provide the particle size distribution. For example, TSI 3550 and AeroTrak 9000 are the currently used nanoparticle surface area detectors [16, 17].

5 Measurement Strategy

The best combination of monitoring technology and measurement solutions must be in place to detect the exposure characteristics of engineered nanomaterials in the workplace with high efficiency, sensitive, and low cost. Currently, there are several solutions for sampling and monitoring nanoparticle exposure, yet no consensus has been reached. However, there are certain principles for the development of nanoparticles sampling and monitoring programs [18].

Information collection: (1) Assess the nanoparticle exposure for collecting the basic information of the production, such as process flow, raw material or intermediate, and tasks. (2) Collect the Material Safety Data Sheet (MSDS) for knowing the physical and chemical characteristics, particle size, morphology, solubility and surface activity, etc. (3) Investigate the layout of workplace, the operation frequency and duration of the production equipment, and the situation of full ventilation or local ventilation for analyzing whether the nanoparticles are leaking due to the ventilation system [19].

Background concentration monitoring: The background concentration of particles in the atmosphere outside the workshop should be measured at first. Prior to work activities, the background concentration of particles in the workshop should be measured. But other operations besides nanomaterial manufacturing can be involved in increasing the particle concentration, such as vacuum pumps, gas burning appliances, workshop forklift trucks, and heat production operations (welding, soldering, etc.) [20, 21].

Initial assessment: According to the production process, CPC or OPC should be applied for detecting the short-term concentration to identify the particle emission sources and determine the concentration range of particles [22].

Main assessment: Based on the purpose of the assessment and the result of the initial assessment, draft the detection scheme and monitor the nanoparticle exposure characteristics of workplace comprehensively in detail, including mass concentration, number concentration, surface area concentration, particle size distribution, particle collection, and composition analysis [23].

Sampling site: The choice of area sampling locations should be representative and should include the sites of the high concentration and the long exposure of workers. Without affecting the operation of workers, the sampled sites should be as close to the workers as possible and the height of detector inlet should be same with the personal breathing zone. While personal sample is applied, the workers with the high exposure concentration and the long exposure times should be chosen preferentially [24].

Sampling period: The normal measurement period should be 8 h in a working day. However, 15 min of sampling can be carried out according to the characteristics of the working process, such as intermittent emissions [24].

Message record: Activities and other interference emissions should be recorded during the measurement. The information such as engineering control, meteorological conditions (especially temperature, humidity, and wind velocity), measurement dates and times, sampling sites, equipment and parameters, data and surveyors, and others should also be recorded. And a sampling layout is drawn.

6 Initial Assessment

The purpose of the initial assessment is to identify the potential nanoparticle emission sources and determine the sampling sites. The basic information of nanomaterials should be collected, then the particle concentration in every position is detected by using CPC or OPC, and the potential emission sources and the positions needed to be monitored emphatically by the comparison of the position concentration and background concentration before and after the production activities are identified. If the potential emission sources are identified, the following items need to be verified:

1. Identify the potential emission sources based on a walk-through survey in the production area and processes.
2. Check the duration and frequency of each operation, and the type of equipment used in the production processes and storage of the nanomaterials.
3. Determine the presence or absence of ventilation and exhaust devices, and check for malfunctions, including whether the ventilation system is using an inappropriate wind speed or whether the pipe is leaking.
4. Identify whether there is any man-made damage to the protective facilities.

7 Main Assessment

1. Particle collection and component analysis

   Collection is a key step to evaluate the exposure characteristics of nanoparticles. It can provide the information about mass concentration by gravimetric method, and the particles collected could be used for morphological and chemical analysis by SEM, TEM, EDX, and ICP-MS, and for toxicological assessment in lab [25].

The most common way to collect the airborne particulate matter is to use the particle sampler to collect the particles on the filter. With aerodynamic cutoff diameters at the inlet of the sampler, particles in a specific particle size range are collected [26]. However,there is no current device offers cutoff point of 100 nm [27]. The air samples should be collected as close as possible to the emission sources, so does the personal sampling, if possible, close to the personal breathing zone (PBZ). The sampling duration should be based on the particle concentration and the duration of the operation associated with the potential airborne release of nanoparticles, which is a generally consecutive 8 h. If the duration of operation is short, a relatively high air sampling flow (approximately 7 L/min) should be required to collect enough particles [28].

In order to collect the particles with a particle size less than 100 nm, low pressure cascade impactor should be chosen. The low pressure cascade impactor has up to 13 impaction plates, which could collect particles of a specific size range on each plate by controlling the nozzle diameter and the interval between the plates. For example, Micro-orifice Uniform Deposition Impactor (Nano-Moudi 122R) by MSP company has 13 stages. The nominal cutoff point of each stage is 10 μm, 5.6 μm, 3.2 μm, 1.8 μm, 1.0 μm, 560 nm, 320 nm, 180 nm, 100 nm, 56 nm, 32 nm, 18 nm, 10 nm, and the size of the particles collected on the plate is less than 100 nm from the ninth impaction plate [29]. However, the low pressure cascade impactor is cumbersome and bulky, which constrains its mobility, just for area sampling.

For achieving the personal sampling of nanoparticles, a mini particle sampler (MPS) was developed by Institut National de L'Environnement Industriel et des Risques (INERIS, France) [30]. It has a small size and light weight that makes it more suitable to personal sampling. This novel tool can very quickly sample nanoparticles on a TEM grid that can be later analyzed with a TEM microscope. While its capacity is restricted, it could not be able to collect enough particles for weighing and toxicological assessment.

2. Measurement of the particle size

   Toxicity studies show that particle toxicity increases as they become smaller [31]. So detecting the size of the particles at workplace is critical to evaluating the occupational exposure risk of nanomaterials.

   The purpose of the particle size detection is to identify the particle size range and the particle numbers in different size ranges (size distribution). The use of SEM or TEM to detect the particles collected on filter from workplace is one way to identify the particle size range; however, it is hard to provide the information about particle size distribution. Therefore, the particle size range and the size distribution are mainly detected in real-time monitoring at workplace by the equipment such as SMPS, FMPS, and ELPI. The particle size monitoring and exposure concentration monitoring should be synchronized in order to further analyze the effects of particle size change on mass concentration, quantity concentration, and surface area concentration [32].

3. Measurement of the particle exposure concentration

   The time integrated mass concentration of particles can be measured by gravimetric method (offline) [33], which is used to evaluate the particle cumulative exposure dose within a certain time range; however, the method could not provide the time-resolved mass concentration that is used for analyzing the variation of particle mass concentration over time. Meanwhile, the real-time monitor, such as OPC, ELPI, and TEOM, could detect the time-integrated mass concentration and time-resolved mass concentration [34]. However, the mass concentration obtained is generally calculated by a specific mathematical model, so the accuracy of the measurement results can hardly meet the requirements of industrial hygiene standards. Therefore, the monitoring mass concentration of nanoparticles should select the suitable scheme according to the needs of the monitoring task.

   In real-time measurement of particle mass concentration, number concentration, surface area concentration, and size distribution should be carried out at the same place simultaneously, and the particle collection should be consistent with real-time monitoring. In this way, the monitoring data can be compared and analyzed in a coordinated way, which is conducive to the comparison of the differences between the methods and the causes of the differences.

   In nanoparticle exposure monitoring, particle sampler (SKC Sampler), particle sizer (SMPS), mass concentration monitor (DUSTTRAK II 8530), number monitor (NANO-5403), and surface area monitor (AEROTRAK 9000) such as monitoring instruments should be placed in a convenient mobile platform. In order to avoid mutual interference, the sampling inlet of various instruments is at least 30 cm, and the height of the sampling port is set at 1.2–1.5 m [24]. According to the precompiled detection scheme, the exposure detection is performed and the items that may affect the detection results are recorded in detail.

4. Quality assurance and quality control

   Due to the lack of calibration standards for most of the nanometer particle measuring equipment, the method is recommended for quality control in order to ensure the effectiveness of the exposure evaluation results:

Use the factory calibrated particle analyzer for reference; Perform the zero check for all particle monitors before each use; Calibrate the sampling pump flow before and after each sampling date;

Submit all the samples to an accredited laboratory for analysis.

5. Data interpretation

Due to the agglomeration of manufactured nanomaterials, the size of nanoparticles in air is not known. It is necessary to use particle sizer to determine particle size and potential emission sources qualitatively. The simultaneous use of CPC and OPC could provide the information of number concentration in different size range. Most CPC has a capacity of detecting the number concentration of particle within a size range of 10–1000 nm; in contrast, OPC could detect the number concentration of particle within a size range of 300–10,000 nm. If the date of CPC and OPC are combined, the nanoparticle number concentration could be determined. For example, a high particle number concentration measured by a CPC, in combination with and a low number concentration measured by OPC, indicates the proportion of small particles (less than 300 nm) is large and the likely presence of nanoparticles. In contrast, a low number concentration measured by CPC and a high concentration measured by OPC show the likely presence of larger particles or the presence of nanoparticle agglomeration and aggregation [35, 36]. Then it could be verified by a TEM or SEM analysis.

That the particle counters could not differentiate the particle sources and component is another crucial problem. Nevertheless, airborne nanoscale particles are present in many workplaces and often originate from multiple sources, such as combustion, exhaust of vehicle, welding, and infiltration of outside air [35]. Therefore the TEM-EDX or SEM-EDX is required to identify the particle shape and component for distinguishing the sources of nanoparticles. However, TEM and SEM analyses can be compromised if there is a particle overload on the filter. Alternatively, if the loading is too sparse, an accurate assessment of the particle characteristics may not be possible [22].

Owing to the existence of the incidental emission source interference, it may lead to an order of magnitude difference in the particle number concentration. For example, a rainy day may lead to more incidental emission, and the welding operation and activation of vacuum pump could increase the airborne particle number. The interference of incidental emission can be ruled out by repeated detection for several days or multiple measurements in different seasons. If the airborne particle concentration is too high that it is almost close to or above the maximum range of CPC, it could result in a huge measurement error and also cause pollution of CPC; in this case, a particle filter should be connected in the front of the CPC inlet to clean the contained CPC until the value of CPC is zero [37, 38]. For the measurement of high-concentration particle emission source, a CPC with dilution function can be adopted, such as high-dilution condensation particle counter (CPC-HD) [39].

Monitoring particle concentration of emission sources is indispensable; the monitoring results reflect the serious exposure of workers. If the particle concentration of emission sources do not exceed the standard, so that the particle concentration of other workplaces do not exceed the standard, and workers' health will not be harmed. On the other hand, the monitoring of emission sources provides support for particle engineering control.

8 Conclusion and Future Trends

In summary, due to the special characteristics of nanomaterials, the traditional exposure assessment methods could not satisfy the requirement of nanoparticle exposure assessment. Although several countries and organizations have recommended several assessment methods, because of the lack of unified assessment indexes, the use of different sampling methods and different test principles between measurement instruments, the data gained are full of low comparability and poor reproducibility. In addition, the health damage mechanism of nanomaterials is unknown yet, and the population epidemiological survey is lacking and the exposure dose–response relationship is unclear; therefore, the studies of nanoparticle measurement methods and the population health effects are urgently needed to provide the standards and the basis to protect the workers related to nanomaterials. The following items are recommended:

1. *Methodological studies*: Nanoparticle exposure measurement methods should be carried out systematically to determine the appropriate assessment indexes, to clarify the agglomeration law of the nanomaterials from different sources, structure and composition, and to clarify the change regularity of nanoparticle concentration under the influence of different climatic conditions, different time and space values, and complex factors.
2. *Instrument optimization studies*: The further optimization of detection and sampling instruments should be put into practice to improve the accuracy and stability of the long-term online measurement, and to achieve the consistency of the detection results between different instruments.

3. *Health effect studies*: Long-term population epidemiological studies are required to identify the dose–response relationship of nanomaterial exposure, to sift the biomarkers of health effects and determine the occupational exposure limit of nanomaterials.

Acknowledgment

This work was supported by the National Key Research and Development Program of China (2016YFE0115500 and 2016YFC0700602) and general program national science foundation of China (21576023).

References

1. ISO T 27687: 2008. Nanotechnologies-Terminology and definitions for nano-objects-Nanoparticle, nanofibre and nanoplate ISO, Geneva
2. ISO T (2007) 80004-1: Nanotechnologies-Vocabulary-Part 1: Core terms. 2007. International Standards Organization, Geneva, Switzerland
3. Pal SL, Jana U, Manna PK, Mohanta GP, Manavalan R (2011) Nanoparticle: An overview of preparation and characterization (2000–2010)
4. Huang C-H, Tai C-Y, Huang C-Y, Tsai C-J, Chen C-W, Chang C-P, Shih T-S (2010) Measurements of respirable dust and nanoparticle concentrations in a titanium dioxide pigment production factory. J Environ Sci Health A 45 (10):1227–1233
5. Eastlake AC, Beaucham C, Martinez KF, Dahm MM, Sparks C, Hodson LL, Geraci CL (2016) Refinement of the nanoparticle emission assessment technique into the nanomaterial exposure assessment technique (NEAT 2.0). J Occup Environ Hyg 13(9):708–717
6. Maynard AD, Kuempel ED (2005) Airborne nanostructured particles and occupational health. J Nanopart Res 7(6):587–614
7. BSI P 6699-3 (2010) Nanotechnololgies-Part 3: Guide to assessing airborne exposure in occupational settings relevant to nanomaterials. BSI, London
8. Grover BD, Kleinman M, Eatough NL, Eatough DJ, Hopke PK, Long RW, Wilson WE, Meyer MB, Ambs JL (2005) Measurement of total PM2. 5 mass (nonvolatile plus semivolatile) with the filter dynamic measurement system tapered element oscillating microbalance monitor. J Geophys Res Atmos 110 (D7)
9. Kaluza S, Balderhaar JK, Orthen B, Honnert B, Jankowska E, Pietrowski P, Rosell M, Tanarro C, Tejedor J, Zugasti A (2009) In: Kosk-Bienko J (ed) Workplace exposure to nanoparticles. European Agency for Safety and Health at Work, Bilbao
10. Marple V, Olson B, Romay F, Hudak G, Geerts SM, Lundgren D (2014) Second generation micro-orifice uniform deposit impactor, 120 MOUDI-II: design, evaluation, and application to long-term ambient sampling. Aerosol Sci Technol 48(4):427–433
11. Marjamäki M, Keskinen J, Chen D-R, Pui DY (2000) Performance evaluation of the electrical low-pressure impactor (ELPI). J Aerosol Sci 31 (2):249–261
12. Gu F, Yang J, Bian B, He A (2008) A model for aerosol mass concentration using an optical particle counter. Chin Opt Lett 6(3):214–217
13. Heim M, Kasper G, Reischl G, Gerhart C (2004) Performance of a new commercial electrical mobility spectrometer. Aerosol Sci Technol 38(S2):3–14
14. Tritscher T, Beeston M, Zerrath AF, Elzey S, Krinke TJ, Filimundi E, Bischof OF (2013) NanoScan SMPS–A novel, portable nanoparticle sizing and counting instrument. In: Journal of physics: conference series. IOP Publishing, Bristol, p 012061
15. Jeong C-H, Evans GJ (2009) Intercomparison of a fast mobility particle sizer and a scanning mobility particle sizer incorporating an ultrafine water-based condensation particle counter. Aerosol Sci Technol 43 (4):364–373
16. Fissan H, Neumann S, Trampe A, Pui D, Shin W (2006) Rationale and principle of an instrument measuring lung deposited nanoparticle

surface area. In: Nanotechnology and occupational health. Springer, New York, pp 53–59

17. Shin W, Pui D, Fissan H, Neumann S, Trampe A (2006) Calibration and numerical simulation of nanoparticle surface area monitor (TSI model 3550 NSAM). In: Nanotechnology and occupational health. Springer, New York, pp 61–69
18. ISO T (2007) 27628. Workplace atmospheres—Ultrafine, nanoparticle and nanostructured aerosols—inhalation exposure characterization and assessment, ISO, Geneva
19. Eastlake A, Hodson L, Geraci C, Crawford C (2012) A critical evaluation of material safety data sheets (MSDSs) for engineered nanomaterials. Chem Health Saf 19(5):1–8
20. Kittelson DB, Watts WF, Johnson JP (2004) Nanoparticle emissions on Minnesota highways. Atmos Environ 38(1):9–19
21. Lee JH, Ahn K, Kim SM, Jeon KS, Lee JS, Yu IJ (2012) Continuous 3-day exposure assessment of workplace manufacturing silver nanoparticles. J Nanopart Res 14(9):1134
22. Methner M, Hodson L, Geraci C (2010) Nanoparticle emission assessment technique (NEAT) for the identification and measurement of potential inhalation exposure to engineered nanomaterials—Part A. J Occup Environ Hyg 7(3):127–132
23. Tsuji JS, Maynard AD, Howard PC, James JT, C-w L, Warheit DB, Santamaria AB (2005) Research strategies for safety evaluation of nanomaterials, part IV: risk assessment of nanoparticles. Toxicol Sci 89(1):42–50
24. Ham S, Yoon C, Lee E, Lee K, Park D, Chung E, Kim P, Lee B (2012) Task-based exposure assessment of nanoparticles in the workplace. J Nanopart Res 14(9):1126
25. Li W, Shao L, Wang Z, Shen R, Yang S, Tang U (2010) Size, composition, and mixing state of individual aerosol particles in a South China coastal city. J Environ Sci 22(4):561–569
26. Duchaine C, Thorne PS, Mériaux A, Grimard Y, Whitten P, Cormier Y (2001) Comparison of endotoxin exposure assessment by bioaerosol impinger and filter-sampling methods. Appl Environ Microbiol 67 (6):2775–2780
27. Maynard AD, Aitken RJ (2007) Assessing exposure to airborne nanomaterials: current abilities and future requirements. Nanotoxicology 1(1):26–41
28. Brouwer DH, Gijsbers JH, Lurvink MW (2004) Personal exposure to ultrafine particles in the workplace: exploring sampling techniques and strategies. Ann Occup Hyg 48 (5):439–453
29. Chen X, Balasubramanian R, Zhu Q, Behera SN, Bo D, Huang X, Xie H, Cheng J (2016) Characteristics of atmospheric particulate mercury in size-fractionated particles during haze days in shanghai. Atmos Environ 131:400–408
30. R'mili B, Le Bihan OL, Dutouquet C, Aguerre-Charriol O, Frejafon E (2013) Particle sampling by TEM grid filtration. Aerosol Sci Technol 47(7):767–775
31. Oberdörster G, Oberdörster E, Oberdörster J (2005) Nanotoxicology: an emerging discipline evolving from studies of ultrafine particles. Environ Health Perspect 113:823–839
32. Powers KW, Brown SC, Krishna VB, Wasdo SC, Moudgil BM, Roberts SM (2006) Research strategies for safety evaluation of nanomaterials. Part VI. Characterization of nanoscale particles for toxicological evaluation. Toxicol Sci 90(2):296–303
33. Morawska L, He C, Hitchins J, Mengersen K, Gilbert D (2003) Characteristics of particle number and mass concentrations in residential houses in Brisbane, Australia. Atmos Environ 37(30):4195–4203
34. Symonds JP, Reavell KSJ, Olfert JS, Campbell BW, Swift SJ (2007) Diesel soot mass calculation in real-time with a differential mobility spectrometer. J Aerosol Sci 38(1):52–68
35. Lee JH, Kwon M, Ji JH, Kang CS, Ahn KH, Han JH, Yu IJ (2011) Exposure assessment of workplaces manufacturing nanosized TiO_2 and silver. Inhal Toxicol 23(4):226–236
36. Han JH, Lee EJ, Lee JH, So KP, Lee YH, Bae GN, Lee S-B, Ji JH, Cho MH, Yu IJ (2008) Monitoring multiwalled carbon nanotube exposure in carbon nanotube research facility. Inhal Toxicol 20(8):741–749
37. Heitbrink WA, Evans DE, Peters TM, Slavin TJ (2007) Characterization and mapping of very fine particles in an engine machining and assembly facility. J Occup Environ Hyg 4 (5):341–351
38. Evans DE, Heitbrink WA, Slavin TJ, Peters TM (2007) Ultrafine and respirable particles in an automotive grey iron foundry. Ann Occup Hyg 52(1):9–21
39. Ji JH, Jung JH, Kim SS, Yoon J-U, Park JD, Choi BS, Chung YH, Kwon IH, Jeong J, Han BS (2007) Twenty-eight-day inhalation toxicity study of silver nanoparticles in Sprague-Dawley rats. Inhal Toxicol 19(10):857–871

INDEX

Qunwei Zhang (ed.), *Nanotoxicity: Methods and Protocols*, Methods in Molecular Biology, vol. 1894,
https://doi.org/10.1007/978-1-4939-8916-4,

Q

R

S

T

U

V

W

Z

CPSIA information can be obtained
at www.ICGtesting.com
Printed in the USA
LVHW061929150119
604021LV00004B/47/P

9 781493 989157